Behavioral Health Services with High-Risk

Infants and Families

Behavioral Health Services with High-Risk Infants and Families

Meeting the Needs of Patients, Families, and Providers in Fetal, Neonatal Intensive Care Unit, and Neonatal Follow-Up Settings

EDITED BY

ALLISON G. DEMPSEY,

JOANNA C. M. COLE,

AND

SAGE N. SAXTON

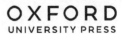

OXFORD
UNIVERSITY PRESS

Oxford University Press is a department of the University of Oxford. It furthers
the University's objective of excellence in research, scholarship, and education
by publishing worldwide. Oxford is a registered trade mark of Oxford University
Press in the UK and certain other countries.

Published in the United States of America by Oxford University Press
198 Madison Avenue, New York, NY 10016, United States of America.

© Oxford University Press 2022

Library of Congress Cataloging-in-Publication Data
Names: Dempsey, Allison G., editor. | Cole, Joanna C. M., editor. | Saxton, Sage N., editor.
Title: Behavioral health services with high-risk infants and families :
meeting the needs of patients, families, and providers in fetal,
neonatal intensive care unit, and neonatal follow-up settings /
[edited by] Allison G. Dempsey, Joanna C.M. Cole, Sage N. Saxton.
Description: New York, NY : Oxford University Press, 2022. |
Includes bibliographical references and index.
Identifiers: LCCN 2022008562 (print) | LCCN 2022008563 (ebook) |
ISBN 9780197545027 (paperback) | ISBN 9780197545041 (epub) | ISBN 9780197545058
Subjects: MESH: Mental Health Services | Maternal-Child Health Services | Perinatal Care |
Intensive Care, Neonatal—psychology | Intensive Care Units, Neonatal
Classification: LCC RG626 (print) | LCC RG626 (ebook) |
NLM WA 305.1 | DDC 618.3/2—dc23/eng/20220610
LC record available at https://lccn.loc.gov/2022008562
LC ebook record available at https://lccn.loc.gov/2022008563

DOI: 10.1093/med-psych/9780197545027.001.0001

9 8 7 6 5 4 3 2 1

Printed by Marquis, Canada

We dedicate this book to Michael Hynan, PhD, a passionate, tireless advocate for NICU infants and their families. Dr. Hynan's early vision helped shape the field of NICU psychology, and his steady wisdom and mentorship helped found the National Network of NICU Psychologists (NNNP).

We also dedicate this book to the memory of Cheryl Ann Milford, Ed.S., our friend, colleague, and NNNP mentor. Ms. Milford was passionate about education and envisioned a comprehensive textbook related to NICU psychology and behavioral health support; it is our great honor to fulfill that dream. Cheryl, you will always be remembered, you will always be treasured, you will always be loved. We miss you every day.

Our hope is that this book, inspired by Dr. Hynan and Ms. Milford, will serve developing and established professionals alike and will continue to improve patient- and family-centered care in both fetal and neonatal settings. In their honor.

AGD, JCMC, and SNS

To Alex, who is a role model for finding joy and living with grace even through the toughest of times—you inspire me every day. And to the amazing interprofessional team with whom I work and the families who allow us into their lives. I count myself lucky to be part of such an incredible community.

AGD

To my incredible fetal and ICU teams and to my fierce perinatal support network. Thank you for your compassion and steadfast dedication. And to the expectant and postpartum parents we serve, thank you for the honor to walk alongside of you as we navigate the uncertainties and complex challenges of parenthood together.

JCMC

To my precious family Rob, Sophia, and Lillian for their ongoing love and constant support; my mentors and colleagues; and to all the children and families who have graciously shared their experience, thank you.

SNS

Dailyn Acosta, PhD, IMH-E*, PMH-C
Neonatal Intensive Care Unit (NICU)
Children's Health/Children's
  Medical Center
Dallas, TX, USA

Ariana Albanese, MS
Department of Clinical Psychology
Drexel University
Philadelphia, PA, USA

Amy E. Baughcum, PhD
Department of Pediatric Psychology
  and Neuropsychology
Nationwide Children's Hospital
Columbus, OH, USA

Sandhya S. Brachio, MD
Columbia University Irving
  Medical Center
New York, NY, USA

Stacey R. Bromberg, PhD
Private Practice
Denver, CO, USA

Joy V. Browne, PhD, PCNS, IMH-E
Department of Pediatrics and
  Psychiatry
University of Colorado School of
  Medicine
Aurora, CO, USA

Melissa Buchholz, PsyD
Department of Psychiatry and
  Pediatrics
University of Colorado School of
  Medicine
Denver, CO, USA

Sakina Butt, PsyD, ABPP-CN
Institute of Brain Protection Sciences,
  Center for Behavioral Health,
  Psychology/Neuropsychology
  Services
Johns Hopkins All Children's Hospital
St. Petersburg, FL, USA

Kristin Carter, MD, MCSC
Ann and Robert H. Lurie Children's
  Hospital of Chicago
Chicago, IL, USA

KristiLynn R. Cedars, PhD
Department of Pediatrics
Sanford Children's Hospital-Fargo
Fargo, ND, USA

Lacy Chavis, PsyD
Department of Psychology
Johns Hopkins All Children's Hospital
St. Petersburg, FL, USA

John Chuo, MD, MS
Attending Neonatologist and Medical
  Director of Telemedicine Children's
  Hospital
Philadelphia, PA, USA
Associate Professor of Clinical
  Pediatrics Perelman School of
  Medicine at the University of
  Pennsylvania
Philadelphia, PA, USA

Nicole Cirino, MD, PMH-C
Department of Psychiatry and
  Department of Obstetrics and
  Gynecology
Oregon Health Science University
Portland, OR, USA

Olivia E. Clark, BA
Loyola University Chicago
Chicago, IL, USA

Joanna C. M. Cole, PhD, PMH-C
Richard D. Wood Jr. Center for Fetal
    Diagnosis and Treatment
Children's Hospital of Philadelphia
Philadelphia, PA, USA

Mary Coughlin, MS, NNP, RNC-E
Caring Essentials Collaborative
Boston, MA, USA

Annelise Cunningham, PhD
Department of Psychiatry
University of Colorado School of
    Medicine
Aurora, CO, USA

Deborah L. Davis, PhD
Author of *Empty Cradle, Broken Heart*
    and *A Gift of Time*
Denver, CO, USA

Teni Davoudian, PhD, ABPP
Center for Women's Health
Oregon Health & Science University
Portland, OR, USA

Jeanne Decker, MSW, LISW-S
Department of Case Management
    and Social Work, The Ohio State
    University Wexner Medical Center
Nationwide Children's Hospital NICU,
    located at The Ohio State University
    Wexner Medical Center
Columbus, OH, USA

Allison G. Dempsey, PhD
Department of Psychiatry
University of Colorado School of
    Medicine
Aurora, CO, USA

Brooke Dorsey Holliman, PhD
Department of Family Medicine
University of Colorado
Aurora, CO, USA

**LaTrice L. Dowtin, PhD, LCPC,
NCSP, RPT**
PlayfulLeigh Psyched
Silver Spring, MD, USA

Beatrice Egboh, MBBS, FAAP
Department of Pediatrics
University of Nebraska Medical Center
Omaha, NE, USA

Mona Elgohail, PhD
Drexel University
Philadelphia, PA, USA

Elizabeth A. Fischer, PhD
Department of Pediatrics, Division
    of Pediatric Psychology and
    Developmental Medicine
Medical College of Wisconsin
Milwaukee, WI, USA

Pamela A. Geller, PhD
Department of Psychological and
    Brain Sciences
Drexel University
Philadelphia, PA, USA

Shannon L. Gillespie, PsyD
Nationwide Children's Hospital
Columbus, OH, USA

Soudabeh Givrad, MD
Department of Psychiatry
Weill Cornell Medicine
New York, NY, USA

Victoria A. Grunberg, MS
Department of Psychiatry
Massachusetts General Hospital/
    Harvard Medical School
Boston, MA, USA

Kathryn E. Gustafson, PhD
Duke University Medical Center
Durham, NC, USA

Sue L. Hall, MD, MSW
Department of Neonatology
St. John's Regional Health Center
Oxnard, CA, USA

Sara C. Handley, MD, MSCE
Department of Pediatrics
Children's Hospital of Philadelphia
Philadelphia, PA, USA

Kara Hansen, MSW
Department of Fetal Health and
Perinatal Services
Children's Mercy
Kansas City, MO, USA

Jennifer Harned Adams, PhD
Center for Maternal Fetal Health
Presbyterian/St. Luke's Medical Center
Denver, CO, USA

Alison R. Hartman, MS
Department of Psychological and
Brain Sciences
Drexel University
Philadelphia, PA, USA

Natalia Henner, MD
Ann & Robert H. Lurie Children's
Hospital of Chicago
Chicago, IL, USA

Sheau-Yan Ho, PhD
Department of Psychiatry
Columbia University Irving
Medical Center
New York, NY, USA

Casey Hoffman, PhD
Department of Child and Adolescent
Psychiatry and Behavioral Sciences
Perelman School of Medicine
University of Pennsylvania
and The Children's Hospital of
Philadelphia
Philadelphia, PA, USA

Jill A. Hoffman, PhD, MSW
Portland State University
Portland, OR, USA

Sunah S. Hwang, MD, PhD, MPH
Section of Neonatology, Department
of Pediatrics
University of Colorado School of
Medicine
Aurora, CO, USA

Michael T. Hynan, PhD
Department of Psychology
University of Wisconsin–Milwaukee
Milwaukee, WI, USA

Jessalyn Kelleher, PsyD
Department of Psychiatry
University of Colorado School of
Medicine
Aurora, CO, USA

Susanne Klawetter, PhD, LCSW
School of Social Work
Portland State University
Portland, OR, USA

Jacquelyn M. Knapp, MD
Department of Psychiatry
Oregon Health & Science University
Portland, OR, USA

Susan Kraemer, PhD
New York University Postdoctoral
Program in Psychotherapy and
Psychoanalysis
New York, NY, USA

Abbey Kruper, PsyD
Department of Obstetrics &
Gynecology
Medical College of Wisconsin
Milwaukee, WI, USA

Jenny Landry, BA
Programs Team
Hand to Hold
Austin, TX, USA

Steven R. Leuthner, MD, MA
Department of Pediatrics
Medical College of Wisconsin
Milwaukee, WI, USA

Kerri Machut, MD
Ann & Robert H. Lurie Children's
Hospital of Chicago
Chicago, IL, USA

Kristina Malik, MD
University of Colorado School of
Medicine
Children's Hospital Colorado
Aurora, CO, USA

Annie Markovits, MSS, LSW
Division of General, Thoracic, and
Fetal Surgery
Children's Hospital of Philadelphia
Philadelphia, PA, USA

Beth M. McManus, PT, MPH, ScD
Health Systems, Management,
and Policy
Colorado School of Public Health
Aurora, CO, USA

Birdie G. Meyer, RN, MA, PMH-C
Postpartum Support International
Speedway, IN, USA

Julie S. Moldenhauer, MD
Children's Hospital of Philadelphia
Philadelphia, PA, USA

Elizabeth D. Morris, LCSW
Center for Fetal Diagnosis and
Treatment and Special Delivery Unit
Children's Hospital of Philadelphia
Philadelphia, PA, USA

David A. Munson, MD
Division of Neonatology
The Perelman School of Medicine at the
University of Pennsylvania and the
Children's Hospital of Philadelphia
Philadelphia, PA, USA

Sarah Nagle-Yang, MD
Department of Psychiatry
University of Colorado School of
Medicine
Aurora, CO, USA

Howard Needelman, MD
Section of Developmental Behavioral
Pediatrics
University of Nebraska
Omaha, NE, USA

Christina Paidas Teefey, MD
General, Thoracic and Fetal Surgery
Children's Hospital of Philadelphia,
Perelman School of Medicine,
University of Pennsylvania
Philadelphia, PA, USA

Brenda Papierniak, PsyD, PMH-C
Perinatal Health Psychology Service
Saint Alexius Women and Children's
Hospital
Hoffman Estates, IL, USA

Chavis A. Patterson, PhD
Department of Neonatology/
Psychiatry
Children's Hospital of Philadelphia/
Perelman School of Medicine,
University of Pennsylvania
Philadelphia, PA, USA

Jennifer J. Paul, PhD
Department of Psychiatry
University of Colorado School of
Medicine
Aurora, CO, USA

**Christena B. Raines, MSN, WHCNP/
PMHNP-BC, PMH-C**
Department of Psychiatry
University of North Carolina at
Chapel Hill
Chapel Hill, NC, USA

**Sarah Robinson, BSN, MSN,
WHNP-BC CNM**
Certified Nurse Midwife
Richard D. Wood Jr. Center for
Fetal Diagnosis and Treatment at
Children's Hospital of Philadelphia
Philadelphia, PA, USA

Kristi Roybal, MSW, MA
Graduate School of Social Work
University of Denver
Denver, CO, USA

**Solimar Santiago-Warner, LCSW
(DSW candidate)**
Morgan Stanley Children's Hospital–
New York Presbyterian
New York, NY, USA

Sage N. Saxton, PsyD
Department of Pediatrics
Oregon Health & Science University
Portland, OR, USA

Melissa Scala, MD
Department of Pediatrics, Division
of Neonatal and Developmental
Medicine
Stanford University
Palo Alto, CA, USA

Verenea J. Serrano, PhD
Department of Psychiatry
University of Colorado School of
Medicine
Aurora, CO, USA

Miller Shivers, PhD
Pritzker Department of Psychiatry and
Behavioral Sciences
Ann & Robert H. Lurie Children's
Hospital of Chicago/Northwestern
University Feinberg School of
Medicine
Chicago, IL, USA

Vincent C. Smith, MD, MPH
Department of Pediatrics Division of
Newborn Medicine
Boston University and Boston
Medical Center
Boston, MA, USA

Diane L. Spatz, PhD, RN-BC, FAAN
Family & Community Health
University of Pennsylvania School of
Nursing with secondary appoint-
ment at Children's Hospital of
Philadelphia
Philadelphia, PA, USA

Zina Steinberg, EdD
Department of Psychiatry and
Pediatrics
College of Physicians and Surgeons,
Columbia University
New York, NY, USA

Rochelle Steinwurtzel, PsyD
Department of Neonatology and
Psychiatry
Columbia University Irving
Medical Center
New York, NY, USA

Whitney Strong-Bak, PhD, LP
Department of Pediatric Psychology
University of Nebraska Medical
Center, Munroe-Meyer Institute
Omaha, NE, USA

Ayelet Talmi, PhD, IMH-E®
Departments of Psychiatry and
Pediatrics
University of Colorado School of
Medicine
Aurora, CO, USA

Mara Tesler Stein, PsyD, PMH-C
The Touchstone Institute for
Psychotherapy and Training
Lincolnwood, IL, USA

Erin Thatcher, BA
The PPROM Foundation
Conifer, CO, USA

Elizabeth Vaught, MA
Retired NICU
Johns Hopkins All Children's Hospital
St. Petersburg, FL, USA

Jonna H. von Schulz, PhD, BCBA
Departments of Pediatrics and
  Psychiatry
University of Colorado School
  Medicine
Aurora, CO, USA

Mollie G. Warren, MD
Department of Pediatric Newborn
  Medicine
Harvard Medical School
Boston, MA, USA

Lana S. Weber, MD
Department of Psychiatry
Oregon Health & Science University
Portland, OR, USA

Tiffany Willis, PsyD
Department of Pediatrics
Children's Mercy Hospital
Kansas City, MO, USA

Grace Winningham, MD
University of Nebraska Medical Center
Omaha, NE, USA

Amy Wrenn, DNP, APRN, CPNP-PC
Department of Pediatrics
Children's Hospital Colorado
Aurora, CO, USA

Anna Zimmermann, MD, MPH
Pediatrix Medical Group, Colorado
Denver, CO, USA

Jeannie Zuk, PhD, RN
University of Colorado School of
  Medicine
Denver, CO, USA

Roles and Practice Issues

INTRODUCTION

HISTORY OF PSYCHOLOGICAL SERVICES IN NEONATAL INTENSIVE CARE

MICHAEL T. HYNAN ■

Nobody, not nobody, is going to stop breathing on me.

—VIRGINIA APGAR (CIRCA 1950S)

That the goal of neonatal care would evolve from getting the baby home in the best possible shape to getting the family home in the best possible shape.

—SHERI NANCE (CIRCA 1990)

Only relatively recently have services provided by psychologists in perinatal care been available. It remains uncommon for a neonatal intensive care unit (NICU) to have a psychologist as a dedicated staff member, although the number of NICU psychologists is increasing. This volume is primarily concerned with perinatal services provided by psychologists. I do, however, make note of the valuable role of social workers as a complement to the care offered by psychologists. Social workers have been available in NICUs since the mid-1960s. The National Association of Perinatal Social Workers (NAPSW) was founded in 1980 to help standardize training and services. The initial focus of perinatal social workers was service delivery in the NICU, but social work services soon spread to antepartum care and follow-up. NAPSW has published an excellent set of standards for a variety of activities, including fertility counseling, bereavement, obstetric settings, adoptions, field education, and surrogacy. Some activities of social workers overlap with those of psychologists, but each discipline has its own set of unique skills. Social workers are often involved in case and crisis management, bedside family support, and discharge planning in the NICU.

Psychologists also work across the whole perinatal spectrum. Follow-up settings have made good use of the testing and evaluation skills that psychologists bring to the table of neonatal medicine, especially developmental assessments of infants. Indeed, many neonatal psychologists had their first experiences in developmental follow-up of high-risk infants. Psychologists' participation in antepartum and fetal care is still in its early stages. Saxton et al. (2020) provide an excellent description of the recent progress of psychologists' involvement in perinatal services. My historical account focuses more on changes that have occurred from the 1960s to approximately 2021.

The changes in neonatal care during the past 40–50 years go hand in hand with the involvement of parents as the infant's caregiver, from early exclusion from the NICU to more recently becoming the primary caregiver, in some cases 24/7. And as parents have become more involved in their infant's care at bedside, psychologists and other behavioral health professionals have used their skills and training to promote the well-being of both families of NICU infants and NICU staff. In this chapter, I describe the evolution of psychological services in perinatal care from the perspective of a clinical psychologist who is also a NICU parent. My primary focus is the various changes that have promoted the well-being of the high-risk family. These changes include architectural improvements in NICUs, acceptance of parent-to-parent support, individualized developmental care, and the recognition that, if possible, infants belong in their parents' arms rather than in isolettes.

CONTEXT: A PERSONAL REFLECTION

When my son, Chris, was born prematurely (30 weeks) in 1980, I felt that I had been hit by an emotional freight train. Then, I was an academic clinical psychologist who knew nothing about NICUs. In the years that followed, I shifted my research focus to the study of post-traumatic stress (PTS) symptoms in NICU parents. Early on, I also wrote a book published in 1987 (*The Pain of Premature Parents: A Psychological Guide for Coping*) to help parents adjust emotionally to the NICU experience. At that time, books written for NICU parents were primarily medical in nature. Through a series of fortuitous incidents and accidents, I learned of an organization called Parent Care: Parents of Premature and High-Risk Infants, International. I joined Parent Care and attended its first national meeting in 1984. There I met many parents (including the authors Helen Harrison and Sheri Nance) along with a select set of nurses, social workers, and neonatologists, all of whom were interested in promoting the physical and emotional health of NICU parents, both during their infant's hospitalization and afterward. Many of these parents and NICU professionals helped me in gathering data for PTS research and in providing stories for my book. I owe many debts of gratitude to these dedicated people. You will learn some of their names in this chapter. I apologize to those whose names I have omitted.

A warning! I have never worked in a NICU. So, I know little from firsthand experience about the nuts and bolts of what a NICU psychologist must do routinely. The other chapters of this book describe the typical activities of psychologists and other behavioral health clinicians in perinatal care. Rather than firsthand experience, my sources include many conversations among NICU psychologists (and social workers, nurses, neonatologists, occupational therapists, etc.) throughout the years. I have also talked with hundreds of parents, primarily at regional and national meetings of groups such as Parent Care. I have benefited greatly from the ethos of the general perinatal community that typically welcomes everyone in a multidisciplinary fashion, even a clinical psychologist/NICU parent.

My activities throughout the years have changed. At the beginning, I was more directly involved in attempting to help high-risk parents adjust emotionally through the guidance in my now outdated book. The book led to invitations to give talks at conferences. As I began to publish PTS studies, I met other researchers and I used the emerging internet technology to build an academic home page housed in my psychology department. The home page allowed others interested in psychology and PTS in the NICU to find me. I believe that my graduate students and I (along with the neonatologists and parents who assisted with data collection) authored the first publication (1996) in the medical and psychological literature that contained "symptoms of posttraumatic stress" and "mothers of infants at high-risk" in the title.

Over time, I began to meet some of the first psychologists working in NICUs. These contacts came through my internet page and chance meetings at conferences I regularly attended—the National Perinatal Association (NPA) annual conference and the Gravens Conference. Some of these psychologists were hired using discretionary funds or grants by chiefs of neonatology, who recognized that psychologists had an added value for the well-being of their NICU parents and staff. Other psychologists, who spent only some of their hours in the NICU, were full-time employees of larger children's hospitals and had obligations in other departments. Many of the first NICU psychologists were creating their own job descriptions. I realized that communication among them could prove beneficial, so I arranged periodic phone calls among them to discuss whatever they wished.

NPA allowed me to work more closely with parents of high-risk infants, along with Erika Goyer, Becky Hatfield, and Kristy Love of the Family Advocacy Network. NPA board membership gave me frequent contacts with wonderful, caring perinatal professionals and parents. In the early 2010s, NPA began to sponsor large multidisciplinary projects (e.g., "Guidelines for the Care of the Late Preterm Infant"). I was fortunate enough to be at a board meeting when neonatologist Dr. Sue Hall proposed a project involving recommendations for psychosocial programs for NICU parents. Sue asked me to co-chair the project with her, and saying "Yes" was one of the best decisions I ever made—not only for the work that was produced but also because Sue is the finest collaborator I have had the pleasure to work with professionally. The project culminated in articles that appeared in a special issue of *Journal of Perinatology* (Hall & Hynan, 2015). These articles continue to be cited widely in the United States and other countries. This issue was one more step toward the evolving concept of the newborn intensive parenting unit (NIPU), which I describe later (Hall et al., 2017).

I am now in my 70s. My son recently turned 40. So, from the perspective of Drs. Dempsey, Cole, and Saxton, I qualify as a historian. Again, the reader should know that what follows is not a traditional historical perspective from someone educated in a medical field. I hope that I can convey, as a NICU parent and friend of professionals, an appreciation of the changes in psychological services that have occurred in perinatal medicine from a parent's perspective and how parents have contributed to this evolution. These psychological services include (a) peer-to-peer support, (b) staff collaboration with parents, and (c) formal psychological assessment and counseling by mental health professionals.

OVERVIEW

In this chapter, I describe the changing culture of neonatal care. In using the term "culture," I am referring to the prevailing goals and values of care during certain time periods. Again, my reference point views culture shifts as reflecting changes in how an infant's parents/caregivers are involved in the overall neonatal care team.

This historical progression includes stages that began with (a) "parents excluded from the NICU" and proceeded to (b) parents as "observers/visitors" during only a few hours of the day, (c) parents welcome for more hours (except during shift changes and rounds) as partial care providers, (d) parents encouraged to be primary care providers for as many hours a day as possible, (e) NICU redesign incorporating single-family rooms to facilitate skin-to-skin contact and comfort of parents 24/7, and (f) a NIPU culture in which the health and emotional well-being of NIPU staff and parents are valued as much as the health of the high-risk infant (Hall et al., 2017).

Neonatologist Dr. Bob Cicco has aptly compared this historical progression in the NICU as being akin to a "medical" house in which neonatology in the early years would get the infant at the front door and the parents were told to show up at the back door in a month after the infant was fixed by the medical team. A decade later, parents were invited to a comfortably decorated living room, where they were called into their infant's large ward and allowed to "visit" for a couple hours while they watched nurses and doctors attend to many infants. Then research showed having parents around helped infants grow. Parents could now go directly into their infant's room without having to ask permission. These rooms were smaller and held fewer infants. Parents were taught to feed their infant and change diapers. There were also a few comfortable chairs available. If the infant was healthy enough, parents could hold their infant in one of these chairs and perhaps go to a special room down the hall to nurse their infant (or nurse behind a portable curtain). Nowadays in the ideal NIPU, the family's room looks like a four-star hotel suite within a village. There is one comfortable living area for most infants and families. Parents can stay the night if they wish. The village contains cooking and laundry facilities, and some meals are provided. Over the infant's stay, the nurses and doctors come into the family's room less frequently, as parents do most of the infant's care. The doctors, nurses, and the rest of the medical staff have told the parents that they (along with the other parents) are the most important caregivers in the building.

Along each step of this progression there has been a growing focus on the emotional health of both NICU families and staff. This focus stems from a growing body of research (Hall & Hynan, 2015) showing (a) the NICU experience is a potentially traumatic one for parents, with elevated rates of perinatal mood and anxiety disorders for both mothers and fathers; (b) high rates of burnout and PTS in NICU staff; (c) correlations of parental emotional distress with impaired growth and development in their children; and (d) parental distress during the perinatal period associated with an increased probability of psychological problems in parents and children later in life.

Early Neonatology Culture: What Is Best for the Infant

The first official NICU in the United States was opened in October 1965 (although one account states 1960) at Yale New Haven Hospital in New Haven, Connecticut. Dr. Louis Gluck was named the Director of Neonatal Services and is credited with being the "father of modern neonatology" in the United States. However, there were "premature nurseries" in the United States before 1965. In the western United States, there was a premature infant center at the University of Colorado General Hospital that opened in 1947 with Dr. Lula Lubchenco and Dr. Joseph Butterfield as early directors. Even earlier, in 1914, Dr. Julius Hess founded the first premature unit at Michael Reese Hospital in Chicago. Hess was a close friend to Dr. Martin Couney, who brought his traveling exposition of premature babies to the United States at the turn of the century.

Two accounts of early neonatology, one from the United Kingdom (Christie & Tansey, 2001) and one from the United States (Philip, 2005), are filled with descriptions of medical advances and infant complications. One can read two-thirds of the way through both lengthy documents before parents are mentioned. The medical advances and complications described in the two accounts include thermoregulation, assisted ventilation, surfactant, oxygen saturation monitors, intraventricular hemorrhage, necrotizing enterocolitis, apnea, retinopathy of prematurity, and neonatal infections. This last concern is one reason that parents were generally restricted from coming into the NICU in the early history of neonatology. Indeed, one neonatal historian (Philip, 2005) writes of pediatric residents seldom being allowed into the NICU in the early years.

In the late 1960s, only approximately one-third of NICUs allowed parents to visit their infants. Klaus and Kennel's (1970) seminal paper on mothers separated from their newborn infants was published the same year as a research study of mothers being "allowed" into the NICU (Barnett et al., 1970). This second publication led to a recognition that (with sanitary precautions) mothers' presence in the NICU did not increase rates of infection in infants. So, the 1970s can be described as a transition from fear that parents would hurt their infants to the possibility that parental presence would be helpful for the bonding process and perhaps even benefit their infant.

Doctors Make the Treatment Decisions

With parents excluded from many NICUs, treatment decisions for most NICU babies were largely controlled by physicians. This created a hierarchical setting that occasionally resulted in severe conflicts, often when neonatologists wished to pursue aggressive treatment against parents' wishes. In some of these cases, the parents expressed that their infant was suffering through medical experiments to prolong life. As a result, parents argued for the termination of treatment and hoped for a peaceful death. In these situations, hospital ethics committees were consulted for advice. An obvious case of this conflict came to light with the publication of a book in 1983, *The Long Dying of Baby Andrew* by Richard and Peggy Stinson, which described the 6-month hospitalization of their infant in 1976 and 1977. The publication of this book, along with the experiences of other parents in similar situations, contributed to the motivation for parents to advocate for an equal role in decision-making for their child's well-being.

Women in Neonatology

Most early neonatologists were concerned with research and focused on the health of infants while hospitalized in NICUs. It has been pointed out to me that female neonatologists were more likely to have interest in both the well-being of the infant's family and the longer term outcomes of NICU graduates. Here is a brief list of noteworthy female neonatologists: Drs. Virginia Apgar (technically an obstetrical anesthesiologist), Mary Ellen Avery, Kathleen Kennedy, Lula Lubchenco, Marie McCormick, Marie Delivoria Papadopolus (frequently referred to as the "mother of neonatology"), Mildred Stahlman, and Betty Vohr.

THE 1980S

Parent Care and Association for the Care of Children's Health

Concern for the emotional well-being of high-risk parents and their families began in the late 1970s. This concern was facilitated by perinatal professionals who recognized that parental involvement in NICU care was beneficial for their infants and that high-risk families needed emotional support during their infant's hospitalization and separation from their child. Groups for parents of premature infants (and other high-risk infants) sprang up in various cities. Sheri Nance (along with five other mothers and a perinatal social worker) started a community group known as Parents of Prematures in Houston, Texas. Membership grew and participants decided to write a book for parents, *Premature Babies: A Handbook for Parents*, in 1982, with Sheri Nance as lead author. The book was advertised in national parenting magazines, and the authors discovered that there were similar groups in other cities (e.g., Concerned Parents Organization, Park Ridge, IL; Neo-Fight, Indianapolis, IN; Pilot Parents of Prematures, Fort Dodge, IA; CHOC Parent-to-Parent, Orange, CA; IVH Parents and Parent to Parent of Miami, FL; Parents and Friends of Special Care Infants, Wichita, KS; Intensive Caring Unlimited, Philadelphia, PA; Neo-Life, Lexington, KY; and Parent Support Group, Boston, MA). The University of Utah in Salt Lake City was home to the first hospital-based NICU parent support group in the United States, Parent-to-Parent, founded in 1975 by Sandy Garrand, RN, and Becky Hatfield, NICU parent.

Leaders of these groups decided to form a national organization called Parent Care: Parents of Premature and High-Risk Infants, International. Parent Care held its first meeting in Salt Lake City, Utah, in 1984. In addition to many parent leaders, attendees included family-friendly nurses, social workers, and notable physicians (including Drs. T. Barry Brazelton, Peter Gorski, Stan Graven, Henry Mangurten, and Richard Marshall). Parent Care held annual meetings until 1996 when lack of finances led it to be merged into the Association for the Care of Children's Health (ACCH), a larger organization founded by Dr. Brazelton and others. Many nonprofits such as Parent Care depended on corporate sponsorship for their continued existence. Dwindling financial support led to the end of ACCH's existence a few years later.

The 1980s bore witness to greater parental participation in perinatal care, especially neonatal care. Another noteworthy book published during this time (1984) was *The Premature Baby Book: A Parents' Guide to Coping and Caring During the First Years* by Helen Harrison with Ann Kositsky. The number of hours that parents were "allowed" into NICUs increased, and parents were encouraged to engage in activities with their infants. The term family-centered care began to be utilized as an ideal model, and the March of Dimes (MOD) continues to be one of the leaders in promoting this concept. Many NICUs began to describe themselves as promoting family-centered care, although some journal articles questioned how well family-centered care was implemented in NICUs.

Individualized Developmental Care

As a graduate student, Dr. Heidelise Als, a developmental and clinical psychologist, observed the behavior of premature infants for countless hours. In the late 1970s, she worked with Dr. Brazelton on creating the Brazelton Newborn Behavior Assessment Scale before focusing her work on preterm infants. Using the Assessment of Preterm Infants' Behavior Scale (Als, 1982), she was able to teach NICU staff how to recognize an infant's unique cues and respond appropriately to optimize self-regulation. Als and colleagues developed the Newborn Individualized Developmental Care and Assessment Program (NIDCAP) in the 1980s. As the NIDCAP program evolved, parents began to learn calming techniques relevant to the developmental stage of their infant.

THE 1990S

A Growing Concern About What Is Best for NICU Families

Four events facilitated the growth of family-centered care in the 1990s: (a) a publication asserting the rights of parents as decision-makers in the NICU, (b) the creation of an institute for family-centered care, (c) the growth of skin-to-skin care, and (d) rethinking the optimal NICU design.

Principles of Family-Centered Neonatal Care

A seminal moment in the evolution of neonatal care occurred with the publication of an article titled "Principles of Family-Centered Neonatal Care" in the journal *Pediatrics* (Harrison, 1993). In quoting a few paragraphs here, I emphasize the impetus created by this article for a recognition of parents' rights both as decision-makers for their infant in the NICU and as equal partners (with professionals) as care providers. Many of the 10 principles refer to professionals and parents "working together" to affect change. The terms "unthinking medical activism" and "poorly drafted laws" in the quote largely refer to the "Baby Doe Rules" legislation (Harrison, 1993):

> Adults have the right to refuse burdensome life-support for themselves. Critically ill newborns, however, cannot say "no" to life-sustaining procedures, no matter how extreme. Parents must once again have the right to refuse excessively painful, burden-some, or unproven therapies on behalf of their infants. Otherwise, these infants can become the unprotected targets of an unthinking medical activism. We urge professionals to work with parents to change laws and policies that promote overtreatment and rob parents of their rights and responsibilities. Medical treatment of critically ill newborns should be driven by compassion and dedication to the welfare of these children and their families, not fear of politically motivated and poorly drafted laws. . . . Part of physician training should include a rotation in a facility or school that cares for children or adults with disabilities. In addition, medical students should have some experience in family settings caring for children or adults with mental and physical handicaps.

We urge perinatal and neonatal professionals to work with parents in advocating for increased public support for children with disabilities and their families and for the prevention of disabilities through universal pre-natal care. (p. 650)

Not only did this *Pediatrics* article have an impact on the future of neonatal care but also Helen Harrison served as a role model for parental advocates for years to come. Harrison was fearless in challenging anyone, including world-famous neonatologists and ethicists, who attempted to limit parents' abilities to advocate for the medical care of their children.

Institute for Patient- and Family-Centered Care

The second facilitator of family-centered care in the 1990s was the founding of the Institute for Patient- and Family Centered Care (IPFCC) by Beverly Johnson, BSN, FAAN, who had previously been an executive with ACCH. IPFCC is con-cerned with all of health care delivery, but Johnson has played a major role in making NICUs family friendly, both in architecture and in practices. She has also been one of the leaders in addressing the issue of parents as *visitors* to the NICU. *Visitors* go to museums where the rules mostly are "Look, but do not touch." *Visitors* as a term also puts parents in a role secondary to NICU staff, with the im-plication that parents do not belong in the NICU full-time. Within all principles of family-centered care, parents play a crucial role as equal members of the care team, growing into the role of leader. Johnson and others have made many NICU staff aware that *visitor* is not a term that should be applied to NICU parents and/ or any family members.

Skin-to-Skin (Kangaroo) Care

Skin-to-skin care in the NICU became more commonplace in Western Europe in the 1990s and began to migrate to the United States. Although there were initial concerns with safety, multiple research studies over decades have shown benefits for the health and development of infants, the emotional well-being of parents, and parent–infant bonding. These studies led hospital administrators to be open to the increased involvement of parents in their infant's care.

Environmental Changes in the NICU

NICUs in the early years were bright and noisy environments. Some neonatologists began investigating whether typical light and sound levels were good for infants' health and development. Early indications were that bright lights and loud sounds interfered with the development of most premature infants. Despite consistent findings, there was initial resistance to changing the NICU "ward environment." Reasons included bright lights provided easy observation of many infants, limited hospital space, optimal nursing efficiency, and reluctance to purchase quieter equipment (White & Whitman, 1992).

An editorial published in *Pediatrics* (White & Whitman, 1992) called for changes in NICU design. Over the years, decibel levels were decreased in the NICU along with constant light. Establishing a circadian rhythm for infants became important. The Gravens Conference has consistently featured the latest research on the effects of environmental changes in NICU care upon the development and health of high-risk infants. Under Dr. Robert White's leadership, the ninth edition of "Recommended Standards for Newborn ICU Design" was recently published (White, 2020). As new NICUs in the United States were built (and older ones remodeled), both Bob White and Bev Johnson were consulted. As a result, NICUs became more welcoming of families in both structure and function. Nowadays, many NICUs have a set of single-family rooms for care so parents can room in with their infant 24/7.

Jerold Lucey, MD

Dr. Jerold Lucey was the editor-in-chief of the prestigious journal *Pediatrics* from 1974 to 2008. On at least two occasions, his decisions on publications in the journal had a notable impact on the evolution of neonatal care. One, he accepted the "Principles of Family-Centered Neonatal Care" (Harrison, 1993) without sending the manuscript for review. The principles were the product of an extensive discussion at a 2-day meeting among NICU parents and professionals. In the issue in which the article appeared, Lucey simply stated that the article needed to be published. In a comment he wrote for the issue, Lucey (1993) stated,

> The discussion was open and frank, and there were several disagreements without resolution. I think both groups learned from this encounter. The parents were asked to rewrite their suggestions, and I agreed to publish these in *Pediatrics.* The article was not to be reviewed or revised by *Pediatrics.* I wanted the parents' article to truly represent *their* viewpoints. Mrs. Harrison spent a year revising the article and widening the input by soliciting views from other parents and groups.
>
> I anticipate this will be a controversial article. It should be recognized for what it is, a sincere attempt to communicate with physicians in a constructive fashion.
>
> In the brave new world we are facing, patients are often referred to as "customer." We are "care providers." It is obviously wise to listen to "customer" viewpoints. I hope that this will be the beginning of a continuing dialogue with concerned parents. In the future we might be able to form a group working together to implement *some* of the parents' suggestions. (p. 724)

This quote certainly reflects earlier tensions between NICU parents and hierarchical decision-makers in the NICU. Dialogues between NICU parents and hospital leadership continue to this day, often with staff "champions" joining parents to promote change.

Lucey made a second executive decision that impacted NICU design. Bob White told me that his editorial published in *Pediatrics* (White & Whitman, 1992) was originally a traditional submission advocating NICU design changes that received a great deal of criticism from reviewers. The reviewers recommended that the manuscript be rejected as "unworkable," among other things. In correspondence about the reviews with White, Lucey decided that the manuscript was acceptable as an editorial.

THE 2000S

Learning from Europe

The changes that began earlier in the United States continued to become more widespread in the 2000s. And, as innovations from Europe became more well-known, NICUs in the United States were more likely to implement the new developments. One innovation became known as "couplet care," which was skin-to-skin care combined with individualized, developmental care. Couplet care was initiated at the Karolinska NICU in Stockholm, Sweden. Couplet care, with 24/7 parental presence, was shown to reduce length of stay and infant morbidity (Ortenstrand et al., 2010).

Interestingly, a nursing shortage in Eastern Europe led to a second innovation in NICU care that continues to be researched. In 1979, a "mother–infant unit" was created at Tallinn Children's Hospital in Estonia. Due to the staff shortage, mothers were trained to provide the majority of care for their high-risk infants. Mothers were able to acquire most of the necessary skills rather quickly, over a matter of a few days. Physicians from Canada observed this unit and later conducted a pilot research study in Canada to determine if this family integrated care (FICare) would be accepted by staff and lead to positive results. It worked (Bracht et al., 2013). The effectiveness of FICare is currently being evaluated at multiple sites throughout the world, including China, a country where parents are still not allowed to enter many NICUs.

Newborn intensive care was transformed in Finland by a program called "Close Collaboration with Parents." This program stresses training as an important first step to prepare NICU staff to interact with NICU parents in creating an atmosphere in which parents ultimately become the decision-makers for their infant's care in the hospital. Close Collaboration was well accepted by staff and led to increased parental presence in the NICU and greater participation in providing care for their infants (Huhtala et al., 2012). Phased research studies have tracked the transformation of NICU care in Finland from the Turku University Hospital to all hospitals in Finland.

Family-Centered Care Becomes Family-Centered Developmental Care

The growth of NIDCAP training led to changes in staff activities to promote parent–infant activities such as breastfeeding and skin-to-skin contact. One of the primary goals of NIDCAP is the support of parents as the optimal caregivers of their infants. NICUs, once proud of the claim of being family-centered, began advertising their care as family-centered developmental care (FCDC). FCDC has also been referred to as neuroprotective care for the infant because it promotes physiologic stability, better infant sleep, and increased growth (Altimier & Phillips, 2016). The first set of standards, competencies, and best practices for infant FCDC has been published by an expert consensus panel (Browne et al., 2020).

PARENT-TO-PARENT SUPPORT

Hospital and Community Based

In the early 2000s, increasingly more hospitals welcomed trained veteran NICU parents as support volunteers, who would meet with new parents in the NICU. Often, if there were sufficient volunteers, parent-to-parent matches could be made that were often based on commonalities in the infant's medical condition. When hospitals were resistant to having parent volunteers come into the NICU, resourceful veteran parents created community-based programs that would make connections with parents. At first, these contacts were made by telephone and then progressed to virtual communication as the technology evolved. A nationwide boost to the movement of supporting NICU parents came from the MOD NICU Family Support Program, which began in 2001. As MOD funding declined, fewer hospitals were able to support the presence of a MOD family support specialist within the NICU; however, MOD continues to provide educational support within the NICU and after hospital discharge along with virtual support services.

Virtual Parent Support

The large network of virtual parent support of other NICU parents that currently exists had its beginnings during the first decade of this century. Some parents who had a child die in the NICU, and other parents of infants with extensive or rare medical complications, created nonprofit organizations and/or foundations as a way of bringing meaning to the trauma of their lives and their infant's existence. Many of these organizations were small in scope and excited to discover other similar organizations. Realizing that they had much to learn from each other, a national organization known as the Preemie Parent Alliance (PPA) was founded by Keira Sorrels of the Zoe Rose Memorial Foundation and five other parent support organizations in 2010. PPA, essentially an umbrella organization composed of a growing number of nonprofits, held yearly meetings and shared information continuously. These smaller organizations also exchanged social media ideas to both communicate their missions and raise funds.

Recognizing that a sizable number of NICU parents did not have premature infants, PPA decided to change its name to the NICU Parent Network (NPN) in 2019 in order to become more inclusive and welcome other parent groups. Some of the groups within NPN coordinate in-hospital NICU parent support representatives. Many groups provide virtual one-on-one and group support services, which have been extremely valuable during the COVID-19 pandemic. NPN and NPA have also collaborated to provide educational presentations. There are currently 48 member organizations within NPN.

Advances in Neonatal Care Have Benefited the Well-Being of Parents

In most instances, implementation of the changes in neonatal care have been evaluated with a variety of forms of research. Many of these research studies have included measures of emotional distress, typically completed by NICU mothers. There is a solid evidence base that all of the intervention described in this chapter (parent-to-parent support, skin-to-skin contact, single-family rooms, family-centered and individualized developmental care, the European interventions, etc.) have reduced emotional distress in NICU mothers (Hall & Hynan, 2015).

A VIEW TO THE FUTURE

As mentioned previously, an NPA work group produced a special supplemental issue of *Journal of Perinatology* titled "Interdisciplinary Recommendation for the Psychosocial Support of NICU Parents" (Hall & Hynan, 2015). In addition to a primary focus on a variety of emotional supports for parents, there was an article addressing education and support for NICU staff. This article was a relatively new addition to the evolution of newborn intensive care. The introduction to the special issue emphasized the concept that staff support was crucial to the evolving culture of newborn intensive care: "In the ideal NICU, psychosocial support of both NICU parents and staff should be goals equal in importance to the health and development of babies" (Hall & Hynan, 2015, p. S1).

The interdisciplinary recommendations included guidance in six areas: family-centered developmental care, peer-to-peer support, NICU mental health professionals, bereavement care, and discharge planning in addition to staff support. These six components of psychosocial support were then combined with

FICare to elucidate the concept of the NIPU. The name NIPU was coined by the Vermont Oxford Network (VON), which invited NPA to collaborate on a presentation at the VON conference in 2016. A combination of NPA and VON members collaborated to write an article introducing the culture of the NIPU (Hall et al., 2017).

NIPU care consists of FICare and the six components of psychosocial support described in the preceding paragraph. In the FICare model, parents are intimately involved in their infant's care. Incremental coaching is done by nurses and other staff members. Mothers, fathers, and partners are mentored to provide almost all the care for their infants, as many hours of the day as possible and a minimum of 6 hours per day (Bracht et al., 2013). Through bedside collaboration, parents gain confidence in providing care for their infants (e.g., bathing and dressing their infant, changing diapers, feeding, proper positioning, giving oral medications, and monitoring and charting their infant's progress). Maximum skin-to-skin contact is encouraged along with participation with the medical team.

Care for parents in the NIPU incorporates Kazak's (2006) pediatric psychosocial preventative health model, which involves three levels of care: universal, targeted, and clinical. Universal care, in the form of parent-to-parent support and psychoeducation groups, is given to all parents. Approximately 40% of NICU parents experience heightened symptoms of psychological distress, but at levels that allow them to still function. These parents would receive additional targeted care by specially trained nursing staff. Listening visits are a good example of targeted care that has received support (Brock et al., 2017). It is estimated that 20–30% of parents have levels of symptoms that would lead to a *Diagnostic and Statistical Manual of Mental Disorders* (American Psychiatric Association, 2013) clinical diagnosis of one of the perinatal mood and anxiety disorders (Hall & Hynan, 2015). Social workers and psychologists would provide formal clinical levels of care to these parents. If possible, clinical care should occur within the NIPU setting.

The number of clinical psychologists who work in NICUs has grown throughout the years. The handful of NICU psychologists that participated in the phone calls 15 years ago has grown to a group of more than 125. These psychologists recently formed the National Network of NICU Psychologists (NNNP). Members of NNNP have published a guide to the competencies and knowledge base that are essential to the practice of NICU psychology (Saxton et al., 2020). NNNP is sponsored by NPA. Many of the authors of chapters in this book are active NNNP members.

CONCLUSION

I wrote most of this chapter in the winter of 2020 during the midst of the COVID-19 pandemic. Currently, the evolution of perinatal care has been sidetracked while health care is in survival mode. Going forward, perinatal care will change in ways that are likely unpredictable. One clarity of the present moment is that distress levels of both NICU parents and staff are at an all-time high. Currently, the future need for greater levels of psychological services in perinatal care is unmistakable.

ACKNOWLEDGMENTS

In writing this chapter, I included information from conversations I have had with caregivers who have a long history of working in perinatal care. They include Brenda Sumrall Smith, PhD, who is a past president of NAPSW and contributor to the published guidelines for perinatal social workers. I also talked with four second-generation neonatologists who have offered suggestions. One is Dr. Bob Cicco from Pittsburgh, Pennsylvania. Bob is a past president of Parent Care, and Dr. John Kennel was his advisor in medical school. Dr. George Little was the first neonatologist in New Hampshire, and he described to me the benefits of being able to set the standards at the Dartmouth NICU with little interference from above. George is well known for being an advocate for parents attending NICU rounds. George includes Drs. Jerold Lucey and Lulu Lubchenco as his mentors and supervisors. A third is Dr. Bob White, who praises his collaboration with Dr. Stan Graven. Bob has taken the lead on creating the design standards for neonatal care, the ninth edition of which was recently published. I also renewed my acquaintance with Dr. John Grausz, one of my son's neonatologists. John established the first NICU in Milwaukee, Wisconsin, and allowed parents and grandparents in the unit 24/7. I remember John encouraging our participation in rounds if we were at bedside. This inclusion of parents was extremely rare in 1980. John completed his pediatric residency at Dr. Louis Gluck's Yale New Haven NICU.

I acknowledge the important contributions of Dr. Barry Lester to the early phone discussions among the NICU psychologists. I also appreciate the editorial assistance of Dr. Lauren Leslie-Hynan.

This chapter is dedicated to the memory of my friends, Ed Chainski, Cheryl Milford, and Jack O'Rourke.

REFERENCES

Als, H. (1982). Toward a synactive theory of development: Promise for the assessment of infant individuality. *Infant Mental Health Journal, 3,* 229–243.

Altimier, L., & Phillips, R. (2016). The neonatal integrative developmental care model: Advanced clinical applications of the seven core measures for neuroprotective family-centered developmental care. *Newborn and Infant Nursing Reviews, 16*(4), 230–244.

American Psychiatric Association. (2013). *Diagnostic and statistical manual of mental disorders* (5th ed.).

Barnett, E. R., Leiderman, P. H., Grobstein, R., & Klaus, M. (1970). Neonatal separation: The maternal side of interactional deprivation. *Pediatrics, 45,* 197–205.

Bracht, M., O'Leary, L., Lee, S., & O'Brien, K. (2013). Implementing family-integrated care in the NICU: A parent education and support program. *Advances in Neonatal Care, 13*(2), 115–126. doi:10.1097/ANC.0b013e318285fb5b

Brock, R. L., O'Hara, M. W., & Segre, L. S. (2017). Depression treatment by non-mental-health providers: Incremental evidence for the effectiveness of listening visits. *American Journal of Community Psychology, 59*, 172–183.

Browne, J. V., Jaeger, C. B., & Kenner, C.; on behalf of the Consensus Committee on Recommended Design Standards for Advanced Newborn Care. (2020). Executive summary: Standards, competencies, and recommended best practices for infant- and family-centered developmental care in the intensive care unit. *Journal of Perinatology, 40*, 5–10.

Christie, D. A., & Tansey, E. M. (Eds.). (2001). *Origins of neonatal intensive care in the UK: A witness seminar held at the Wellcome Institute for the History of Medicine, London, on 27 April 1999.* http://www.neonatology.org/pdf/WellcomeVolume9NeoUK.pdf

Hall, S. L., & Hynan, M. T. (Guest Eds.). (2015). Interdisciplinary recommendations for the psychosocial support of NICU parents. *Journal of Perinatology, 35*, S1–S36.

Hall, S. L., Hynan, M. T., Phillips, R., Lassen, S., Craig, J. W., Goyer, E., & Cohen, H. (2017). The neonatal intensive parenting unit: An introduction. *Journal of Perinatology, 37*(12), 1259–1264.

Harrison, H. (1993). The principles for family-centered neonatal care. *Pediatrics, 92*(5), 643–650.

Harrison, H., & Kositsky, A. (1984). *The premature baby book: A parents' guide to coping and caring during the first years.* St. Martin's Griffin.

Huhtala, M., Korja, R., Lehtonen, L., Haataha, L., Lapinleimu, P., Rautava, P.; PIPARI Study Group. (2012). Parental psychological well-being and behavioral outcomes of very low birth weight infants at 3 years. *Pediatrics, 129*(4), e937–e944.

Hynan, M. T. (1987). *The pain of premature parents: A psychological guide for coping.* University Press of America.

Kazak, A. E. (2006). Pediatric psychosocial preventative health model (PPPHM): Research, practice, and collaboration in pediatric family system medicine. *Family Systems Health, 24*, 381–395.

Klaus, M. H., & Kennell, J. H. (1970). Mothers separated from their newborn infants. *Pediatric Clinics of North America, 17*, 1015–1037.

Lucey, J. (1993). Parent dissatisfaction with neonatal intensive care unit and suggestions. *Pediatrics, 92*(5), 724.

Nance, S. (1982). *Premature babies: A handbook for parents.* Arbor House.

Ortenstrand, A., Westrup, B., Bronstrom, E., Sarman, I., Akerstrom, S., Brune, T., Lindberg, L., & Waldenstrom, U. (2010). The Stockholm Neonatal Family Centered Care Study: Effects on length of stay and infant morbidity. *Pediatrics, 125*(2), e278–e285.

Philip, A. G. S. (2005). The evolution of neonatology. *Pediatric Research, 58*, 799–815.

Saxton, S. N., Dempsey, A. G., Willis, T., Baughcum, A. E., Chavis, L., Hoffman, C., Fulco, C. J., Milford, C. A., & Steinberg Z. (2020). Essential knowledge and competencies for psychologists working in neonatal intensive care units. *Journal of Clinical Psychology in Medical Settings, 27*, 830–841. https://doi.org/10.1007/s10880-019-09682-8

Stinson, R., & Stinson, P. (1983). The long dying of Baby Andrew. Little, Brown.

White, R. D.; on behalf of the Committee to Establish Recommended Standards for Newborn ICU Design. (2020). Recommended standards for newborn ICU design, 9th edition. *Journal of Perinatology, 40,* 2–4.

White, R. D., & Whitman, T. L. (1992). Design of ICUs. *Pediatrics, 89,* 1267.

2

ROLES, ACTIVITIES, AND OPPORTUNITIES OF BEHAVIORAL HEALTH CLINICIANS IN DELIVERING CONTINUITY OF CARE

TIFFANY WILLIS, LATRICE L. DOWTIN, DAILYN ACOSTA, AND KARA HANSEN ■

Continuity of care is vitally important and allows families to feel safe and supported in a frequently changing environment. Mental health services across perinatal/neonatal settings can address parental mental health concerns, infant development, and infant–parent relationships. This chapter discusses the roles of a behavioral health clinician (BHC) in providing continuity of care from pregnancy through post-discharge follow-up of the infant.

INTEGRATED VERSUS CONSULTATION–LIAISON SERVICE MODELS

When establishing behavioral health services in perinatal/neonatal settings for pregnant patients and high-risk infants, health care organizations can utilize an integrated or a consultation–liaison (C/L) service delivery model. Typically, an integrated service model includes having a BHC, such as a psychologist or clinical social worker, who may attend unit meetings (e.g., bedside rounds, interdisciplinary rounds, and care meetings), is kept abreast of infant status, responds directly to the infant's or family's mental health needs, and has an active presence on the team. In contrast, the C/L model consists of a BHC who is involved with the family upon referral by the medical team. The BHC often serves other areas of the hospital and may not have any prior knowledge regarding the infant or the family. After receiving a consultation referral, the BHC consults with the team and provides intervention to the family. However, the BHC would not be a constant pillar within the unit. The implementation of both delivery models can vary across settings.

Fetal Care Center

Fetal care centers (FCCs) designed to monitor and treat pregnant people and their fetuses are growing without haste (Dempsey et al., 2021). Some provide comprehensive services from fetal diagnosis through initial neonatal intensive care intervention across disciplines, whereas others may provide services anywhere along the continuum.

A focus on perinatal mental health as a specialty in FCCs has increased following recommendations from several national organizations (e.g., the American Academy of Pediatrics and the American College of Obstetricians & Gynecologists). Expectant parents in FCCs are at high risk for developing a perinatal mood and anxiety disorder (PMAD) or needing additional psychological support related to coping with a fetal diagnosis (Cole et al., 2018). Because of this, it is recommended that a BHC be included as an integrated member of the health care team (Dempsey et al., 2021) to provide screening, assessment, and evidence-based psychological and behavioral interventions to parents. Furthermore, BHCs in FCCs create opportunities for program development, staff education, and support. This programmatic collaboration builds a bridge of communication between FCCs, neonatal intensive care units (NICUs), and follow-up settings.

NICU

Whereas social workers have long been a part of the NICU support staff, the recognition for needing psychologists in the NICU has grown since the 1970s (Saxton et al., 2020). Currently, there are both integrated and C/L NICU psychologists in select hospitals globally. Ideally, BHCs in the NICU should offer services from a family-centered approach, which allows for the inclusion of parental support, even though the infant is the identified patient (Hynan et al., 2015). In some instances, the BHC in the NICU also provides service in the NICU follow-up clinic, allowing for continuity of care. Continuity of care increases patient cooperation across settings and enhances the therapeutic alliance between clinician and patient (Haggerty, 2003).

NICU Follow-Up Clinic

When a high-risk infant is discharged from the hospital, they are often followed by medical providers in a specialty clinic referred to as a NICU follow-up clinic. In these clinics, BHCs continue to provide support utilizing a family-centered care approach. Infants who are NICU graduates are at high risk for developmental concerns (i.e., cognitive, socioemotional/behavioral, language, and motor). Socioemotional intervention provided by BHCs can enhance the parent–child relationship and improve subsequent development. Furthermore, engagement with a BHC allows families to gain knowledge and skills about developmental care, behavioral challenges, and/or neurodevelopmental concerns (Saxton et al., 2020).

SCREENING AND ASSESSMENT

PMADs and Screening

One study found that pregnant people with a diagnosis of a fetal anomaly have an increased likelihood of experiencing depression (22%), anxiety (31%), and traumatic distress symptoms (39%) compared to the general pregnant population, 11% of whom experience perinatal depression (Long et al., 2019). Likewise, NICU parents have a three times increased risk of experiencing a PMAD (S. Hall et al., 2015). This risk for a mental health crisis can continue post NICU discharge and can directly affect the infant's well-being, both medically and developmentally. PMADs can interfere with a caregiver's ability to bond and create a secure attachment with their infant, thus disrupting healthy developmental, cognitive, and emotional outcomes (S. Hall et al., 2015). Research has shown that this disruption during a critical period of development can cause lifelong consequences, even into future generations (S. Hall et al., 2015). Therefore, screening for PMADs in the FCC, NICU, and NICU follow-up clinic is imperative.

Early identification through screening, support, resources, and treatment decreases the severity and length of a mental health episode (Austin & Kingston, 2016). The Edinburgh Postnatal Depression Scale (EPDS) is the most widely accepted screening tool for perinatal and postpartum depression. The EPDS is freely accessible online and translated in 18 different languages. The tool can be administered quickly and has high validity and reliability, including three questions that assess anxiety (Zhong et al., 2014). Whereas there is no universally recommended time frame for administering mental health screening in the perinatal period, it is recommended that screening be completed at least once during pregnancy and postpartum, at minimum (American College of Obstetricians and Gynecologists, 2018). Screening has been shown to effectively identify parents who are experiencing current symptoms of depression and anxiety (Maliszewska et al., 2016), which makes it a key part of a person's pregnancy and postpartum experience.

A positive EPDS score indicates the need for further assessment and referral. It is important to note that the EPDS was created for the general pregnant and post-partum population, without taking into account the distress that occurs for many parents in a fetal care, NICU, and/or NICU follow-up setting. Ideally, parents who screen positive on the EPDS are referred to a BHC within the hospital system for further assessment and treatment (Hynan et al., 2015). Seeing a BHC within the health care setting correlates with patients rating their therapeutic alliance with their BHC higher than their therapeutic alliance with previous therapists (Corso et al., 2012). It is worth noting that screening should only be implemented when it is also possible to conduct risk assessment and provide appropriate intervention and/or referrals in a timely manner.

Assessment of Family/Family System

It is important that within the first week of the NICU stay or within the first few appointments in an FCC, a BHC performs an evaluation of the family's history, existing resources, and needs. It is also important that both parents receive a screening for emotional distress. With this early assessment, a BHC can engage necessary support services and make appropriate referrals. If a family needs clinical support, they should be referred to an internal BHC (which is ideal) or community-located mental health professional for individual, couple, or family therapy. Assessment of a pregnant or postpartum parent's mental health is best completed by a BHC with training specific to perinatal mental health. The assessment is completed with the parent and ideally their partner or primary support person. The BHC's goal is to gather information about the parent's birth story, primary support systems (e.g., family, culture, spirituality, and profession), personal strengths and weaknesses, past experiences with health care, social determinants of health, trauma history, current or past substance use, and prescription drug use—all indicators of a thorough perinatal mental health assessment (Maliszewska et al., 2016). The BHC will attempt to gain an understanding of how the parent was functioning prior to pregnancy. This provides insight into the onset of symptoms, which may help with diagnosis and treatment planning.

As with any assessment process, it is important that the BHC have appropriate training and understanding of assessment protocols, as well as psychometrics. It is imperative to pay close attention to issues of confidentiality and privacy, time and resources needed, and logistics of implementation and to have a clear plan delineating how screening and assessment results will be handled, including in instances of acute crisis identified during the assessment process.

Developmental Surveillance, Screening, and Assessment

NICU follow-up clinics throughout the United States vary in how they serve NICU graduates. However, there are some basic consistencies found in most follow-up clinics, including developmental surveillance, screening, and assessment. In some NICU follow-up clinics, BHCs offer dyadic therapy to support bonding and attachment by addressing the mental health needs of the parent as well as the socioemotional and developmental needs of the infant. In order to address the totality of the impact of the NICU experience, it is recommended that all aforementioned services be made available to families receiving care in a NICU follow-up clinic.

The American Academy of Pediatrics (AAP, 2006) recommends that all providers of child health care conduct developmental monitoring (also called surveillance), in addition to developmental screening for young children. Developmental monitoring is an informal process that involves verbal inquiry with parents to discuss the child's milestones and developmental progress, whereas developmental screening is a more formal process that utilizes standardized developmental screening tools to identify developmental areas of strength and concern. This type of screening is especially important for NICU graduates because they are at greater risk for delays, and early identification of areas of concern can aid in ensuring families are engaged in adequate early intervention services.

Developmental assessment in the NICU follow-up clinic is also important because it helps direct intervention. Developmental screening helps identify areas of concern, whereas assessment evaluates developmental functioning and aids in creation of recommendations for treatment and intervention when there is a developmental delay identified. There are variations regarding recommendations for when infants should receive their first neurodevelopmental assessment. Some literature suggests it should occur within the first year, whereas others suggest waiting until toddler age when language is more developed (Kuppala et al., 2011). The AAP recommends that infants, particularly those born weighing 1,500 grams or less, should participate in follow-up evaluations at 1 and 2 years of age, at minimum (Kilpatrick et al., 2017). The AAP also recommends both developmental and behavioral measures be used to identify early developmental and learning difficulties for NICU graduates (DeBattista, 2018). In addition, there are several dyadic assessments that shed light on the strength of the attachment relationship and provide insight to help engage the parent in a healthy relationship and improve bonding (Givrad et al., 2021). Standard attachment assessments include the Marshack Interaction Method, Early Relational Assessment, and the Crowell. Results from these assessments can help inform the intervention, and these assessments can be used throughout therapy to evaluate progress.

The *Diagnostic Classification of Mental Health and Developmental Disorders of Infancy and Early Childhood* manual (DC:0–5; Zero to Three, 2016) is commonly used for the diagnosis of children from birth to age 5 years. In its diagnostic criteria, this manual takes into consideration the age and developmental expectations of infants and young children and is most appropriate when providing a diagnosis in a NICU follow-up clinic setting. It allows for diagnosis of neurodevelopmental delays, social and emotional problems, as well as problems within the relationship between the child and their primary caregiver. Some diagnoses in the DC:0–5 do not directly correlate to the *International Classification of Diseases* (ICD; World

Health Organization, 2019) billing system; however, there is a cross-walk to the fifth edition of the *Diagnostic and Statistical Manual of Mental Disorders* (DSM-5; American Psychiatric Association, 2013), which is used in psychology and psychiatry to diagnose pathology in children and adults. Once a DC:0–5 diagnosis is cross-walked to a DSM-5 diagnosis, it can be correlated with an ICD code and used for billing because most insurance companies require an ICD code for reimbursement.

CONSULTATION, INTERVENTIONS, AND TREATMENT

Fetal Care Center

Psychoeducation is the most used intervention to address perinatal mental health conditions in the prenatal stage (Long et al., 2019). Psychoeducation, incorporating components of evidence-based interventions, is an effective tool for helping people cope with symptoms of perinatal mental health conditions (Byatt et al., 2013). Helping parents understand the fetal diagnosis, what they can anticipate for the remainder of their pregnancy, and normalizing what they may experience emotionally are often therapeutic.

In addition to psychoeducation, various models of therapy can support expectant parents. Crisis counseling addresses the urgent needs of expectant parents and families who have received difficult news about their developing baby. Supportive counseling can provide acknowledgment, affirmation, and validation. Family or couples therapy may be appropriate depending on how the family is coping (Hynan et al., 2015). Cognitive–behavioral therapy (CBT) and interpersonal therapy (IPT) are commonly used evidence-based methods for treating patients with PMADs (Hynan et al., 2015).

In the fetal care setting, the BHC gives special attention to grief, redefining pregnancy and parental expectations, and interpersonal relationships, including the bond between the developing baby and parents. Introducing and teaching the practice of mindfulness is also an effective intervention (Hynan et al., 2015). The BHC introduces the concept of mindfulness and can teach some basic tenets of the practice, such as stillness and deep breathing. If the parent's mental health needs go beyond the scope of practice for the BHC within the confines of a brief therapeutic or C/L model, referrals can be made to psychiatry for a medication evaluation and/or a perinatal mental health provider for longer term/more intensive therapeutic services. Ideally, such services can be offered directly in the FCC by an integrated BHC who has adequate training and expertise.

NICU

The NICU BHC can provide trauma-informed, family-centered, developmental care for infants and families during their hospitalization. Areas for intervention and consultation in the NICU may involve (a) addressing caregivers' experiences of emotional distress; (b) engaging in dyadic work to support the parent–infant relationship and parenting practices; (c) providing education, consultation, and advocacy regarding the NICU environment and unit design, and its impact on infant neurodevelopment; and (d) supporting, educating, and consulting with the NICU staff (S. L. Hall et al., 2015).

The BHC may provide infant mental health interventions to the infant and family drawn from multiple approaches and modalities, including CBT, psychodynamic theory, family and couples therapy, and IPT (Hynan et al., 2015). At some institutions, the parent will have a separate medical chart, in which documentation may be most appropriate. However, in a children's hospital setting, documentation will likely occur in the chart of the infant who is the identified patient. Caution should be exercised regarding documenting the details of the parent's mental health. Information that will be helpful to supporting and interacting with the family or treating the patient is within reason to document. The BHC should remain well informed on hospital-wide and community resources that would support further assessment and treatment of parental emotional distress that goes beyond the scope of the family's experience of the infant's NICU hospitalization or ongoing medical needs.

Dyadic work with families may center on (a) providing support around positive parenting in the context of a medical diagnosis or the NICU setting, (b) facilitating and exploring infant mental health topics that address aspects of the evolving parent–infant bond, and (c) supporting developmental neuroprotective practices of daily caregiving. Additional recommendations for infant- and family-centered developmental care practices are delineated in the *Report of the First Consensus Conference on Standards, Competencies and Best Practices for Infant and Family Centered Developmental Care in the Intensive Care Unit* (Consensus Committee, 2019).

With a focus on protecting and supporting infant neurodevelopment, the BHC is also uniquely positioned to advocate, support, and educate on NICU environmental practices and unit design standards that are evidenced-based and neuroprotective. The Consensus Committee has provided the most recent updates to the unit design recommendations in the *Recommended Standards for Newborn Intensive Care Unit Design 9th Edition,* which focuses on optimizing unit design to facilitate medical care for the infant while also supporting the needs of the family and the staff (Consensus Committee, 2020).

Similar to the FCCs, BHCs can also facilitate care through the consultation, education, and direct support of the NICU staff, who may experience burnout, compassion fatigue, moral distress, secondary traumatic stress, and/or other forms of distress (S. L. Hall et al., 2015).

NICU Follow-Up Clinic

BHCs in NICU follow-up clinics should have training and supervised experience in infant and young child development, ideally with an emphasis on medical complexities. Integration of a BHC in a NICU follow-up clinic is advisable because it helps address an array of needs beyond the child's medical disposition (Feehan et al., 2019). BHCs in this setting serve as an extension of the medical team and can help screen, evaluate, and treat various presenting concerns, including developmental, behavioral, parent–child relationships, and perinatal mental health (Feehan et al., 2019).

BHCs can engage with a family in multiple ways in the NICU follow-up clinic. The pediatrician can consult the BHC during a medical visit if a relevant concern is raised during the medical portion of the visit. For example, if the parent shares with the pediatrician that they are having difficulty getting their child on a consistent sleep schedule, the BHC can meet with the parent during the visit and provide solution-focused, practical guidance and psychoeducation to improve the child's sleep routine. The BHC can choose to follow up at the child's next medical visit and/or schedule a separate follow-up visit with the family prior to their next scheduled medical visit.

Consultations can be a one-time encounter, consist of follow-up visits, or translate to ongoing therapy with the BHC. In a true integrated care setting, the BHC can see the child and parent within the NICU follow-up clinic setting, and progress notes, treatment goals, and recommendations are documented and accessible to the entire medical team providing care to the child. Although this approach is recommended, some clinics have a co-located model in which integration of services is not present and teams work as referral partners. In these settings, the BHC may be unable to see the parent and child in real time (during the medical appointment), and thus documentation and recommendations are not readily accessible to the medical team. The latter model is less preferred, but for some, it is a first step toward developing an integrated care model.

One of the major benefits to having a BHC in the NICU follow-up clinic is that it increases access to care for those at highest risk but who may be least likely to access psychology support service (Feehan et al., 2019). Indeed, with African American families being at greatest risk for infant mortality and having perinatal depression at a rate three times that of their counterparts, but least likely to seek therapy, having a BHC in the NICU follow-up clinic helps ensure that a subset of families who would otherwise go without services receive them (Feehan et al., 2019).

PROGRAM DEVELOPMENT AND EVALUATION

Program Development

Program development in an FCC, NICU, or NICU follow-up clinic begins with investment from the medical directors regarding the importance of mental and emotional well-being for families and infants. There are many articles supporting the need for mental health professionals in these settings; many of these can be found on the National Perinatal Association (NPA) website (https://www.nationalperina

tal.org). Once administrative buy-in is acquired, there are four main areas of development across all settings that may occur: family support, developmental care,
staff education and support, and quality improvement (Hynan et al., 2015). When
implementing behavioral health services in a fetal or neonatal setting, the existing
services will determine which area of development will serve as a priority. Utilizing
NPA's NICU self-assessment tool is an excellent way to determine a unit's strengths
and areas for growth and development. After completing this NICU self-assessment,
program development can be adjusted and/or initiated, as indicated.

FAMILY SUPPORT

FCCs and NICUs are two distinct units; however, there is significant overlap in
the family support that is needed. The focus in both settings is prevention and intervention of mental health sequela, parent–infant/fetal bonding, education, and
peer connection. It is important that families have the resources they need to cope
with the trauma of their experience. Peer-to-peer support is one form of support that is often available to families. Some NICUs and FCCs have family groups
that are more casual and include educational information, as well as provide
families the opportunity to receive support and provide support to one another.
Other institutions have a more formal mental health, provider-led group therapy.
Many hospitals also offer a one-on-one parent support program in which current
families are partnered with a veteran mentor family that can offer advice and support from a "lived" perspective. It is also important that families have a respite
space either on the unit or in the hospital where they can have solitude, quiet, and
decompress after or before a difficult procedure, surgery, or a challenging medical
report. Families should also have access to activities such as arts and crafts that
can be made for their infant's bedside social gatherings (e.g., a family lunch event
or ice cream social). These types of events allow families to engage in self-care and
promote social engagement.

Spiritual care services is another important support service that should be made
available to families. Chaplains are spiritual leaders who can pray for and with
families and help them strengthen their faith, as well as process questions that
challenge their faith as a result of their infant's NICU admission or fetal diagnosis.
Last, program development should include access to palliative care services. In an
FCC, NICU, and NICU follow-up clinic, there are risks for mortality. Palliative
care services provide families access to individuals who can support them across
the continuum of care as they endeavor into a world of having a fragile, medically complex, high-risk child. Palliative care support is an extension of the support from the BHC because palliative care can help guide decision-making from
a medical perspective as well as coordinate with the medical team regarding comfort care and end-of-life procedures and preferences.

DEVELOPMENTAL CARE

Developmental care in the NICU and NICU follow-up clinic setting is vitally
important. Infants in the NICU consequently forfeit regular engagement and

interaction with people and their environment; as a result, development can be impacted. It is important that providers are aware of this and create programming and initiatives, as well as provide education about how to address barriers to adequate development. Child life specialists are excellent resources and should be involved in the care and treatment of infants in the NICU. They can help engage infants in social and emotional play, as well as developmental games and activities. In addition, more formal developmental services such as speech, occupational, and physical therapies should be made available for infants who qualify for these interventions. Services such as music therapy and infant massage support healthy brain development, along with socioemotional development. Last, a developmental care team that evaluates the NICU environment for factors that influence development, such as sound decibels, cycled lighting, and positioning, is helpful to ensure that infants are exposed to the most conducive environment for their development.

STAFF EDUCATION AND SUPPORT

Physicians, nurse practitioners, nurses, fellows, residents, and any fetal care and NICU staff should receive regular training on topics that relate to the care of pregnant people and developing infants. Training should be a part of the orientation process for new staff and conducted regularly at conferences or educational updates throughout the year (S. Hall et al., 2015). It is important for those caring for families to received training on the power of relationships, the impact of attachment and bonding, PMAD symptoms, trauma-informed care, family-centered care, culture and diversity, and death and dying (S. Hall et al., 2015). When staff are educated on these topics, it positions them to provide more holistic care. Health care providers in high-stress, high-trauma environments often experience vicarious trauma. It is important that they also have a safe place to debrief about their experiences and gain support for their own distress. This form of support can serve as a protective factor against compassion fatigue and burnout (S. Hall et al., 2015). BHCs, with their training and education around providing emotional support, are well-positioned to serve in this role for staff.

RESEARCH AND QUALITY IMPROVEMENT

Given that psychology in perinatal/neonatal settings is still a developing field, it is important that research and quality improvement (QI) initiatives are embedded in the program development process. Research and QI topics can take various directions depending on the unit, clinic, and the providers' specific interests. Research and QI can be utilized in the program evaluation process by evaluating the effectiveness of interventions, the service of psychology, or other implemented initiatives. These data can be helpful in justifying the role of psychology in the perinatal/neonatal setting and can help provide necessary feedback to adjust BHCs' service delivery to meet the needs of infants and families.

Program Evaluation

According to Newcomer et al. (2015), program evaluation is the process of methodically analyzing a program's outcomes, participation, adherence to policies and structures, ongoing feasibility, modification, and continuation. For evaluations to be helpful in the decision-making process, the collected data must be consistent and gathered using tools and measures that have high validity and reliability (Newcomer et al., 2015). Proper program evaluation should be established at the outset, during planning, and throughout implementation (also referred to as program monitoring). At a minimum, it would be beneficial for mental health programs designed for expectant parents and high-risk infants to explore disparities in access to care, adherence to program policies (e.g., screening and assessment accuracy and timeliness), satisfaction with communication among and between staff and parents, and effectiveness of education. When health care inequities are identified, program administrators should seek consultation from field experts who are knowledgeable about minimizing such disparities.

Program evaluation is best conducted by a multidisciplinary team so that all facets of service delivery can be considered in the evaluation process. Input from a variety of disciplines not only widens the perspective of what data or information to gather but also aids in the implementation of the evaluation so that the workload does not rely on one individual or a single discipline.

ADVOCACY

Advocating for the integration of BHCs in the perinatal/neonatal setting is imperative to the well-being of families. It is important to determine who are the decision-makers in the institution and then prepare a formal proposal for integrating mental health services in the FCC, NICU, and NICU follow-up settings. Including information regarding the current rate of PMADs in the general population compared to families of hospitalized infants and those carrying high-risk pregnancies will be a critical component in the proposal. It is also important to include information on the impact of developmental care, family-centered care, and perinatal and infant mental health needs for infants and families in the NICU and post discharge. In addition, information on the benefits of developmental surveillance and assessment in the follow-up clinic setting should be included in the proposal. Establishing a job description, which can be found on the NPA website under "Psychologists in the NICU," might be helpful to include in the proposal in addition to information about billing. Hospitals need to know how to pay for mental health services. Many hospitals offset a portion of the BHC's salary by billing for their services using Health and Behavior codes for inpatient services and Psychotherapy codes for outpatient services; however, this can vary by institution. There is a need for improved reimbursement models because all state Medicaid agencies have not opened the Health and Behavior codes used for services provided in these settings. Hospitals also supplement with grant funding, philanthropy monies, and/or through the departmental budget. Psychology and other behavioral health services for families with high-risk pregnancies and medically complex children in the FCC, NICU, and NICU follow-up setting are a growing area, but advocacy for continued expansion and financial backing is necessary.

CONCLUSION

BHCs provide an important service to families throughout the perinatal and neonatal continuum. Although an integrated BHC is the preferred model, at minimum a C/L provider trained in perinatal mental health, infant/child development, and delivery of services within medical settings is recommended to adequately meet the mental health, developmental/behavioral, and relational needs of infants and their parents across the continuum of care. BHCs provide vital services, such as screening, assessment, and therapeutic intervention, which improve mental health and developmental outcomes for infants and families. All FCC, NICU, and NICU follow-up clinics should have a BHC who can develop programming that supports the infant, child, parent, and family experience and evaluates the outcomes of the programming through research and quality improvement projects. The push for BHCs in these settings is central to ensuring the highest potential is reached for infants and their families alike.

REFERENCES

American Academy of Pediatrics. (2006). Identifying infants and young children with developmental disorders in the medical home: An algorithm for developmental surveillance and screening. *Pediatrics, 118*(1), 405–420. doi:10.1542/peds.2006-1231

American College of Obstetricians and Gynecologists. (2018). ACOG Committee Opinion No. 757: Screening for perinatal depression. *Obstetrics & Gynecology, 132*(5), e208–e212.

American Psychiatric Association. (2013). *Diagnostic and statistical manual of mental disorders* (5th ed.).

Austin, M. P., & Kingston, D. (2016). Psychosocial assessment and depression screening in the perinatal period: Benefits, challenges and implementation. In A.-L. Sutter-Dalley, N. M.-C. Glangeaud-Freudenthal, A. Guedeney, & A. Riecher-Rossler (Eds.), *Joint care of parents and infants in perinatal psychiatry* (pp. 167–195). Springer.

Byatt, N., Biebel, K., Friedman, L., Debordes-Jackson, G., Ziedonis, D., & Pbert, L. (2013). Patient's views on depression care in obstetric settings: How do they compare to the views of perinatal health care professionals? *General Hospital Psychiatry, 35*(6), 598–604.

Cole, J. C. M., Olkkola, M., Zarrin, H. E., Berger, K., & Moldenhauer, J. S. (2018). Universal postpartum mental health screening for parents of newborns with prenatally diagnosed birth defects. *Journal of Obstetric, Gynecologic & Neonatal Nursing, 47*(1), 84–93. https://doi.org/10.1016/j.jogn.2017.04.131

Consensus Committee. (2019, November). *Report of the First Consensus Conference on Standards, Competencies and Best Practices for Infant and Family Centered Developmental Care in the Intensive Care Unit.* https://nicudesign.nd.edu/assets/350964/website_manuscript_complete_document_w_references_november_2019_1_.docx.pdf

Consensus Committee. (2020). *NICU recommended standards.* University of Notre Dame. Retrieved December 11, 2020, from https://nicudesign.nd.edu

Corso, K. A., Bryan, C. J., Corso, M. L., Kanzler, K. E., Houghton, D. C., Ray-Sannerud, B., & Morrow, C. E. (2012). Therapeutic alliance and treatment outcome in the primary care behavioral health model. *Families, Systems, & Health, 30*(2), 87.

DeBattista, A. (2018). HRIF clinic organization: A statewide approach. In H. Needelman & B. J. Jackson (Eds.), *Follow-up for NICU graduates* (pp. 207–219). Springer.

Dempsey, A. G., Chavis, L., Willis, T., Zuk, J., & Cole, J. C. M. (2021). Addressing perinatal mental health risk within a fetal care center. *Journal of Clinical Psychology in Medical Settings, 28*(1), 125–136. https://doi.org/10.1007/s10880-020-09728-2

Feehan, K., Kehinde, F., Sachs, K., Mossabeb, R., Berhane, Z., Pachter, L. M., Brody, S., & Turchi, R. M. (2019). Development of a Multidisciplinary Medical Home Program for NICU graduates. *Maternal and Child Health Journal, 24*(1), 11–21. doi:10.1007/s10995-019-02818-0

Givrad, S., Dowtin, L. T. L., Scala, M., & Hall, S. L. (2021). Recognizing and mitigating infant distress in neonatal intensive care unit (NICU). *Journal of Neonatal Nursing, 27*(1), 14–20. https://doi.org/10.1016/j.jnn.2020.09.009

Haggerty, J. L. (2003). Continuity of care: A multidisciplinary review. *British Medical Journal, 327*(7425), 1219–1221. https://doi.org/10.1136/bmj.327.7425.1219

Hall, S., Hynan, M., Phillips, R., Press, J., Kenner, C., & Ryan, D. J. (2015). Development of program standards for psychosocial support of parents of infants admitted to a neonatal intensive care unit: A national interdisciplinary consensus model. *Newborn and Infant Nursing Reviews, 15*(1), 24–27. doi:10.1053/j.nainr.2015.01.007

Hall, S. L., Cross, J., Selix, N. W., Patterson, C., Segre, L., Chuffo-Siewert, R., Geller, P. A., & Martin, M. L. (2015). Recommendations for enhancing psychosocial support of NICU parents through staff education and support. *Journal of Perinatology, 35*(1), S29–S36. doi:10.1038/jp.2015.147

Hynan, M. T., Steinberg, Z., Baker, L., Cicco, R., Geller, P. A., Lassen, S., Millford, C., Mounts, K. O., Patterson, C., Saxton, S., Segre, L., & Stuebe, A. (2015). Recommendations for mental health professionals in the NICU. *Journal of Perinatology, 35*(1), S14–S18. doi:10.1038/jp.2015.144

Kilpatrick, S. J., Papile, L. A., & Macones, G. A. (2017). *Guidelines for perinatal care.* American Academy of Pediatrics.

Kuppala, V. S., Tabangin, M., Haberman, B., Steichen, J., & Yolton, K. (2011). Current state of high-risk infant follow-up care in the United States: Results of a national survey of academic follow-up programs. *Journal of Perinatology, 32*(4), 293–298. doi:10.1038/jp.2011.97

Long, M. M., Cramer, R. J., Jenkins, J., Bennington, L., & Paulson, J. F. (2019). A systematic review of interventions for healthcare professionals to improve screening and referral for perinatal mood and anxiety disorders. *Archives of Women's Mental Health, 22*(1), 25–36.

Maliszewska, K., Świątkowska-Freund, M., Bidzan, M., & Preis, K. (2016). Relationship, social support, and personality as psychosocial determinants of the risk for post-partum blues. *Ginekologia Polska, 87*(6), 442–447.

Newcomer, K. E., Hatry, H. P., & Wholey, J. S. (Eds.). (2015). *Handbook of practical program evaluation*. Wiley.

Saxton, S. N., Dempsey, A. G., Willis, T., Baughcum, A. E., Chavis, L., Hoffman, C., Fulco, C. J., Milford, C. A., & Steinberg, Z. (2020). Essential knowledge and competencies for psychologists working in neonatal intensive care units. *Journal of Clinical Psychology in Medical* Settings, *27*, 830–841. https://doi.org/10.1007/s10 880-019-09682-8

World Health Organization. (2019). *International statistical classification of diseases and related health problems* (11th ed.).

Zero to Three. (2016). *Diagnostic classification of mental health and developmental disorders of infancy and early childhood: DC:0–5*.

Zhong, Q., Gelaye, B., Rondon, M. E., Sánchez, S. J., García, P., Sánchez, E. V., Barrios, Y. E., Simon, G. C., Henderson, D., May Cripe, S., & Williams, M. A. (2014). Comparative performance of patient health questionnaire-9 and Edinburgh Postnatal Depression Scale for screening Antepartum Depression. *Journal of Affective Disorders, 162*, 1–7. https://doi.org/10.1016/j.jad.2014.03.028

3

QUALITY IMPROVEMENT AND RESEARCH ACROSS FETAL AND NEONATAL CARE SETTINGS

PAMELA A. GELLER, ARIANA ALBANESE,
VICTORIA A. GRUNBERG, JOHN CHUO,
AND CHAVIS A. PATTERSON ∎

In recent decades, there has been a surge in research focusing on parental mental health and psychosocial issues within fetal and neonatal care settings. This growth mirrors the increased national attention to parental mental health and psychosocial factors across these care settings. A recent historical review showed continuing trends of exponential growth of publications addressing the emotional responses and psychosocial well-being of parents and families across neonatal care settings (Geller, Albanese, et al., 2021). In large part, this growth in attention and published research reflects the (a) substantial evidence that parental psychological well-being is significantly associated with child's behavioral, emotional, linguistic, and cognitive development (Huhtala et al., 2012); (b) technological medical advances that have permitted a wider scope of neonatal care beyond infant physical health outcomes; and (c) expansion and diversification of disciplines involved in service delivery across neonatal intensive care units (NICUs), fetal care centers (FCCs), and neonatal follow-up clinics. In particular, the presence of psychologists and other clinical scientists on treatment teams who have training in clinical research design and methods creates unique opportunities for projects aimed to enhance behavioral health services for families and staff functioning, as well as promote new knowledge in the field.

Although there has been tremendous advancement in efforts to address parental and familial mental health and psychosocial functioning in this arena, there is still a long way to go and the field is ripe for improvement. As such, the FCC, NICU, and neonatal follow-up settings provide a vast and unique frontier for important and novel investigation. Investigative efforts are necessary to further identify psychosocial needs of parents, refine and develop evidence-based care for families, better assist with staff education and support, create an evidence base to provide information critical to advocate for staffing and policy changes, and extend knowledge to propel the field forward.

In this chapter, we discuss two investigative disciplines—research and quality improvement (QI)—and present their distinctions as well as their synergies and application within fetal and neonatal care settings. The chapter begins with a brief overview to distinguish these disciplines and highlight typical approaches/models within each. This is followed by presentation of key areas that warrant research exploration related to behavioral health issues in fetal and neonatal care settings and an overview of practical considerations for research application in these settings.

DIFFERENTIATING RESEARCH PROJECTS FROM QUALITY IMPROVEMENT PROJECTS

As QI techniques have become more extensive and sophisticated over time, there are some gray areas in which research and QI methodology show overlap (Finkelstein et al., 2015); however, although research and QI investigations share a number of similarities, there are several key features that set them apart. Table 3.1 illustrates key features of research and QI and provides exemplar projects within each category. Distinctions are also described below.

In terms of studies conducted in NICU treatment settings, research studies are concerned with *identifying* treatments that are efficacious, whereas QI studies focus on *delivery of* efficacious treatment. The gold standard model of intervention research is the randomized controlled trial (RCT), which aims to test the efficacy of a treatment against a control condition. The goal of efficacy studies is to determine whether a specific treatment will improve physical or mental health outcomes compared to placebos or alternative treatments. However, in this study design, random assignment limits other sources of bias that may impact results, which in turn increases confidence that the observed results are due to the treatment being studied. QI projects alternatively focus on implementation, or the "real-world" treatment effectiveness in medical practice. QI studies use SMART aims (i.e., specific, measurable, achievable, relevant/realistic, and time-based/timely) to create a goal that is carefully planned, clear and trackable, and that intends to improve an outcome by implementing change in the health system that will optimize delivery of treatments already proven to be efficacious in a well-controlled research setting. Results in research studies typically are not analyzed and determined until the end of the study, whereas data are constantly being monitored in QI, searching for statistical shifts in outcomes.

Interventions in research designs remain constant throughout the study time period, whereas QI interventions can evolve over time based on monitored data and observations in the experimental setting. Randomization (random assignment to a study condition) is deployed in controlled trials in research and in planned experimentation in QI (Finkelstein et al., 2015). Specifically, randomization is

Table 3.1 DISTINCTIONS AND SIMILARITIES OF QUALITY IMPROVEMENT
AND RESEARCH

	Research	Quality Improvement
Intent	OPTIMIZE THE HEALTH OF INDIVIDUALS AND POPULATIONS	
General project goals	Development of new knowledge to prove or disprove *a hypothesis* to explain biological mechanisms and/or identify efficacious methods of treatment or health care delivery. Knowledge is usually generalizable across different scenarios.	Development of new knowledge to solve *a specific problem* regarding the quality of health care delivery. Knowledge usually needs to be modified according to local context in order to be useful.
Approach to clinical management	*Efficacy of treatment*: Does the treatment under investigation work better than placebo under ideal conditions?	*Effectiveness of treatment*: What does the health care system have to do in order to implement efficacious treatment and get the expected results?
Premise	Hypotheses are generated to determine mechanistic relationships between variables (i.e., impact of physical separation of parents from infant on family bonding).	Theories are generated to identify interventions that improve the quality of health care delivery (safe, effective, equitable, efficient, patient-centered, timely) in order to impact important outcomes (i.e., integrating research-backed bonding techniques into practice for NICU families).
Controls	Designed to identify associations among variables while controlling for cofounders	Designed to coexist with cofounders in order to close existing gaps between ideal and real practices and outcomes
Setting	SINGLE OR MULTISITE	
Hypotheses and use of data	Data are collected for later analysis of interactions between an outcome and influencing factors—in support or to disprove a *single hypothesis.*	Data are collected for real-time analysis of interactions between outcomes and interventions, and the interventions are adopted, adapted, or abandoned in the course of the project—*multiple hypotheses* are generated over iterative PDSA experiments.
Subject risk	Variable risks and benefits—often unknown	None or minimal

Table 3.1 Continued

	Research	Quality Improvement
Ethics board approval	Approval is provided by the IRB of the institution in which the head of the study (primary investigator) practices. All IRBs are held to a universal standard of human protection outlined by the Declaration of Helsinki. The approval process can be lengthy.	Approval is provided by ethics board in the local institution. Members may vary slightly from one institution to the next.
Informed consent	Required	Not typically required, but institutional IRB dependent
Exemplar projects	FNI randomized controlled trial (Welch et al., 2012) *Hypothesis*: Increasing the amount of bonding and calming activities for the mother–infant dyad during a preterm infant's NICU stay will improve behavioral and emotional outcomes for the mother and neurodevelopmental and emotional outcomes for the infant. *Goal*: Compare the efficacy of the novel FNI, a program that promotes mother–infant bonding and dyad well-being via facilitated engagement in calming activities, to standard care (the typical treatment mothers and infants receive during a NICU stay). *Method*: Randomized controlled trial wherein families are randomly assigned to either standard care or FNI and assessments are "blinded" (individuals collecting data are unaware of whether participants are in the standard care or FNI group).	Implementation of efficacious FNI interventions in two NICUs *Problem*: Compliance with best practices (FNI interventions is at 50%). *SMART aim*: Improve compliance with FNI practice guidelines in two NICUs by 10% within 12 months. *Method*: In each NICU, a driver diagram will be created by a multidisciplinary stakeholder team. Process measures related to the drivers for each unit will be tracked in a family of control charts in order to assess the effectiveness of interventions and determine whether they require change using iterative PDSA cycles. Balance measures will be tracked similarly to understand unintended consequences.

FNI, Family Nurture Intervention; IRB, institutional review board; NICU, neonatal intensive care units; PSDA, Plan–Do–Study–Act.

applied to determine the assignment of factor combinations or the order of performing some step in the project (Moen et al., 2012). A multitude of statistical methods can be used to analyze data obtained in a research study depending on the research question(s), whereas QI projects predominantly utilize statistical control charts. In terms of models of inquiry employed, QI projects might implement plan–do–study–act (PDSA) cycles, which involve testing changes and iterating upon change in response to observed consequences of the change.

As different as research and QI are, ultimately they depend on each other to achieve a common goal—healthier patients and families. Whereas research may provide information about mechanistic relationships between variables and evidence of treatment efficacy, QI work allows providers to effectively integrate these findings into real-world practice. In order to determine whether one's project is best classed as QI or research, investigators in fetal and neonatal care settings should answer the questions provided in Box 3.1. Of note, although institutional review board (IRB) approval processes vary between QI and research, with human-subjects research approval generally proving more lengthy and intensive, it is highly encouraged that investigators submit their QI projects to the local IRB because approval procedures may vary between institutions.

IMPORTANT TOPICS AND DIRECTIONS FOR RESEARCH

A range of topics, questions, variables, and aspects of care are currently the focus of clinical and research attention in fetal and neonatal care settings and would be beneficial to address as the field moves forward. The selection of topics and potential areas of investigation presented in this section reflect areas of current importance and could be the focus of QI or research projects, including sociodemographic considerations, NICU family experience, longitudinal research, guidelines for psychosocial care, and psychosocial interventions. Consideration of the goals, questions, and scope of the specific project, as outlined in the previous section, would determine which approach best addresses the study objectives.

Sociodemographic Considerations

The majority of extant data on parents during the perinatal period, including NICU parents, focus on mothers. Ideally, data should be obtained from fathers and partners as well as mothers to extend current knowledge about this often neglected group. Inclusion of siblings and extended family members (e.g., grandparents) in studies is also lacking. Broader definitions of the family system beyond the traditional family structure should be considered, such as single parents, same-sex parent(s), adoptive, and surrogate families. Moreover, consideration of intersectionality and concerted efforts toward inclusivity in terms of race, ethnicity, language, religion, spirituality, culture, and socioeconomic status are necessary to obtain accurate data about the population of families who receive services across fetal and neonatal care settings.

Box 3.1

ACTIONABLE CHECKLIST

Answer the questions below by marking an option in the column that best corresponds to your project. Tally each column total (the number of response options selected in that column) to get a sense of whether your project is best understood as QI or Research. Of note, counsel should always be sought from your institution's review board as requirements may vary from site to site.

	Research	**Quality Improvement**

Checklist Question 1: Are you focusing on proving/disproving a hypothesis or solving a problem?

	☐ Hypothesis	☐ Problem

Checklist Question 2: Does your treatment or clinical intervention pose more than minimal risk to patients/families or present a question of whether there may be unknown risks to patients/families?

	☐ Yes	☐ No

Checklist Question 3: Are you trying to demonstrate *efficacy* or *effectiveness*?

	☐ Efficacy	☐ Effectiveness

Checklist Question 4: Are you trying to show mechanistic relationships between variables?

	☐ Yes	☐ No

Checklist Question 5: Does the study control for confounders?

	☐ Yes	☐ No

Checklist Question 6: Are data collected over time and used to modify interventions in real time?

	☐ No	☐ Yes

Checklist Question 7: Is your study protocol "fixed" (i.e., no major adjustments to procedures will be made in accordance with gained experience)?

	☐ Yes	☐ No

Total	**Research:**	**Quality Improvement:**

Multisite studies that involve collaboration among institutions with fetal and neonatal care services throughout the United States and internationally are sorely lacking. A related consideration is the creation and utilization of databases specific to behavioral health and psychosocial variables or the extension of such variables to existing medical databases, such as the Children's Hospitals Neonatal Consortium; the Neonatal Research Network, which includes 15 medical centers where data are collected on newborns and common practices; and the Vermont Oxford Network, which is an organization that allows for collaborative QI projects within NICUs (Horbar et al., 2010). Existing databases also focus on the infant rather than the parents and family system. Capturing both parent and child data is essential to characterizing the needs of these families and establishing best practices. Databases with an expanded focus would allow for a more universal collection of psychosocial variables to promote collaboration, and the benefit of aggregating data across sites and across fetal and neonatal care settings would be impactful to understanding the association between the medical and psychosocial realms.

NICU Family Experience

It is well understood that the NICU is a stressful environment for patients and families, given the fast-paced medical setting, array of sights and sounds, and emergent nature of the infant's condition (Geller et al., 2018). Existing research indicates that parents commonly respond to the NICU experience and their altered parenting role with anxiety, sadness, anger, perceived lack of control, fear, uncertainty, guilt, and grief. Elevated levels of depression, anxiety, and trauma symptoms have been documented in 40–50% of NICU parents (Hynan et al., 2013), and the associated impairments in parent–child interactions and bonding have significant implications for child prognosis and neurocognitive development. Given the interrelated nature of child health and parental psychosocial functioning, conceptualizing the "patient" as the infant–caregiver dyad would enhance future QI and research projects for families.

Current NICU literature tends to focus on maternal mental health, maternal–infant attachment, and infant neurocognitive development (Grunberg et al., 2019) and examines two variable relationships as opposed to multiple, interrelated relationships. Because infant, parental, and family factors are connected in complex ways, appropriate statistical techniques (e.g., structural equation modeling) and methodological designs that can include a variety of factors (e.g., parental couple relationship and family resources) to understand these relationships would be a valuable next step in the research. Research also tends to focus on the psychological reactions of mothers of preterm infants admitted to the NICU soon after birth and does not routinely include fathers and partners, or infants born both preterm and full-term with diverse medical complications. These studies provide valuable information, but the results are limited in terms of broader generalizability because of the restricted samples and limited family factors studied. QI and research projects have tended to focus on parental mental health in the NICU, and only recently has parent–infant attachment gained more momentum. Future QI programs that screen for and enhance parent–infant interactions throughout hospitalization would help extend the research and help parents create a meaningful parental role while in the NICU.

Longitudinal Research Across Fetal and Neonatal Settings

With the identification of some medical diagnoses occurring prenatally (e.g., in FCCs), there is important longitudinal research that can extend across fetal, neonatal, and post-discharge settings. To better understand long-term child outcomes, organizations such as the North American Fetal Therapy Network (NAFTNet; https://www.naftnet.org) conduct and share information about ongoing research. Studies examining myelomeningocele, gastroschisis, twin-to-twin transfusion syndrome, and congenital diaphragmatic hernia are just a few that are highlighted on NAFTNet's website. These projects begin in FCCs, and data collection continues longitudinally across settings.

Examining the experience of parental trauma, rates of anxiety, depression, and post-traumatic stress disorder (PTSD), and psychosocial needs over the course of the perinatal period (including the birth experience) and across settings would yield information to assist with identification of parental and familial risk and resilience factors for treatment targets as well as the extension of knowledge. Such information could inform delivery of preparatory guidance for parents, what they might expect at various stages, and techniques that might be used to reduce overall trauma and its adverse sequelae (e.g., psychoeducation, mindfulness-based stress reduction, anxiety management, and other therapeutic approaches).

Infant brain development is a dynamic biopsychosocial process that starts in the prenatal environment and continues throughout development (O'Mahony et al., 2017). Prenatal and antenatal environments can impact fetal neurodevelopment through hypothalamic–pituitary–adrenal dysregulation, inflammatory processes, and genetic vulnerabilities (Jacques et al., 2019). Psychosocial predictors of fetal and infant outcomes include the influence of adverse life events, chronic tension and stress, and quality of relationships between mothers and partners (Yim et al., 2015). Maternal exposure to adversity during prenatal and antenatal periods can impact biological stress responses and health behaviors (e.g., substance abuse) and, in turn, child neurodevelopmental trajectories (Raineki et al., 2017). Therefore, targeting chronic maternal stress, depression, and health behaviors in fetal centers may be important for prevention and early intervention to optimize infant health outcomes.

Infants admitted to a NICU can have a variety of diagnoses and comorbid functional impairments that may affect parent–infant relationships as well as infants' own neurocognitive and socioemotional development. Infant health severity (e.g., birth weight and length of hospitalization), parental mental health (e.g., depression, anxiety, and PTSD), and parent–infant interaction impact infant neurocognitive and socioemotional development (Grunberg et al., 2019). Children born preterm exhibit more problems with attention, executive function, language, spatial skills, and fine and gross motor functions compared to normal birth weight controls, and these problems can be exacerbated by parental mental health issues (Anderson et al., 2003). Conduct disorders, attention-deficit/hyperactivity disorder, externalizing symptoms (e.g., delinquency), internalizing symptoms (e.g., anxiety, depression, and phobias), and social issues (e.g., victim of bullying) are more prevalent among children born preterm than full-term (Bhutta et al., 2002). With the implications that prenatal, antenatal, and postpartum environmental exposures and experiences have for infants and families, more longitudinal research that begins during the prenatal period when problems are first identified in FCCs and continues well beyond NICU discharge as the child ages is clearly warranted.

Although research has investigated neurobiological factors directly related to infant brain development, with particular attention to infants born extremely preterm (i.e., ≤28 weeks of gestation), and the individual contributions of parental mental health, maternal–child interactions, and also parental education, income, and intellectual ability to child neurocognitive, behavioral, and socioemotional development (Grunberg et al., 2019), research is limited with regard to additional family variables that may be relevant (e.g., parenting alliance and time that parents have for themselves) and how biopsychosocial systems interact to explain long-term child development. A better understanding of familial adjustment could positively impact infant development and lead to more effective family interventions and outcomes.

Hospitals and community health care providers have recognized the value of continuity of care for families because of the stressors associated with the postdischarge period. After being discharged from the hospital, families no longer have psychosocial and 24-hour medical support available to them and have to manage ongoing medical appointments as well as cope with concerns related to their child's long-term development from home. Developing and implementing services post-discharge to support this transition can help alleviate anxiety, provide education and skills to manage their child's illness, instill self-efficacy, and provide ongoing psychosocial support. More research and QI projects that examine, develop, and implement services for families post-discharge may help alleviate stress and promote child development.

Guidelines for Psychosocial Care

An important advancement in the field was the systematic process to create interdisciplinary recommendations for psychosocial care in the NICU and neonatal follow-up (see Hall et al., 2015). Included in a special issue of *Journal of Perinatology* are recommendations specific to mental health screening and treatment (Hynan & Hall, 2015); however, a gap still exists in terms of systematic evaluation of the adoption of recommendations among NICUs throughout the United States. Relevant research would include questions such as Are the various recommendations for NICUs feasible? and To what degree are they being implemented? To address these questions, a national assessment of programs could be conducted to evaluate the extent to which programs are adhering to specific recommendations related to staffing and assessment, for example. When recommendations are being implemented, a survey of the clinical interventions could be conducted, as well as whether or not adherence to these recommendations is associated with improved outcomes for infants and their families. With the recognition of the multidisciplinary nature of staffing within fetal and neonatal settings (see Chapter 5, this volume), future research might also involve a role delineation study of staff involved with behavioral health service provision.

NICU Psychosocial Interventions

Short-term interventions that incorporate evidence-based skills to address parental depression, anxiety, and trauma have been developed for the NICU. Interventions have also focused on maternal–infant attachment by facilitating calming interactions, in addition to maternal–infant co-regulation. In fact, Melnyk and colleagues (2006) developed an RCT (Creating Opportunities for Parental Empowerment) to improve parent–infant interactions and parental mental health and enhance infant development and behavior. Furthermore, practices to promote neurodevelopment in the NICU, including protected sleep, pain and stress assessment and management, individualized care, activities of daily living (positioning, feeding, and skin-to-skin/kangaroo care), and family-centered care, have been effective in promoting infant growth and development (Butler & Als, 2008). With most psychosocial interventions focusing on the caregiver's or infant's individual needs, researchers have recently advocated for an infant mental health perspective, focusing on the importance of the emerging caregiver–infant relationship (Browne et al., 2016). Infant mental health intervention models focus on the parent–infant relationship and directly address potentially traumatic experiences of both members of the dyad. This model may promote developmental, behavioral, and relational functioning; improve the parent–child relationship; and increase parental self-efficacy and infant responses to parents' care.

Changing the Structure of Fetal and Neonatal Settings Through Research and Quality Improvement

To enhance psychosocial care in fetal and neonatal settings, directing investigative efforts toward the environment, staffing, and methods of service delivery is warranted. These settings, like the hospital itself, involve systems with the goal of providing family-centered health care to improve the health outcomes of mothers, infants, and families. To that end, the system consists of individuals or groups of people interacting and performing tasks, following certain processes (either self-created or standardized in the unit), using enabling tools. Therefore, implementing QI changes in fetal and neonatal settings requires a keen understanding of the people, process, and tools associated with the settings and how they interact. For example, patient daily rounds typically happen at the bedside in the morning and are attended by the clinicians and nurses. Typically, there is a standard rounding process whereby relevant clinical information is transmitted, discussed, and followed up by formulating the care plan. The tools utilized could be the electronic medical record and image viewers. If health care providers would like more family engagement, the current system would not work because it was not originally designed for that purpose. In order to modify the system, systematic employment of experienced based co-design could be examined (see https://www.pointofcarefoundation. org.uk/resource/experience-based-co-design-ebcd-toolkit) and include family members as active members of a redesign team. The result could be the addition of a telemedicine system that allows them to join hospital rounds remotely from their home or workplace and that also includes the processes that would alert them that rounds are starting. The addition of regular tele-mental health services is also a potential structural change for psychosocial service delivery that can evolve through research (see the section titled Research Questions Related to the COVID-19 Pandemic).

As an example of this changing structure, the neonatal intensive parenting unit (NIPU) is a concept developed by Hall, Hynan, and colleagues in 2017 that is a potential direction for QI and research to modify the structure of the NICU. The philosophy behind the NIPU is a major shift in paradigm, from an infant-focused intensive care unit to a broader family-focused infant and parenting unit. Hall and colleagues believe that in their current state, NICUs are not set up to provide the appropriate emotional support for parents who have infants in the NICU. Literature has provided evidence that the emotional stress and intensity parents experience while their infant is in a NICU have a deleterious effect on the neurocognitive development of their newborn (Schore, 2001). The design of the NIPU takes into account the emotional burden parents endure and creates a family-centered and family-integrated care environment that offers education, support, and resources to both families and staff.

Hall and colleagues (2017) derived the following six themes from the "Interdisciplinary Recommendations for the Psychosocial Support of NICU Parents" (Hynan & Hall, 2015) as the building blocks for the NIPU: (a) family-centered developmental care, (b) peer support, (c) mental health support, (d) palliative and bereavement care, (e) post-discharge support, and (f) staff education and support. The goal is to provide guidance to centers in their creation of programs and services to enhance the relationship between parent(s) and infant, parent(s) and staff, and staff with staff. A more inclusive environment would be established in which families and staff worked together in different ways. In such an environment, infants would have better neurodevelopmental outcomes, families would have their mental health needs met, and staff would feel supported and less fatigued in their work.

Staff Burnout and Support

While attention to mental health resources and family support and education has increased in fetal and neonatal settings, research attention directed toward support for health care providers is also growing. Compassion fatigue and burnout rates among health care providers in these settings have ranged from 7.5% to 54.4% (Profit et al., 2014). Providers are also at risk for acute distress disorder, secondary traumatic stress syndrome, and PTSD related to the emotional impact of their work. Staff burnout or trauma can influence provider–patient relationships as well as patient care. Recently, providers doing research or QI in this field have implemented training and education programs, staff support, and interventions (e.g., mindfulness and peer consultation) to support providers (Lan et al., 2014; Lorrain, 2016). However, this work is limited, and more research and QI initiatives that focus on provider self-care, coping skills, communication techniques, education, and social support from colleagues and loved ones are needed. Initiatives related to mind–body techniques and interpersonal effectiveness skills would help providers learn to manage their own stress and communicate their needs. Promotion of reciprocal communication with families and team building among multidisciplinary teams would help create mutual respect and coordinate care to implement effective family-centered care (Hynan, 2020). Research and QI focused on promoting well-being among staff and providers would enhance emotional and physical health as well as efficient and effective patient care—work that became needed more urgently with the onset of the COVID-19 pandemic (Hynan, 2020).

Research Questions Related to the COVID-19 Pandemic

The COVID-19 pandemic necessitated a number of changes to the provision of health care in fetal and neonatal settings, and accordingly it presented an opportunity to study the impact of the public health crisis on psychosocial–emotional functioning for infants and their families. The increased use of tele-mental health presents challenges and opportunities that are also ripe for research (Geller, Spiecker, et al., 2021).

IMPLEMENTATION OF TECHNOLOGY

As public health guidelines called for strict social distancing to prevent the spread of the COVID-19 beginning in 2020, many health care services transitioned from in-person delivery to a telehealth format. In this model, appointments, consultations, and other services are held via video conferencing or telephone call. Telehealth adoption prior to COVID-19 was modest (Olson et al., 2018), with significant barriers removed temporarily due to the pandemic, resulting in an exponential increase in adoption. As a result, data are being collected and allow for retrospective and prospective analysis. The SPROUT (Supporting Pediatric

Research in Outcomes and Utilization of Telehealth) Telehealth Evaluation and Measurement or STEM framework provides a guide to evaluate a telehealth program by identifying variables in each of four domains (clinical health outcome, quality and cost of health care delivery, individual experience, and program performance and implementation indicators) from the perspective of family/patient, clinician, health system, and payor. These variables can be used as target metrics in research and QI designs (Chuo et al., 2020). For example, research might examine how telehealth has impacted clinical health outcomes and quality of health care delivery for women, infants, and families.

Tele-mental health, defined as the delivery of psychotherapeutic care via remote technology, in the FCC and NICU in general had previously been used as an equitable method of accessing populations in medically underserved areas and of following up with parents of preterm infants post-NICU graduation via tele-home care (Aziz et al., 2020). As an example, tele-mental health clinical outcomes could be assessed using scores on a formal depression measure or NICU parental stress scales.

Telehealth services health delivery quality can be measured by the number of no-shows or rescheduled tele-sessions, personal experience as measured by the telehealth usability and/or the patient assessment of communication in telehealth questionnaires, and program performance indicators as number of visits completed per month. Recent data suggest existing disparities in technology adoption showing that tele-mental health could remove barriers to attendance (e.g., time and expense of travel) but raises other barriers (e.g., the necessity of consistent internet access, child care for siblings, and safe quiet space to talk) (Katzow et al., 2020; Makkar et al., 2020). Such findings could help providers better understand the risks and benefits of utilizing tele-mental health care with FCC and NICU patients and their families on a regular basis during non-pandemic times. Other promising uses of telehealth include video-assisted monitoring and integration of supplementary technology to aid in effective care (Makkar et al., 2020) and the use of NICU cameras that enable parents to see their infants from afar (Guttmann et al., 2020).

PRE- AND POST-COVID-19 SCREENINGS OF PSYCHOLOGICAL DISTRESS FOR NICU FAMILIES

Whereas existing work has examined the impact of NICU hospitalization on family member distress, future research might compare data collected on indices of distress prior to COVID-19 to data collected after the crisis began. Given the multitude of stressors created by the crisis (physical health risk, social isolation, and employment and financial loss), it is important to understand the ways in which the COVID-19 crisis may impact family members of a patient experiencing a NICU hospitalization. Such work has been initiated by researchers at the Children's Hospital of Philadelphia, who are using an online survey to collect data on depression and trauma symptoms from parents of NICU patients. These data will be compared to data on the same variables collected prior to the pandemic and will begin to elucidate the impact of the COVID-19 crisis on the level of distress experienced by family members of NICU patients.

IMPACT ON INFANTS AND BONDING

Given the elevated risk status of NICU infants, special care must be taken to keep the infants protected from the spread of the COVID-19 virus. This involves stringent use of personal protective equipment when in close proximity to the infants, as well as restricting the number of visitors and family members to the unit. Although medically necessary, these practices drastically change the infant's experience of the world around them. For example, infants have limited exposure to live human faces given the use of face masks. In addition, their contact with family members and other caretakers is limited. Given the importance of physical contact and facial expressions for bonding, a key area of research might involve an examination of the impact of the COVID-19 crisis on infant bonding and other developmental outcomes.

PRACTICAL CONSIDERATIONS

Given that inpatient fetal and neonatal settings are fast-paced, highly complex, and often changing medical environments, it can be difficult to integrate research. As discussed in this section, a number of potential barriers to implementation are important to consider when developing a research or QI initiative within these inpatient settings, as well as in outpatient neonatal follow-up settings.

Inpatient fetal care and critical care settings for neonates/infants are constantly adapting to meet patients' medical needs. Such intensive care settings can make it difficult to set times to meet with family members given that they are not the patients, have ongoing responsibilities outside of the hospital, and may be focused on being a new parent to their infant. It is essential for researchers and QI staff who are conducting inpatient research projects to be flexible given that the infant could need emergency medical care at any moment. In addition, within NICUs, parents are protective of and want to spend time alone with their child during this time of crisis. For example, staff can provide parents with options to come and go from a study group, as needed, or problem solve with them on how they can be involved in research or QI projects. It becomes more important to facilitate buy-in to the service or study and provide psychoeducation on the benefits of participating for them and their child. Finally, bringing research or services to families at the bedside—including through the use of technology and using multidisciplinary collaboration, whenever possible—can help increase participation and engagement.

Participant or parental burden is of the utmost importance when designing research or QI projects. Families of NICU infants are usually highly stressed and overburdened with the amount of responsibilities they are managing (e.g., other children, work, family members, sick child). Therefore, researchers and providers implementing QI protocols should limit the amount of time and energy asked of families. For example, they should carefully choose measures that are the most clinically meaningful for QI initiatives and choose abbreviated measures for research. This can help reduce the burden and increase parental engagement and interest in participating. Early parenthood is already a stressful time, so limiting the amount of additional stress or burden for families is essential both ethically and clinically.

The FCC, NICU, and neonatal follow-up programs are unique in that psychological services and research more directly involve the family, as opposed to the infant. Research and QI projects are needed to advocate for family-centered care and psychosocial services, but legal and financial complications can arise. For example, documenting parent information can be challenging when one only has access to the infant's chart. Therefore, it can be helpful to include the impact of the research or service on the child to help advocate for family services in those settings. Gathering only key information that is necessary from families and demonstrating the positive impact on the child's neurodevelopmental outcomes and prognosis may be key for facilitating greater funds for family services in these settings and improving clinical outcomes for children and families.

Greater prioritization of funding for psychosocial research in the perinatal period is needed, not only to support parental mental health and well-being but also to optimize infant socioemotional and neurocognitive development. The presence of mental health providers in the FCC and NICU settings is relatively new despite research showing the high number of families experiencing clinically significant levels of psychological distress. Research in neonatal follow-up settings is also in its infancy. With limited numbers of dedicated mental health providers in these settings, nearly all of their time is allocated to clinical work, which makes it challenging to conduct research or QI. Additional support is needed to help offset this burden and create more opportunities to expand research in fetal and neonatal settings. Using trainees/students and volunteers can make the integration of QI and research in clinical settings more feasible, but this may present its own challenges; for example, trainee and family availability in the NICU may not overlap to allow for easy recruitment, screening/assessment, or intervention delivery. More external funding would provide greater opportunities for large-scale projects that can include project-dedicated staff members on the team who could more effectively develop and implement research and QI initiatives.

CONCLUSION

Recent decades have witnessed momentum in fetal and neonatal settings in terms of research focused on psychosocial, socioemotional, and mental health issues in expectant parents and families of hospitalized infants. More investigation—both QI and research studies—is needed to better assist this population of parents, improve clinical outcomes for both parents and infants, and propel the field forward.

There remain many gaps in knowledge such that the FCC, NICU, and post-discharge settings (including the neonatal follow-up clinic and patients' homes) provide ample opportunity for conducting psychosocial research.

To move the field forward, it is important that investigative efforts in fetal and neonatal settings include studies with certain characteristics. For example, it is important that studies are guided by scientific theory as well as the most current clinical information. Research and QI designs that include longitudinal approaches and use of standardized assessment tools with established psychometric properties for the population can help extend extant knowledge in the field. Prospective investigations following infants and their families from fetal to neonatal settings as well as post-discharge will promote better understanding of risk and protective factors as well as critical associations among key variables. Collaboration and the coordination between inpatient and outpatient settings and with follow-up care is essential not only for continuity of care but also for cross-validation across these multiple settings to accurately characterize the trajectories of infants and their families.

The expanding presence of psychologists and other clinical scientists on treatment teams can help facilitate QI and research studies. Projects involving parent screening and assessment of potential risk and protective factors, as well as evaluation of existing practices and programs and the introduction of novel care applications, can help create an evidence base to guide the field. Newer technology and greater acceptance of telemedicine and tele-mental health offer unique opportunities for innovative research. In addition, increased adoption of these technologies due to the COVID-19 pandemic will allow for the opportunity to better study their impact. Systematic integration of research and QI studies into clinical practice can help generate key evidence that can be used to support advocacy initiatives around appropriate staffing (e.g., hiring dedicated mental health providers), promoting parental psychosocial issues as a national funding priority, and driving policy change to improve the experience of NICU hospitalization during the perinatal period and optimize outcomes for infants and their families.

REFERENCES

Anderson, P., Doyle, L. W.; Victorian Infant Collaborative Study Group. (2003). Neurobehavioral outcomes of school-age children born extremely low birth weight or very preterm in the 1990s. *JAMA, 289*(24), 3264–3272.

Aziz, A., Zork, N., Aubey, J. J., Baptiste, C. D., D'alton, M. E., Emeruwa, U. N., Fuchs, K. M., Goffman, D., Gyamfi-Bannerman, C., Haythe, J. H., LaSala, A. P., Madden, N., Miller, E. C., Miller, R. S., Monk, C., Moroz, L., Samsiya, O., Ring, L. E., Sheen, J. J., ... Friedman, A. M. (2020). Telehealth for high-risk pregnancies in the setting of the COVID-19 pandemic. *American Journal of Perinatology, 37*(8), 800–808.

Bhutta, A. T., Cleves, M. A., Casey, P. H., Cradock, M. M., & Anand, K. J. (2002). Cognitive and behavioral outcomes of school-aged children who were born preterm: A meta-analysis. *JAMA, 288*(6), 728–737.

Browne, J. V., Martinez, D., & Talmi, A. (2016). Infant mental health (IMH) in the intensive care unit: Considerations for the infant, the family and the staff. *Newborn and Infant Nursing Reviews, 16*(4), 274–280.

Butler, S., & Als, H. (2008). Individualized developmental care improves the lives of infants born preterm. *Acta Paediatrica, 97*(9), 1173–1175.

Chuo, J., Macy, M. L., & Lorch, S. A. (2020). Strategies for evaluating telehealth. *Pediatrics, 146*(5), e20201781.

Finkelstein, J. A., Brickman, A. L., Capron, A., Ford, D. E., Gombosev, A., Greene, S. M., Iafrate, R. P., Kolaczkowski, L., Pallin, S., Pletcher, M. J., Staman, K. L., Vazquez, M. A., & Sugarman, J. (2015). Oversight on the borderline: Quality improvement and pragmatic research. *Clinical Trials, 12*(5), 457–466.

Geller, P. A., Albanese, A., Russo, G., Hartman, A., & Patterson, C. (2021). *Evolution of psychosocial care for parents in the NICU: An historical analysis.* Unpublished manuscript.

Geller, P. A., Bonacquisti, A., & Patterson, C. A. (2018). Maternal experience of neonatal intensive care unit hospitalization: Trauma exposure and psychosocial responses. In M. Muzik & K. L. Rosenblum (Eds.), *Motherhood in the face of trauma: Pathways of healing and growth* (pp. 227–247). Springer.

Geller, P. A., Spiecker, N., Cole, J. C., Zajac, L., & Patterson, C. A. (2021, August). The rise of tele-mental health in perinatal settings. In *Seminars in Perinatology* (Vol. 45, No. 5, p. 151431). WB Saunders.

Grunberg, V. A., Geller, P. A., Bonacquisti, A., & Patterson, C. A. (2019). NICU infant health severity and family outcomes: A systematic review of assessments and findings in psychosocial research. *Journal of Perinatology, 39*(2), 156–172.

Guttmann, K., Patterson, C., Haines, T., Hoffman, C., Masten, M., Lorch, S., & Chuo, J. (2020). Parent stress in relation to use of bedside telehealth: An initiative to improve family-centeredness of care in the neonatal intensive care unit. *Journal of Patient Experience, 7*(6), 1378–1383.

Hall, S., Hynan, M., Phillips, R., et al. (2017). The neonatal intensive parenting unit: an introduction. *Journal of Perinatololgy, 37*, 1259–1264. https://doi.org/10.1038/jp.2017.108

Hall, S. L., Cross, J., Selix, N. W., Patterson, C., Segre, L., Chuffo-Siewert, R., Geller, P. A., & Martin, M. L. (2015). Recommendations for enhancing psychosocial support of NICU parents through staff education and support. *Journal of Perinatology, 35*(1), S29–S36.

Horbar, J. D., Soll, R. F., & Edwards, W. H. (2010). The Vermont Oxford Network: A community of practice. *Clinics in Perinatology, 37*(1), 29–47.

Huhtala, M., Korja, R., Lehtonen, L., Haataja, L., Lapinleimu, H., Rautava, P.; PIPPARI Study Group. (2012). Parental psychological well-being and behavioral outcome of very low birth weight infants at 3 years. *Pediatrics, 129*(4), e937–e944.

Hynan, M. T. (2020). Covid-19 and the need for perinatal mental health professionals: Now more than ever before. *Journal of Perinatology, 40*(7), 985–986.

Hynan, M. T., & Hall, S. L. (2015). Interdisciplinary recommendations for the psychosocial support of NICU parents [Special issue]. *Journal of Perinatology, 35*(S1).

Hynan, M. T., Mounts, K., & Vanderbilt, D. (2013). Screening parents of high-risk infants for emotional distress: Rationale and recommendations. *Journal of Perinatology, 33*(10), 748–753.

Jacques, N., de Mola, C. L., Joseph, G., Mesenburg, M. A., & da Silveira, M. F. (2019). Prenatal and postnatal maternal depression and infant hospitalization and mortality in the first year of life: A systematic review and meta-analysis. *Journal of Affective Disorders*, *243*, 201–208.

Katzow, M. W., Steinway, C., & Jan, S. (2020). Telemedicine and health disparities during COVID-19. *Pediatrics*, *146*(2), e20201586.

Lan, H. K., Subramanian, P., Rahmat, N., & Kar, P. C. (2014). The effects of mindfulness training program on reducing stress and promoting well-being among nurses in critical care units. *Australian Journal of Advanced Nursing*, *31*(3), 22–31.

Lorrain, B. (2016). Reflective peer consultation as an intervention for staff support in the NICU. *Newborn and Infant Nursing Reviews*, *16*(4), 289–292.

Makkar, A., McCoy, M., Hallford, G., Foulks, A., Anderson, M., Milam, J., Wehrer, M., Doerfler, E., & Szyld, E. (2020). Evaluation of neonatal services provided in a level II NICU utilizing hybrid telemedicine: A prospective study. *Telemedicine and E-Health*, *26*(2), 176–183.

Melnyk, B. M., Feinstein, N. F., Alpert-Gillis, L., Fairbanks, E., Crean, H. F., Sinkin, R. A., Stone, P. W., Small, L., Tu, X., & Gross, S. J. (2006). Reducing premature infants' length of stay and improving parents' mental health outcomes with the Creating Opportunities for Parent Empowerment (COPE) neonatal intensive care unit program: A randomized, controlled trial. *Pediatrics*, *118*(5), e1414–e1427.

Moen, R. D., Nolan, T. W., & Provost, L. P. (2012). *Quality improvement through planned experimentation* (3rd ed.). McGraw-Hill.

Olson, C. A., McSwain, S. D., Curfman, A. L., & Chuo, J. (2018). The current pediatric telehealth landscape. *Pediatrics*, *141*(3), e20172334.

O'Mahony, S. M., Clarke, G., Dinan, T., & Cryan, J. (2017). Early-life adversity and brain development: Is the microbiome a missing piece of the puzzle? *Neuroscience*, *342*, 37–54.

Profit, J., Sharek, P. J., Amspoker, A. B., Kowalkowski, M. A., Nisbet, C. C., Thomas, E. J., Chadwick, W. A., & Sexton, J. B. (2014). Burnout in the NICU setting and its relation to safety culture. *BMJ Quality & Safety*, *23*(10), 806–813.

Raineki, C., Bodnar, T. S., Holman, P. J., Baglot, S. L., Lan, N., & Weinberg, J. (2017). Effects of early-life adversity on immune function are mediated by prenatal environment: Role of prenatal alcohol exposure. *Brain, Behavior, and Immunity*, *66*, 210–220.

Schore, A. N. (2001). Effects of a secure attachment relationship on right brain development, affect regulation, and infant mental health. *Infant Mental Health Journal*, *22*(1–2), 7–66.

Welch, M. G., Hofer, M. A., Brunelli, S. A., Stark, R. I., Andrews, H. F., Austin, J., & Myers, M. M. (2012). Family nurture intervention (FNI): Methods and treatment protocol of a randomized controlled trial in the NICU. *BMC Pediatrics*, *12*(1), 1–17.

Yim, I. S., Stapleton, L. R. T., Guardino, C. M., Hahn-Holbrook, J., & Schetter, C. D. (2015). Biological and psychosocial predictors of postpartum depression: Systematic review and call for integration. *Annual Review of Clinical Psychology*, *11*, 99-137.

4

SYSTEMS INTERVENTIONS AND PROGRAM DEVELOPMENT

SUSANNE KLAWETTER, JILL A. HOFFMAN, KRISTI ROYBAL, AND SUNAH S. HWANG ■

Perinatal mood and anxiety disorders (PMADs) are common and serious complications of pregnancy that negatively affect parent and child health and developmental outcomes. PMADs affect 15–20% of the general population, and those who experience pregnancy complications or socioeconomic disadvantage are at higher risk for these conditions (Lomonaco-Haycraft et al., 2019). PMADs often go undiagnosed and untreated, leading to increased risk for adverse parent, infant, and child outcomes such as maternal suicide and self-harm, preterm birth, low birth weight, decreased use of preventive maternal and infant health care, and behavioral and developmental disorders among infants and children (Lomonaco-Haycraft et al., 2019; Luca et al., 2019). In addition, PMADs are associated with societal costs such as decreased parent workforce participation and high health care utilization. One estimate places the societal costs of undiagnosed and untreated PMADs at $32,000 over 6 years per parent–infant dyad (Luca et al., 2019).

Integrated behavioral health care, or integrated care, is a promising strategy to address PMADs and other behavioral health needs of high-risk infants and families (Lomonaco-Haycraft et al., 2019). The Agency for Healthcare Research and Quality (AHRQ, n.d.) defines integrated care as the blending of care "in one setting for medical conditions and related behavioral health factors that affect health and well-being." Across a variety of medical settings, integrated care reduces barriers to behavioral health services and improves health care quality and outcomes. Research points to unique barriers and opportunities for the integration of behavioral health services in perinatal, neonatal, and pediatric care settings that must be taken into consideration when planning and implementing systems-level interventions and programs. The following provides a brief overview of integrated care in the previously mentioned settings, along with a discussion of systems approaches and program opportunities to support the behavioral health needs of patients and families.

INTEGRATION OF BEHAVIORAL HEALTH SERVICES INTO MEDICAL SETTINGS

Integrated behavioral health care recognizes that both behavioral and medical factors contribute to overall health. Primary and behavioral health care systems often function independently of one another, resulting in fragmented and inadequate care. In integrated care models, primary care and behavioral health providers collaborate to provide coordinated, evidence-based care in primary care settings. Integrated care reduces gaps, inefficiencies, and costs associated with independently functioning medical and behavioral health care systems, resulting in higher quality, patient-centered care that improves overall health (AHRQ, n.d.).

Integrated care is an emerging approach in perinatal, neonatal intensive care unit (NICU), and pediatric primary care settings given the relationships between parental mental health, parent–infant bonding, and infant health and developmental outcomes. Research suggests that integrated care in these settings may help overcome complex barriers to behavioral health treatment such as uncoordinated behavioral and medical care, behavioral health stigma, and psychosocial factors that prevent patients from accessing care (Lomonaco-Haycraft et al., 2019). During the perinatal period, behavioral health services integrated in routine obstetric care are associated with increased screening, improved uptake of behavioral health services, and reduced PMAD symptoms (Lomonaco-Haycraft et al., 2019). A study of integrated care in a pediatric setting suggests that embedded or co-located behavioral health services may reduce barriers to behavioral health treatment such as logistical challenges, stigma, and fears of child protective services involvement (Young et al., 2019). Studies also demonstrate that integrated care approaches in NICU settings lead to improved parental mental health and strengthened parent–infant interactions (Welch et al., 2016).

Although integrated care has potential to better support the overall wellbeing of high-risk infants and families across medical settings, attention must be given to the barriers and facilitators to integration. A recent cross-national systematic review identified provider- and systems-level factors that contribute to the success of integration of behavioral health services (Wakida et al., 2018). These include (a) knowledge and skills about mental health screening, diagnosis, and treatment; (b) attitudes about the acceptability, appropriateness, and credibility of integrated care; (c) motivation to integrate care; (d) management/leadership to oversee the integration process; and (e) financial considerations such as funding and insurance reimbursement mechanisms for behavioral health services.

Continuity of Care in Fetal, Labor and Delivery, NICU, and Neonatal Follow-Up Settings

Given the large body of evidence demonstrating the risk for PMADs during pregnancy, at the time of birth, and during the postpartum course, consistent and continuous behavioral health support should be integrated into the perinatal spectrum of care. The following sections highlight three clinical care approaches: (a) universal screening for PMADs at several time points during the perinatal period; (b) continued behavioral health support by the same team of behavioral health providers from pregnancy through the first year postpartum; and (c) co-location of behavioral health services with obstetric, primary care, and infant care (Kendig et al., 2017).

CONSISTENT SCREENING FOR PMADs ACROSS THE PERINATAL SPECTRUM
The American College of Obstetricians and Gynecologists (ACOG, 2018) recommends universal screening for PMADs during the prenatal period with a validated screening tool, at least once during pregnancy, and at the postpartum follow-up appointment. Whereas these screening practices may be adequate for the general population, individuals who experience complicated pregnancies and births may require additional behavioral health support. Despite greater risks for adverse behavioral health outcomes across the perinatal spectrum for individuals impacted by complicated pregnancies and births, these clinical settings lack consistent screening for PMADs.

There is little published literature on the prevalence, consistency, and adopted protocols of universal PMAD screening in fetal care centers, during postpartum hospitalization, and in the NICU on a large scale. In a local effort based in an Oklahoma NICU, investigators identified barriers to universal depression screening of parents in the NICU. Barriers included difficulties making initial contact with mothers to complete screening, lack of culturally appropriate resources such as interpreters, lack of resources to have consistent availability of a unit-based psychologist, referral barriers related to insurance coverage, and access to behavioral health providers (Vaughn & Hooper, 2020). Clearly, a multi-tiered approach addressing patient-, family-, health system-, community-, and broader policy-level factors will be required. However, universal screening is a critical first step in addressing the mental health needs of parents impacted by high-risk pregnancies and births.

CONTINUITY OF BEHAVIORAL HEALTH SUPPORT FROM PREGNANCY THROUGH THE FIRST YEAR POSTPARTUM
In addition to PMAD screening, individuals who screen positive during pregnancy, birth hospitalization, and postpartum must have access to consistent behavioral health care. Often, medical and behavioral health care is siloed within these three perinatal periods, leading to gaps in care during critical transition periods. For instance, pregnant individuals who screen negative

for PMADs by their obstetrician early in pregnancy may subsequently screen positive if approached by specialists at a fetal care center following a diagnosis of a congenital anomaly. The results of the new screening assessment may not be relayed to the obstetrician, who will continue to treat this pregnant individual for obstetric care in conjunction with the maternal fetal medicine specialist. Furthermore, upon delivery and NICU admission, the mechanisms to communicate parental behavioral health status from providers in the fetal care center to the neonatal care team may be lacking. Given the importance of parent engagement in the NICU in neonatal outcomes, addressing parental behavioral health is critical for both parent and infant outcomes. Some fetal care centers and NICUs provide continuous behavioral health support by using the same individual or a small team of providers (e.g., social workers, psychologists, and/or other mental health providers) to engage parents from initial diagnosis of medically complex pregnancies through birth and NICU hospitalization (Dempsey et al., 2021). Research on the impact of such programs on parent and infant health outcomes as well as health care cost and utilization is still needed. Moreover, continued behavioral health support after the infant's discharge from the NICU to home will likely be required. However, the prevalence of availability, accessibility, and parental acceptance of such services is not yet well known at a population level.

CO-LOCATION OF BEHAVIORAL HEALTH SUPPORT SERVICES WITH MATERNAL AND INFANT HEALTH CARE

Given the competing priorities of pregnant individuals and parents, particularly in the presence of medical complications for themselves or their infants, provision of behavioral health services should be easily accessible and feasible. Maternal attendance at the first postpartum outpatient visit is suboptimal, especially among mothers with socioeconomic disadvantage (Sudhof & Shah, 2019). For parents with infants in the NICU, engagement in both medical and behavioral health care may be even lower than for parents with healthy term infants (DiBari et al., 2014). However, integrated care provided where parents already access parent or infant health care may improve engagement with and acceptance of behavioral health support (Lomonaco-Haycraft et al., 2019). In situations of parental substance use disorders, co-location of behavioral health care, primary care, prenatal care, addiction treatment, and infant care is now considered the optimal way to deliver comprehensive dyadic care for parents and infants. Similarly, prolonged NICU hospitalization affords chances for behavioral health providers to engage parents in the NICU, thus increasing opportunities for parents to spend critical time with their infant. Studies demonstrate that NICUs striving to integrate parents into the medical and developmental care of preterm infants have lower rates of PMADs and higher rates of parenting efficacy (Franck & O'Brien, 2019). These findings illustrate the tremendous opportunities to positively impact high-risk infants and families through the integration of parental emotional support into routine NICU care.

SYSTEMS CHANGE THEORIES

The integration of PMADs screening, continuous behavioral health support, and co-located services across perinatal health care settings is often the result of significant systems change efforts. Although each health care system is complex and has unique needs, several theoretical frameworks can be used to support systems through major change processes, including Lewin's change theory, diffusion of innovation theory, and whole systems change.

Lewin's Change Theory

Health care leadership and staff play a critical role in identifying a problem or gap, identifying solutions, and moving change. Lewin's change theory is a three-step theory of planned change that is widely accepted and used in nursing practice, nursing education, and health care operations (Shirey, 2013). The three steps in Lewin's framework are unfreezing, moving, and refreezing. With *unfreezing*, perinatal and behavioral health care leadership and staff identify when change is needed and prepare to make change by identifying solutions, addressing resistance to proposed change, and garnering support for the change. Next is a process known as *moving*, in which leadership and staff initiate a plan of action to make change and attend to the fears and uncertainty that accompany change through clear communication and stakeholder engagement. Finally, change is institutionalized to ensure sustainability in a process called *refreezing*.

For instance, in a NICU setting, leadership and staff may identify that although parents are screened for PMADs, they do not receive behavioral health services when needed. Leadership and staff may subsequently identify potential solutions, such as co-located services or adjustments to the referral process. After addressing potential challenges and garnering support, a select group of leadership and staff would then implement their proposed changes (e.g., instituting a warm handoff referral protocol), making sure to communicate with stakeholders throughout the process. Finally, if the implementation of the new protocol results in improved uptake of behavioral health services, the changes can be made a permanent part of the NICU's referral process. This planned change framework is best suited for top-down change initiatives guided by formal leadership. In an ever-changing health care landscape, successful implementation of this framework depends on the stability of and time available to the behavioral and medical systems as they pursue change.

Diffusion of Innovation Theory

Diffusion of innovation theory explains how, over a period of time, an innovative idea, practice, or product spreads and is adopted by members of a social system

(Rogers, 2003). Innovations such as utilizing a team approach to support continuity of care from pregnancy through the first year postpartum would typically not be adopted by all members of a system at the same time. Instead, *innovators* and *early adopters* implement changes first, followed by the *early majority*, *late majority*, and *laggards*. The earliest adopters within and across perinatal and behavioral health care settings serve as opinion leaders, spreading word of the innovation to members of later adopters and building a critical mass for widespread adoption. Five key factors determine the successful adoption of an innovation (Rogers, 2003): (a) *relative advantage*, or the extent to which the innovation is perceived as better than what it will replace; (b) *compatibility*, or the extent to which the innovation aligns with the values, beliefs, and needs of potential adopters; (c) *complexity*, or the perceived difficulty of innovation use; (d) *triability*, or the degree to which the innovation can be tested prior to adoption; and (e) *observability*, or the visibility of the results of an innovation's adoption. For instance, co-located behavioral health services for parents within a pediatric primary care setting may be perceived as superior to the current siloed structure and align with the values, beliefs, and needs of health care professionals. However, the perceived complexity of implementing this change, along with challenges in testing co-located services prior to adoption, may hinder this type of innovation from being utilized. When proposing a systems-level change, understanding the target population is critical, as is understanding the factors that affect rates of adoption so that communication processes can be tailored to motivate adoption.

Whole Systems Change

The final theoretical framework discussed in this section, whole systems change, highlights the nonlinear and unpredictable nature of change. Although changes may occur within NICU settings (e.g., establishing a new PMADs screening policy), these changes will not necessarily lead to desired outcomes (e.g., increased screens completed or increased number of parents connected to mental health services). Furthermore, this framework highlights the self-organizing nature of health care systems, meaning that any changes to one part of the system will lead to subsequent change in other areas of the system, whether intended or not (Edwards et al., 2011). For instance, establishing PMAD screenings within the NICU may prompt other departments to implement relevant screening measures with their patients, potentially leading to an increase in the number of mental health referrals that may stretch the capacity of community behavioral health providers. These principles make interdisciplinary work with diverse stakeholders and sectors an important part of systems change. Including multiple perspectives from parents, hospital administrators, behavioral health providers, nurses, social workers, physicians, and others involved in perinatal care can help identify potential unintended consequences of changes before they occur. Continuing with the PMAD screening example presented previously, community behavioral health providers should be included in the change process, along with hospital staff and parents, in order to understand community capacity constraints.

Whole systems change also emphasizes the multiple levels at which change occurs, from micro-level changes (e.g., improved skills in identifying PMADs at the patient level or changes in specific screening policies at a particular clinic) to meso-level changes (e.g., regional legislative changes related to providing care, such as requiring timely follow-up for patient care between perinatal providers) and macro-level changes (e.g., federal legislation related to professional practice, such as requiring a certain number of PMAD screens during prenatal and postpartum care). Identifying the levels at which change will be implemented or anticipated is an essential piece of the change process (Edwards et al., 2011).

Education, policy and legislation, professional practice, and resources serve as the foundation on which systems change is built and help organize the shape of each system. Challenges in any of these areas, such as inadequate training on how to conduct screening or policies that prevent sharing of patient information across providers, can hinder change within and across these multiple levels (i.e., micro, meso, and macro). Identifying challenges and opportunities across each of these areas (i.e., education, policy and legislation, professional practice, and resources) within health care systems can be helpful in addressing potential barriers early in the change process. Leadership, advocacy, partnerships, and knowledge exchange can support or hinder these foundational components of systems change. As such, they are also important areas to examine when attempting to implement systems and cross systems change (Edwards et al., 2011). For example, leadership within a pediatric primary care office may serve as a barrier to implementing co-located behavioral health services; however, a community parent advocacy organization that partners with many of the families served by this particular office has the potential to support changes to the current structure. Successful systems change relies on identifying and understanding each of these change aspects.

NEEDS ASSESSMENT

Prior to the implementation of systemic change, it is important to identify the needs that exist within each system that relate to providing behavioral health services for high-risk infants and families. A needs assessment identifies the scope and nature of a particular challenge or area for growth within a system, identifies what is working and not working, and describes potential solutions. Needs assessments are inextricably linked to program development and program change, helping develop relevant outcomes for tracking progress (Grinnell et al., 2016).

A needs assessment begins with identifying an assessment team that includes representation from all key stakeholders (e.g., nurses, social workers, psychologists, physicians, parents, and administrators). Although to create a well-rounded team it is important to include stakeholders from various fields, those connected to administration across the perinatal and behavioral health care systems are critical to overall systemic buy-in and long-term change. After the team has been formed, it identifies and defines the goals and purpose of the assessment (e.g., to identify behavioral health needs of NICU families), guiding questions and data collection procedures, as well as additional stakeholders and systems with whom to consult. Once the team has established logistical details, it implements the needs assessment, analyzes and interprets the data, and communicates findings to stakeholders. Findings then shape further program development and evaluation, such as whether to move forward with co-located behavioral health services. Communication with assessment team members during the assessment process is critical so that key stakeholders maintain awareness of the status of the project (Grinnell et al., 2016).

PROGRAM EVALUATION

Although a needs assessment can inform program change and development, a program evaluation is needed to assess whether a program or policy is working as intended and to improve and refine the program. Depending on the system's needs, a program evaluation may assess program implementation, effectiveness or efficiency, cost-effectiveness, or overall impact. Thus, clear identification of the overall purpose of the evaluation is essential to useful program evaluations (Grinnell et al., 2016).

The steps in conducting a program evaluation are similar to those of a needs assessment. First, an interdisciplinary team is created to carry out the evaluation and identify additional stakeholders to engage throughout the process. Next, the team outlines all of the program's or policy's key components along with its intended outcomes. Once each component has been detailed, the evaluation team makes decisions about the specific type of evaluation, guiding questions, and evaluation design. After all methodological details are established, data collection begins, followed by analysis and dissemination of findings to stakeholders (Grinnell et al., 2016).

Cherry and colleagues (2016) described the development and evaluation of a postpartum depression (PPD) screening program for parents with infants in the NICU. Although the purpose of the program was to connect NICU parents with behavioral health services, their evaluation focused on the program implementation barriers in order to inform other settings considering similar work. This example highlights the fact that not all program evaluations must focus on outcomes but can also assess program implementation processes. Their program evaluation identified numerous obstacles encountered during the screening process, including establishing contact with parents, administering the screener, and providing referrals. The authors also highlight the importance of involving a variety of stakeholders in the evaluation process, including parents, medical staff, behavioral health providers, and administrators.

DEMONSTRATING VALUE

Value is a central consideration in systems intervention and program development in health care settings that serve high-risk infants and families. Value, as it is described here, refers to a comprehensive assessment of costs, benefits, and the quality of a behavioral health intervention or program such that value is determined by how much it costs to achieve a desired outcome such as reduced PMADs. Rising health care costs, expanded insurance coverage for behavioral health care, multiple payers (e.g., insurance providers), cost shifting, and accountability for outcomes create a complex environment in which to assess value and require critical discernment around what behavioral health programs are most valuable (Sudhof & Shah, 2019). As a result, integrated care programs must be able to demonstrate their value and justify the existence of behavioral health programs and services.

Economic Studies and Cost-Effectiveness Analysis

Economic studies offer a systematic way to assess the value of behavioral health care. Economic study is an umbrella term referring to the assessment of health care service costs and consequences. Among different types of economic studies, cost-effectiveness analysis (CEA) is commonly used to assess and compare the value of health care services. CEA may be defined as the "costs per designated outcome (e.g., unit of effectiveness) between alternative strategies" (Dukhovny & Zupancic, 2011, p. c70). CEAs are particularly relevant to economic evaluations of behavioral health programs because they express value in terms of clinical outcomes. For example, a CEA of a peer support-based behavioral health program designed to address PPD among Canadian mothers articulated outcomes in terms of cost of the program per case of PPD avoided (Dukhovny et al., 2013).

The International Society for Pharmacoeconomic and Outcomes Research (ISPOR) provides guidelines for conducting and reporting CEA alongside clinical trial studies (Husereau et al., 2013). Although not all behavioral health interventions or programs will undergo clinical trial study, these guidelines may inform the development and evaluation of behavioral health programs in fetal, neonatal, and NICU follow-up settings. Using ISPOR guidelines, CEA should assess effectiveness with measures of clinical outcomes and health care utilization using patient-reported data. Behavioral health programs should integrate CEA plans into the program design and evaluation early so that optimal measures and time points for analysis can be incorporated prospectively. Although retrospective economic studies are feasible, prospective evaluation allows for more accurate estimates of costs and consequences. Various perspectives, or points of view, may be important to consider depending on program context, but CEA conducted from a societal perspective offers the most comprehensive information necessary for determining value (Husereau et al., 2013). Thus, CEA of behavioral health programs should include broader costs borne by society (e.g., missed productivity, family costs, or costs incurred by education or child welfare systems).

Time horizons, or the time period over which costs and effectiveness are assessed, are another component of CEA (Husereau et al., 2013). For instance, a behavioral health program with significant implementation costs but that delivers long-term clinical benefits and a reduction in health care utilization may be worth its initial investment. Time horizons are especially useful in determining the value of behavioral health programs in fetal, neonatal, and NICU settings given the cascading effects of parental mental health on parent and child outcomes. Ideally, lifetime time horizons facilitate the most accurate and comprehensive CEA. More realistically, studies should set time horizons as far as possible based on the theoretical knowledge related to study constructs and taking the particularities of each study into account. Computer modeling or decision analysis can also lengthen time horizons when it is not possible to use lifetime time horizons.

Payment Models

FEE-FOR-SERVICES

Payment models are a critical part of the context in which health care's value is determined. Thus, payers for services are considered key stakeholders when conducting economic evaluations, along with health care systems, institutions, patients and families, providers, and society (Dukhovny & Zupancic, 2011). In the United States, fee-for-service models have historically dominated payment model approaches in health care. In fee-for-service models, health care services are disaggregated and reimbursed, based on a predetermined rate, per service (Sudhof & Shah, 2019). For instance, a payer may reimburse for individual psychotherapy provided on-site in a NICU based on a rate per session to treat a particular mental health disorder such as depressive disorder in the context of the postpartum transition using a specific treatment modality (e.g., cognitive–behavioral therapy). Determining the actual cost of this behavioral health service, however, can be quite complicated and should include provider costs and training, institutional operating costs, as well as hidden patient costs such as travel and missed work time for parents beyond that spent participating in infant care in the NICU, as well as child care costs incurred for children other than the hospitalized infant while parents participate in services. Benefits of a fee-for-service model involve its theoretically straightforward approach to determining service costs. A particular service is associated with a price, and the "purchase" of multiple services costs the sum of each individual service. In fee-for-service models, providers are rewarded for services delivered and not necessarily for the parental and neonatal outcomes produced as a result of those services.

VALUE-BASED CARE

Value-based care offers an alternative payment model approach to fee-for-service models. Reflective of contemporary health care policy trends, value-based care rewards quality health care services that improve the overall health and well-being of patients and the overall public health. In a value-based care model, providers are rewarded for outcomes that improve health rather than for the delivery of services (Sudhof & Shah, 2019). This shifts the development, implementation, and evaluation of health care services toward including cost as just one important element alongside outcomes when determining value. Value-based care should also include an assessment of equity, or how services create, perpetuate, or avoid reducing disparities.

Continuing with the individual psychotherapy example, a value-based care model would consider comprehensive and long-term costs avoided by preventing and providing early treatment of depression. Examples could include costs associated with reduced NICU length of stay and infant rehospitalizations, increased use of infant preventive care, and outcomes associated with improved parent–child attachment such as increased breastfeeding and improved child developmental and behavioral outcomes. In a NICU setting, payers could reimburse behavioral health services that include PMADs screening, psychoeducation, peer support, and other early treatment efforts, along with more intensive services when indicated. Behavioral health programs could also consider pursuing a bundled care approach in which behavioral health services are connected to parent and infant medical care. Furthermore, value-based care would promote investigation of population-level outcomes and disparities, as well as work to disrupt negative health trends and suboptimal outcomes through improved services, implementation, and evaluation.

Value-based care places a high priority on patient-reported outcomes and experiences (e.g., patient-satisfaction measures), coordinated care, and innovation (Sudhof & Shah, 2019). Behavioral health programs seeking high-value care should consider team-based approaches, integrated services in patient-accessible settings, and optimizing use of technology (Dukhovny et al., 2013; Sudhof & Shah, 2019). Throughout these efforts, behavioral health services should use an equity lens to ensure disparities are identified, investigated, and addressed. Value-based care payment models reflect contemporary trends and hold potential to improve patient and public health while remaining accountable for costs and limited resources (Sudhof & Shah, 2019). Health care systems that serve high-risk infants and families can move toward integrated behavioral health care while recognizing practical resource constraints and optimizing patient well-being through adopting value-based care approaches.

CONCLUSION

Integrated care reflects an exciting approach to respond to behavioral health needs along perinatal and pediatric spectrums of care. Fetal, NICU, and neonatal follow-up providers can optimize the implementation success of integrated care through understanding fundamentals of systems change, conducting needs assessments and program evaluations, and working to demonstrate the value of integrated behavioral health services. It is well established that increased risk for PMADs and other behavioral health concerns exists during pregnancy, birth, and postpartum. However, these time periods also present rich opportunities for fetal, NICU, and neonatal follow-up settings to reimagine services and positively impact health and developmental outcomes among high-risk infants and families.

REFERENCES

Agency for Healthcare Research and Quality. (n.d.). *What is integrated behavioral health?* https://integrationacademy.ahrq.gov/about/integrated-behavioral-health

American College of Obstetricians and Gynecologists. (2018). Screening for perinatal depression: ACOG Committee Opinion No. 757. *Obstetrics & Gynecology, 132*(5), e208–e212.

Cherry, A. S., Blucker, R. T., Thornberry, T. S., Hetherington, C., McCaffree, M. A., & Gillaspy, S. R. (2016). Postpartum depression screening in the Neonatal Intensive Care Unit: program development, implementation, and lessons learned. *Journal of Multidisciplinary Healthcare, 9*, 59–67. https://doi.org/10.2147/JMDH.S91559

Dempsey, A. G., Chavis, L., Willis, T., Zuk, J., & Cole, J. C. M. (2021). Addressing perinatal mental health risk within a fetal care center. *Journal of Clinical Psychology in Medical Settings, 28*, 125–136. https://doi.org/10.1007/s10880-020-09728-2

DiBari, J. N., Yu, S. M., Chao, S. M., & Lu, M. C. (2014). Use of postpartum care: Predictors and barriers. *Journal of Pregnancy, 2014*, 530769. https://doi.org/10.1155/2014/530769

Dukhovny, D., Dennis, C. L., Hodnett, E., Weston, J., Stewart, D. E., Mao, W., & Zupancic, J. A. (2013). Prospective economic evaluation of a peer support intervention for prevention of postpartum depression among high-risk women in Ontario, Canada. *American Journal of Perinatology, 30*(8), 631–642. https://doi.org/10.1055/s-0032-1331029

Dukhovny, D., & Zupancic, J. A. F. (2011). Economic evaluation with clinical trials in neonatology. *NeoReviews, 12*(2), e69–e75. https://doi.org/10.1542/neo.12-2-e69

Edwards, N., Rowan, M., Marck, P., & Grinspun, D. (2011). Understanding whole systems change in health care: The case of nurse practitioners in Canada. *Policy, Politics & Nursing Practice, 12*(1), 4–17. https://doi.org/10.1177/1527154411403816

Franck, L. S., & O'Brien, K. (2019). The evolution of family-centered care: From supporting parent-delivered interventions to a model of family integrated care. *Birth Defects Research, 111*, 1044–1059. https://doi.org/10.1002/bdr2.1521

Grinnell, R. M., Gabor, P. A., & Unrau, Y. A. (2016). *Program evaluation for social workers: Foundations of evidence-based programs* (7th ed.). Oxford University Press.

Husereau, D., Drummond, M., Petrou, S., Carswell, C., Moher, D., Greenberg, D., Augustovski, F., Briggs, A. H., Mauskopf, J., & Loder, E.; on behalf of the ISPOR Health Economic Evaluation Publication Guidelines—CHEERS Good Reporting Practices Task Force. (2013). Consolidated Health Economic Evaluation Reporting Standards (CHEERS)—Explanation and elaboration: A report of the ISPOR Health Economic Evaluation Publication Guidelines Good Reporting Practices Task Force. *Value Health, 16*(2), 231–250. https://doi.org/10.1016/j.jval.2013.02.002

Kendig, S., Keats, J. P., Hoffman, M. C., Kay, L. B., Miller, E. S., Moore Simas, T. A., Frieder, A., Hackley, B., Indman, P., Raines, C., Semenuk, K., Wisner, K. L., & Lemieux, L. A. (2017). Consensus bundle on maternal mental health: Perinatal depression and anxiety. *Obstetrics & Gynecology, 129*(3), 422–430. https://doi.org/10.1097/AOG.0000000000001902

Lomonaco-Haycraft, K. C., Hyer, J., Tibbits, B., Grote, J., Stainback-Tracy, K., Ulrickson, C., Lieberman, A., van Bekkum, L., & Hoffman, M. C. (2019). Integrated perinatal mental health care: A national model of perinatal primary care in vulnerable populations. *Primary Health Care Research & Development, 20*, E77. https://doi.org/10.1017/S1463423618000348

Luca, D. L., Garlow, N., Staatz, C., Margiotta, C., & Zivin, K. (2019). *Societal costs of untreated perinatal mood and anxiety disorders in the United States* [Issue brief]. https://www.mathematica.org/our-publications-and-findings/publications/socie tal-costs-of-untreated-perinatal-mood-and-anxiety-disorders-in-the-united-states

Rogers, E. M. (2003). *Diffusion of innovations* (5th ed.). Free Press.

Shirey, M. R. (2013). Lewin's theory of planned change as a strategic resource. *Journal of Nursing Administration, 43*(2), 69–72. https://doi.org/10.1097/NNA.0b013e318 27f20a9

Sudhof, L., & Shah, N. T. (2019). In pursuit of value-based maternity care. *Obstetrics & Gynecology, 133*(3), 541–551. https://doi.org/10.1097/AOG.0000000000003113

Vaughn, A. T., & Hooper, G. L. (2020). Development and implementation of a postpartum depression screening program in the NICU. *Neonatal Network, 39*(2), 75–82. https://doi.org/10.1891/0730-0832.39.2.75

Wakida, E. K., Obua, C., Rukundo, G. Z., Maling, S., Talib, Z. M., & Okello, E. S. (2018). Barriers and facilitators to the integration of mental health services into primary healthcare: A qualitative study among Ugandan primary care providers using the COM-B framework. *BMC Health Services Research, 18*(1), Article 890. https://doi. org/10.1186/s12913-018-3684-7

Welch, M. G., Halperin, M. S., Austin, J., Stark, R. I., Hofer, M. A., Hane, A. A., & Myers, M. M. (2016). Depression and anxiety symptoms of mothers of preterm infants are decreased at 4 months corrected age with Family Nurture Intervention in the NICU. *Archives of Women's Mental Health, 19*(1), 51–61. https://doi.org/10.1007/s00737-015-0502-7

Young, C. A., Burnett, H., Ballinger, A., Castro, G., Steinberg, S., Nau, M., Bakken, E. H., Thomas, M., & Beck, A. L. (2019). Embedded maternal mental health care in a pediatric primary care clinic: A qualitative exploration of mothers' experiences. *Academic Pediatrics, 19*(8), 934–941. https://doi.org/10.1016/j.acap.2019.08.004

5

INTERDISCIPLINARY BEHAVIORAL HEALTH TEAMS

CHAVIS A. PATTERSON, MONA ELGOHAIL,
ALISON R. HARTMAN, VINCENT C. SMITH,
AND PAMELA A. GELLER ■

Advances in technology, including fetal surgical procedures, have allowed for more complex medical interventions to be available in utero, which can increase the likelihood of delivering infants at a much younger gestational age. With advancing neonatal care, the age of viability has improved (Ho & Saigal, 2005). Medical teams are now able to intervene in utero to identify, address, and correct certain congenital anomalies, malformations, and disruptions in the normal process of fetal development. Medicine is also embracing a more inclusive, patient- and family-centered approach to care. Multidisciplinary teams across fetal care, obstetrics, neonatal intensive care unit (NICU), and NICU follow-up clinic (NFC) settings that offer emotional support to families have grown to include psychology, social work, child life specialists, and chaplains. In some hospitals, perinatal psychiatry is also available to caregivers who have an infant in the NICU. These disciplines take an active role in helping parents manage the perinatal mood and anxiety disorders (PMADs) that often accompany the stress that parents experience, both while the fetus is in utero and postpartum.

INTERDISCIPLINARY BEHAVIORAL HEALTH TEAM

The behavioral health team partners with staff to offer training and tools to support the mental health of patients and their families who spend time in fetal care centers, NICUs, or NFCs due to complications during their pregnancy or following the birth of their child. Whereas well-funded NICUs are able to hire a wider range of specialists, smaller NICUs may seek resources to provide training for their medical and nursing staff so that they can best support patients and their families at bedside. Hall and colleagues (2016) Hynan and Hall (2015) created a NICU self-assessment tool that compares available mental health resources of a NICU to an ideal NICU that is fully resourced. Documents that accompany the assessment tool offer strategies for building a strong mental health program within NICUs, which include hiring a psychologist. It outlines how to cover the costs through billing, institutional support, grants, and philanthropic donations. For licensed providers, billing is a clear way to generate revenue for these services.

BEHAVIORAL HEALTH TEAM MEMBERS

The model of patient- and family-centered care, which has gained popularity in recent decades, has shed light on the intense emotional challenges that patients and their families experience in perinatal settings. This has led to more mental health professionals embedded in these settings. Many organizations and foundations offer informal and/or formal opportunities to learn about working with patients and their families in these settings. In particular, Postpartum Support International offers a perinatal mental health certification that is available to all providers who complete the requisite coursework, years of experience, and qualifying examination. In perinatal settings, behavioral health team members serve as advocates for and liaisons between the pregnant patient, the pediatric patient's family (neonate/infant), and the medical team. They facilitate communication between the family and the medical team regarding any aspect of the patient's medical care, from intake admission to post-hospital discharge and beyond.

Psychologists, social workers, chaplains, and child life specialists can help patients and their families identify their needs, strengths, coping skills, and sources of support. In their initial assessment, social workers interview families to identify specific mental health needs that would be better suited for psychology, religious practices to include spiritual care, and siblings to involve child life specialists. This assessment may also include referral to other psychosocial services offered within the hospital (e.g., lactation specialists and language interpreter services). Additional responsibilities include bereavement assistance; participation in care team conferences and family meetings; facilitation of communication between staff, patients, and patients' families; and facilitation of support groups. The aforementioned services can be available to patients and their families during prenatal care or during any point in their hospitalization, such as when receiving a diagnosis, prior to or during procedures, during decision-making, and at end of life. In addition, psychologists and social workers serve as a resource to staff. They may provide education to colleagues regarding parental mental health, parenting, and stressors, as well as community resources. They may also discuss burnout, self-care, institutional racism, and workplace satisfaction among staff members through seminars, lectures, or workshops.

Psychologists

Psychologists in these settings are licensed and have either a PhD or PsyD degree in clinical psychology or early childhood development. They have completed a pre-doctoral internship and, often, a post-doctoral fellowship. There is no specific certification needed for psychologists to work in perinatal settings; however, a training background in interdisciplinary health care settings is essential. Although not often required, some hospitals may seek out psychologists who have received board certification in clinical health psychology, clinical child and adolescent psychology, or clinical neuropsychology from the American Board of Professional Psychology (Saxton et al., 2020).

ASSESSMENT

Assessment and screening are central to the role of NICU psychologists. Psychologists conduct clinical assessments of perinatal patients and couples to assess for mental health concerns during the antepartum and postpartum periods (see the following section) and provide intervention and referrals as needed. Given the increased risk for developmental delays, psychologists also administer developmental assessments to infants in the NICU. Based on the results and in collaboration with other care team members, a developmentally focused treatment plan is created for staff to follow. This plan will also include infant–caregiver attachment strategies to help mitigate potential developmental issues. In NFC settings, psychologists administer and interpret neuropsychological assessments in order to evaluate the developmental trajectories throughout childhood, differentially diagnose, and provide referrals to additional early intervention services as needed.

SCREENING

In addition to providing assessment services to infants, psychologists work to address the needs of family members within the context of a patient- and family-centered care model. Ideally, psychologists should universally screen caregivers for emotional distress, at-risk behaviors, and psychological disorders both prior to and following birth. Screening caregivers for perinatal mood and anxiety disorders (PMADs) is of particular importance in these high-stress settings. Mothers and their partners are at increased risk for PMADs, which may be highly debilitating for them and are linked with poor infant and family outcomes. It is important to include partners because, unfortunately, they are often overlooked. Psychologists can evaluate and interpret these screenings and, upon further clinical assessment, can provide differential diagnoses, interventions, and referral services as needed (Hynan et al., 2013).

PSYCHOTHERAPY

Psychologists in perinatal settings also provide short-term interventions, including bereavement and palliative care counseling, for families, couples, and individuals who are experiencing acute distress or interpersonal difficulties. Depending on their training and theoretical orientation, psychologists may deliver short-term cognitive–behavioral therapy, mother–baby interactions therapy, interpersonal therapy, couples or family systems-based therapy, and/or mindfulness-based interventions, when needed. In conjunction with social work colleagues, psychologists may provide support, education, and psychosocial care for staff members, with the acknowledgment that working in these settings, particularly fetal care, obstetrics, and the NICU, can be emotionally taxing and lead to staff burnout (Hall et al., 2019).

RESEARCH

In addition to their specialized training in clinical assessment and intervention, research methodology and design are central to psychologists' training. Therefore, as well as providing clinical care, psychologists in perinatal settings seek to advance the field through research and dissemination. In this capacity, psychologists may deploy quantitative and/or qualitative research to better understand the experiences of families or staff members in their respective settings. Using quality improvement or research-based techniques, they engage in many lines of research, such as work to develop or assess new interventions for expectant parents, infants, children, and/or families; improve family-centered care; investigate the efficacy of various staff practices; evaluate staff–family interactions; or assess quality of care.

Social Workers

Social workers play a central role in the care of patients, their families, and staff in all hospital settings. Master's-level social workers may move between different settings within the hospital or may be embedded in the fetal care center, NICU, or NFC. The National Association of Perinatal Social Workers (NAPSW, 2005) recommends that every family be offered social work services as standard of care. Many of these families endure intense emotional stress due to the fact that their developing fetus or newborn infant has a life-threatening illness. In addition to medical expenses, these families also experience financial difficulties as a result of taking time off from work for multiple prenatal care appointments, to be with their infant at home or hospital bedside, relocating to be closer to the hospital, and having to pay for daily expenses (i.e., child care for siblings, food, parking, gas, and lodging).

Social workers in the hospital setting have earned a master's degree in social work (MSW) and may be required to have obtained licensure from a state licensing board (i.e., Licensed Social Worker [LSW]) (National Association of Social Workers, 2005). Furthermore, some perinatal settings may require a Licensed Clinical Social Worker (LCSW) degree. Obtaining an LCSW credential, the highest level of licensure available to social workers, requires completing 2 or 3 years of supervised clinical experience and passing a state licensure exam. Special training, beyond what is required for a master's degree and/or licensure, is not often required of social workers who work in perinatal settings. They may also receive a case management certification in health care. In addition, the NAPSW offers training and mentorship opportunities for exposure to these settings.

Social workers connect families with benefits, services, and resources, as needed, both within the hospital and in the community. As such, social workers have an in-depth knowledge of specialists' roles within the hospital and resources in the community (e.g., housing and transportation, financial and insurance, mental health, and addiction intervention). Social workers collaborate with a diverse array of disciplines and agencies to ensure adequate care is provided for patients and their families. Social workers are often responsible for coordinating continuity of care and follow-up plans after postpartum and NICU discharge.

Social workers in perinatal settings, particularly those that do not have a doctoral-level psychologist on staff, may also provide supportive mental health services. Social workers may provide counseling to address parenting skills, stress management, family conflict, difficult medical decisions, and bereavement. Social workers may also screen parents for psychological distress or factors that put them at risk for distress in order to make appropriate referrals. In some cases, LCSWs or other experienced social workers may provide brief psychotherapeutic interventions or supportive counseling to parents and other family members who are experiencing acute emotional distress. These services may mitigate the negative downstream effects of early hospitalization on the infant and family. Importantly, social workers may be a first point of contact in instances of suspected interpersonal partner violence and child abuse or neglect. In some circumstances, social workers may liaise between hospital staff and Child Protective Services or domestic violence programs.

Child Life Specialists

Child life specialists in perinatal settings collaborate with parents to develop and implement a personalized care plan to address the needs of older siblings during the perinatal period. They work with pregnant women with prolonged antepartum stays and/or with activity restrictions and those who are at home to support attachment with siblings. The goal of these care plans is to minimize the adverse effects of the maternal and neonatal hospitalization on siblings and promote healthy integration of these stressful experiences. This involves developmentally appropriate preparation, coping skills, therapeutic play, and expressive modalities (Brown & Chitkara, 2014). Parents are encouraged to use age-appropriate, honest, and concrete explanations without euphemisms when speaking with young children to help them understand what is happening to their mother and newborn sibling. They are also encouraged to honor the role of an older sibling when discussing their family narrative. Siblings who are supported by their family in a developmentally appropriate manner are better able to cope with the stress of the expected or unanticipated hospitalization.

Chaplains

Chaplains provide valuable spiritual and emotional guidance in the fetal care and NICU settings, and families may lean on chaplains with spiritual struggles or when faced with difficult decision-making. Chaplains can work with families to provide meaning and purpose to a difficult situation by using the family's faith or spirituality to guide them. They can provide comfort, hope, and courage to explore areas of conflict when a family believes its faith is being tested. They help patients and/or their families process their feelings, thoughts, and concerns, as well as facilitate meaning making about the health challenges they or their infants are facing. Chaplains provide religious consolation and incorporate religious rituals and traditions as appropriate, such as prayer, sacraments, memorial services, and infant naming ceremonies.

OTHER TEAM MEMBERS OFFERING SUPPORTIVE CARE

Nurses

Advanced practitioners and beside nurses are often the health care providers who interface most frequently with women in the fetal care and obstetric clinics, as well as infants and their families in the NICU. In the obstetrics setting, nurses not only physically care for women but also advocate to protect their desired wishes for their birth experiences and assist them with important self-care throughout their inpatient admission, lactation onset, and early postpartum transition. In this way, nurses can help reduce the risk of trauma during labor and birth, normalize the experience, and celebrate the birth. In addition, nurses can help women prepare for the difficult emotional experience of leaving the hospital while their newborn remains in the NICU by teaching them about the discharge process throughout the provision of care (Association of Women's Health, Obstetric and Neonatal Nurses, 2015).

In the NICU, nurses focus on the physical and psychosocial well-being of patients and their families. Nurses can model bonding behaviors, helping families become more comfortable with seeing, touching, holding, and caring for their infant despite all of the medical equipment surrounding them. As the "gatekeepers" of all provision of care, nurses advocate for the infant and their family, as well as coordinate care across services to allow for best possible infant outcomes (Hallowell et al., 2019). For example, as gatekeepers they advocate for providers to cluster care so that infants are only touched every 3 hours to allow for optimal rest time. They also educate families and keep them updated about their infant's care, helping promote optimal communication between the care team and NICU families.

Attending Physicians

In the majority of clinical settings, the attending physician is considered the leader of the care team. The primary role of the physician is to help develop and execute a medical care plan. In situations in which the fetal or neonatal diagnosis is not known, the physician is expected to facilitate the development of a differential diagnosis and a plan to determine a final diagnosis. When the diagnosis is known, the physician is expected to develop and/or oversee the treatment plan, anticipate crises, and revise the treatment plan when changes arise.

Providing supportive care is another facet of their responsibility. Physicians are empathetic to the emotional struggles families endure while remaining impartial to the medical decisions families make. Due to the nature of having complications during pregnancy or medically compromised infants, parents are often dealing with more stress and uncertainty than they have experienced in the past. The staff members who work with and support these families pay an emotional toll of being supportive. As such, another compelling but less discussed role of physicians is supporting staff to ensure that they have the care that they need to work in these high-stress and emotionally charged environments. A simple place to begin is to focus on ensuring that all of the team members have their basic needs met for hydration, food, hygiene, and rest. After basic needs are met, the next goal is to foster an environment in which the members of the medical team can discuss their concerns about medical management, patient interactions, errors, and challenging situations as well as recent experiences in a safe space to process their feelings with one another. This can help address the emotional and mental well-being of the entire medical team.

Compassion and understanding from leadership can help build a culture of wellness that includes sharing and acceptance. The physician may set the tone and help foster an environment in which it is acceptable to discuss a wide array of feelings. This can help create a culture in which psychological first aid can be provided in a supportive way for those who are in need. Psychological first aid is an evidence-informed approach to assist individuals who have distress following a stressful event; it can be used to help foster coping and adaptive functioning following stressful events. It is critical that we move away from a culture of shame and blame and toward a culture of psychological safety in which one can learn from one's errors and receive support from colleagues.

Palliative Care Specialists

A number of institutions have formed a palliative care team (PCT) to deliver palliative care to families with a child who has a life-threatening illness. A PCT can be composed of representatives from all disciplines who work in the hospital, including physicians, fellows, nurse practitioners, nurses, social workers, chaplains, child life specialists, psychologists, music therapists, and art therapists. The PCT may assess the needs of the patient and family and then determine which team member would be the best fit for support, with each playing an individualized role in collaboration with the team. Physicians on the PCT have had formal pediatric palliative care training through fellowship. Other interdisciplinary team members may have had further training as part of their general education, which may include bereavement work.

The PCT works with providers and staff in perinatal settings to provide emotional, social, spiritual, and bereavement support to families as they manage the stress that accompanies having a child with a life-threatening illness. In the fetal care center, consults are requested by the maternal fetal medicine physicians when they encounter a pregnant patient who is carrying a fetus with a life-threatening diagnosis. A perinatal palliative care birth plan is constructed to care for the family throughout the pregnancy and in preparation for the birth (Cole et al., 2017). If the infant is anticipated to survive beyond the first day or two, team members will typically consult a hospital-wide palliative care team to help support the family in thinking through the next options for care in collaboration with the neonatology team that is caring for their infant. Similarly, in the NICU, a plan of neonatal care is constructed in collaboration with the infant's care team.

Genetic Counselors

Genetic counselors play an integral role in fetal care and NICU settings but typically are not assigned to NFCs. They complete an initial screening that is used to determine whether additional genetic testing is recommended for the patient and/or their family, as well as which additional specialist(s) should be involved in the care. Once genetic testing results are available, genetic counselors are often the first to reach out to families to provide education, nondirective counseling about care options, facilitation of informed decision-making, and help coordinate appropriate follow-up care. In addition, they provide related psychosocial assessment and intervention as needed, such as crisis intervention, grief and bereavement counseling, and pregnancy management. As with services mentioned previously, genetic counselors help identify families' needs and provide referrals to appropriate support services. It is not uncommon for genetic counseling services to start in the fetal care center and continue into the NICU and after discharge (e.g., to discuss autopsy postmortem or to provide additional options regarding subsequent pregnancy risks).

Lactation Specialists

International Board-Certified Lactation Consultants (IBCLCs) work with mothers to help them achieve their personal breastfeeding goals for their infants. Grounded in evidence-based, scientific understanding of human milk production and committed to providing personalized, holistic care, IBCLCs walk with families on their lactation journeys. This involves providing education about breastfeeding and pumping, as well as practical assistance with creating a pumping schedule to maximize breast health, milk production, breastfeeding positions, proper latch techniques, oral care, and skin-to-skin contact (i.e., kangaroo care). Consultants teach parents about the importance of skin-to-skin contact, which supports the physical and psychological well-being of both infant and parent, including improving the bonding and attachment between them.

Developmental Therapists

Developmental therapists include occupational therapists, physical therapists, and speech–language pathologists with specialized training in infant development. They assess the oral, motor, and feeding skills of the infant, as well as their ability to move and engage with others and engage in their environment. Once the needs of the infant have been identified, developmental therapists work with NICU families and their care team to create individualized care plans and environments to help infants increase muscle tone and control. Developmental therapists provide parent education and training on how to care for their infants in a way that continues the individualized care plan outside of sessions and extends to NFC. The specialists may be involved in ongoing assessments and treatment to meet the specific needs of the infant while creating meaningful opportunities for bonding between parents and their infant. These plans of care are included in the chart and can usually be accessed in NFC to allow for continuity of care across settings and coordination with early intervention services post discharge.

Language Interpreter Services

For parents with infants who have increased medical needs, there is a great deal for them to understand about managing the infants' medical conditions in utero, during labor and birth, during their NICU hospitalization, and especially upon discharge from the NICU. Fundamentally, this requires clear communication between parents and the care team to ensure optimal health outcomes for maternal and infant health. However, high-quality communication is not possible when parents and care team providers do not speak the same language. In these situations, it is most ethical to utilize language interpreter services, as mandated by U.S. law and national guidelines (Juckett & Unger, 2014). Care team providers should not wait for the request for language interpreters to come from parents, as parents may erroneously fear being perceived as a nuisance or a burden in making such a request.

Qualified interpreters provide in-person, video, or telephonic interpreting services. This ensures meaningful access and effective, complete, accurate, impartial, and confidential communication between the hospital staff and the patient and/or patient representative who are limited English proficient and/or Deaf or hard of hearing.

TEAM BUILDING ACROSS DISCIPLINES AND BUILDING RELATIONSHIPS WITH FAMILIES

With so many disciplines involved in the care, it is important to explore how they can come together as a team to work collaboratively to support families through one of the toughest periods in their lives. This section outlines some thoughts about creating a cohesive work group in such high-stress environments. In developing a strong workforce, time and attention should be paid to team building, role definition, team dynamics, and partnering with families.

Team Building

Team building requires intention and willing participation by all members. In order for a team to function most effectively, its members must select a strong leader and work together toward common goals (Katzenbach & Douglas, 1993). The leader sets the tone, determines directions, and course corrects the team as needed. It is important for the leader to get to know all of the team members (Katzenbach & Douglas, 1993). By knowing and understanding the members, the leader will be able to maximize the team's function. Given the importance of each team member's work to the overall goal, it is important that all of the contributions of team members be acknowledged and valued by leadership (Adair, 1986).

Team building helps team members understand that it is ultimately about the achievements of the team and less about the individual contribution. Team building strategies aim to foster and strengthen connections between members (Adair, 1986). In order for team building to work, there must be a culture of effective communication between the team members (Shuffler et al., 2011). The team members need to be able to discuss both positive and negative aspects of the work. It helps to be able to provide both positive and negative feedback from a constructive learning point of view. This can be accomplished in a variety of ways, including working on team projects, doing team-building activities, and sharing challenging experiences. Given the diverse nature of many teams, leaders must recognize the value of different approaches and points of view, even as they work toward a common goal. Another strategy for team building is to have clear objectives and roles for each of the team members (Shuffler et al., 2011). This will allow each member to understand the goals of their work and what part they are expected to play. Team members are likely to be engaged with one another and the work when they understand the context of a particular activity or individual contribution as part of a larger objective.

Clinical Handoffs

It is imperative that the fetal care, obstetric, NICU, and NFC medical teams coordinate care to help ensure optimal continuity of care and consistent messaging for the families. Clinical handoffs involve the transfer of patient care or health information from one health care provider to another or from one health care facility to another. This transfer may include pertinent patient information and knowledge as well as responsibility for ongoing care. As such, an effective handoff is a vital step in maintaining quality clinical care and a culture of safety within the fetal care center, obstetrics unit, NICU, and NFC. The effectiveness of the handoff process is contingent upon the quality and completeness of the information (Arora, 2020).

The handoff process is dynamic and vulnerable to interference, disruptions, and variable skill levels of the participants (Arora, 2020). Furthermore, there is evidence from the literature to support the claim that shift handoffs are characterized by a high level of information corruption and lack of structure (Pezzolesi et al., 2013). For patients, this often means altered or delayed treatment plans, unclear diagnoses, and frequent medication errors (Forster et al., 2003). Implications for the medical staff include emotional distress and clinical uncertainty due to the lack of clear instructions on care management (Cleland et al., 2009). Given the stated vulnerability of handoffs and the ramifications of severe consequences for both patients and staff when it is done poorly (Pezzolesi et al., 2013), it is imperative that handoffs be done safely and effectively. Arora and Farnan (2020) suggest that effective handoffs contain verbal communication, written communication, and transfer of responsibilities. They also suggest that handoffs have a standard format, written template, and locale with limited distractions.

Interdisciplinary Referrals

Ongoing formal and informal assessments monitor the needs of the pregnant patient and infant. During the course of treatment, interdisciplinary teams may be requested. Psychology, social work, spiritual care, lactation, or other services may be introduced as warranted for the pregnant patient. For the infant, a medical evaluation or developmental assessment may prompt the team to request additional services, such as occupational therapy, physical therapy, and/or speech and language pathology. When these referrals are made, providers are able to access the electronic health record to see the history of illness and course of treatment, helping streamline care.

Role Negotiation

In establishing a well-run team, it is important to communicate one's role to both the team and the family. Although governed under different licensing bodies, social work, psychology, chaplaincy, child life, music therapy, and art therapy each have a strong mental health component.

Because not all perinatal settings are exactly the same and may have various compositions in number of individuals and types of interdisciplinary teams, it is important to identify strengths, reduce redundancy, and streamline care.

Encouraging staff to work at the top of the scope of their license establishes their role on the team and takes full advantage of their area of expertise. This is also important to reduce conflicts within the team and avoid potential harm to the patient and their family. Although this might take some time to navigate in the beginning, as with all group formations (Tuckman, 1965), the benefits certainly outweigh the challenges along the way.

Team Dynamics

Team dynamics play an important role in building and sustaining a cohesive work group. Brodsky and colleagues (2013) believe that reducing silos, involving representatives from multiple disciplines in decision-making, and always thinking about process improvement represent the basic tenets to building a strong team. These strategies are not routinely taught to providers, and it is incumbent on each institution to recognize the benefits. Hall and colleagues (2015) showed that staff appreciate training that enhances skills when working with families in crisis. In addition to offering skills, it has the potential to reduce staff burnout. For these trainings to be successful, they need to be interdisciplinary and draw from best practices, which might include topics of cultural humility, openness to feedback, and risk assessment. In a research project offering such training, Hall and colleagues (2019) reported that staff had significant improvement in both knowledge and attitudes after the training.

Building Relationships with Families

Due to the complexity of fetal care and NICU/NFC environments and in order to manage medically complex pregnancies and medically ill infants, it is paramount that the aforementioned teams work collaboratively with the family. Time and attention should be paid to the psychosocial experience and its impact on both the families and staff as systems theory suggests. In supporting the families, one must begin the process by engaging parents and families, viewing them as part of the interdisciplinary team. Engagement, if possible, should be established during the perinatal period. Families should meet with staff during the pregnancy to review the birth plan and acknowledge some of the potential challenges ahead. Hynan and Hall (2015) described three principles of communication that are important to incorporate with families to develop a trusting relationship: (a) Acknowledge and clarify a parent's concern, (b) share medical information on a regular basis, and (c) be empathetic when delivering bad news to a family.

In the fetal care, NICU, and NFC environments, meeting the family where they are upon entry can go a long way in establishing a trusting relationship. Setting up an initial family meeting to introduce the family to the particular perinatal environment is one way to do this. During the meeting, members of the care team, such as the social worker, the attending physician, and the nurse or advanced practice provider, discuss with the family how the team functions and time is allowed for the family to process their experience so far. It is important to explain any differences in care and interventions that may be in place in the new setting. If the pregnant patient or infant has transferred care from one hospital to another, it is important to identify changes in care as well as differences in hospital policies and procedures. The team should explain the rotation of physicians who will be caring for the mother or infant and emphasize the hospital's policy on partnering with the family. Teams should indicate that because of the acuity of the fetal or neonatal infant's condition, the plan of care may change once it has been set, due to the changing nature of pregnancy and acutely ill infants. Be clear about the most efficient ways to reach and communicate with staff if/when questions arise. Throughout prenatal care and during introductory meetings, the team should allow time for the family members to talk about their journey to this point. By showing this type of empathy, staff are acknowledging trauma that the family may have already experienced. The team can also obtain valuable information about how the family manages stress, sets expectations, and asks for available resources. Finally, the team should schedule follow-up meetings with the medical team for more in-depth reviews of the medical plan of care. The behavioral health team members can follow up with the family to assess their needs and put in place the appropriate resources.

Assessing Families and Caregivers for Mental Health Support

Partnering with the family also includes understanding and assessing the caregiver for any mental health support needed. Hynan et al. (2013) and Bush et al. (2020) reported that parents' mental health conditions can have a negative impact on their infant's neurodevelopment. A growing number of institutions currently screen parents during pregnancy, postpartum, and in follow-up care. Recently published studies indicate notable mental health distress in caregivers (e.g., Cole et al., 2016; Moreyra et al., 2021). Screening can also be used to identify level of care needed and thereby direct the efforts of behavioral health teams. For example, A. Baughcum (personal communication, July 2020) screened 171 parents in the NICU using a NICU version of the Psychosocial Assessment Tool and a model by Pai et al. (2008). Baughcum reported that 66.7% of caregivers scored in the range for "universal support" (i.e., mild distress), 26.3% scored in the range for targeted support (i.e., moderate distress), and 7% scored in the clinical range, showing signs of acute distress and requiring a high level of support. Resources available to each of these caregiver subgroups would be determined by the institution and their available resources. These resources could include social work, music therapy, psychology, chaplain services, as well as recommendations for a psychiatric evaluation and inpatient admission, when warranted. Purdy et al. (2015) encouraged screening in NFCs because they reported that mothers of preterm infants experience higher levels of depression compared to mothers of term infants. In many institutions, this type of universal screening is now considered a best practice.

Handling Disagreements

Inherent with all relationships are times when disagreements arise. These disagreements can be the result of miscommunication, misinformation, style of communication, and/or errors in care. Miscommunication, misinformation, and/ or errors in care can cause a fracture in the care team–family alliance, resulting in a disagreement and loss of trust with the family. This is even more likely when a clinical mistake is made, often resulting in heightened emotions and stress levels, or when the pregnancy or infant's trajectory has changed unexpectedly.

The care team is interdisciplinary, with the disciplines coming together to organize a plan of care for each pregnant patient and infant. Although it is incumbent on the primary physician to work with the multiple disciplines and organize and explain the care plan to the family, this sometimes does not happen in a way that the family finds helpful. This miscommunication or misinformation can be compounded by the fact that the care plan is a living plan that can change as the patient's status changes.

Although a structure of checks and balances is set up to avoid errors, at times they do occur and, to a greater extent, jeopardize the care team–family alliance. It is important in these situations to report the error to the family as soon as possible and, as a team, take responsibility for the error and maintain transparency. It is the responsibility of the team leader involved in the patient's clinical care to clarify that the team has made an error and one person will not be identified. When an error does occur, the team leader should communicate to the family where the breakdown occurred and that there are steps being taken to implement a process to ensure the error does not happen again. It should be made clear to the family that every error is taken extremely seriously and each is reported to hospital leadership. Some of this documentation and activity may contain information that is protected under confidentiality statutes. When communication issues or errors occur, families usually ask to change providers, request a second opinion, or even request a transfer to another institution. Patients and/or caregivers may also pursue litigation. Using the skills and resources of the behavioral health team, these fractures in care team–family alliance can often be ameliorated.

When handling disagreements, it is important to involve the behavioral health team early to act as a mediator between the staff and family. Often, the family's expression of anger, frustration, and/or anxiety stems from a deeper-rooted emotion linked to exhaustion, feelings of helplessness, anxiety, loss, issues of trauma, and/or institutional racism. A behavioral health perspective can assist the entire team in navigating through these challenges in order to arrive at the best outcome for everyone.

One way to be proactive and mitigate disagreements is to plan for and expect them. Although it is the hope that disagreements will not occur, they are difficult to avoid given the high stress levels and the nature of the work. Managing expectations and being conservative in response to patient and caregiver questions often reduce disagreements. This sets the stage for open discussion when there is a difference of perspective and opinion between the family and the care team. Simulation training offers staff another modality to practice difficult conversations. Janice-Woods Reed and Sharma (2016) had neonatal–perinatal fellows deliver difficult news to actors representing caregivers. The fellows reported feeling more comfortable delivering bad news following the training. The authors felt that this training enhanced the communication skills of the fellows.

Blackall et al. (2009) use moments of disagreements as opportunities to reassess and improve the care team–family alliance. Their 5-point model focuses on competence, connection, control, contribution, and collaboration. The care team must highlight the *competencies* that the family brings to the environment. The team must search for ways to *connect* with the family around the care of the infant. Blackall et al. recommend that providers move away from the idea of *control* to collaboration, in terms of the situation and reaction of the family. They must take time to address the team's *contribution* to the impasse. Finally, they must *collaborate* to bring the family back in as a part of the care team, re-establishing trust and open communication.

CONCLUSION

The behavioral health care team can be an asset when providing a high level of care for each infant in perinatal settings. Optimal care requires that providers have a deep understanding of their own role, including biases and their professional strengths and limitations. They must also understand the roles of their colleagues and the role of the team as a whole. They should expect and prepare for conflicts between team members and with the patient and/or family in these high-stress and emotionally charged settings. However, when disruptions occur, re-engagement with the patient and/or family is always possible. In times of conflict, teams should capitalize on the expertise of psychologists and social workers. Relying on their expertise can help repair, maintain, and strengthen the care team–family alliance and promote good health outcomes for the patient and family.

REFERENCES

Adair, J. E. (1986). *Effective teambuilding*. United Kingdom: Gower.

Arora, V., & Farnan, J. (2020). Patient handoff. UptoDate. https://www.uptodate.com/contents/patient-handoffs

Association of Women's Health, Obstetric and Neonatal Nurses. (2015). Mood and anxiety disorders in pregnant and postpartum women. *Journal of Obstetric, Gynecologic, & Neonatal Nursing, 44*, 687–689.

Blackall, G. F., Simms, S., & Green, M. J. (2009). *Breaking the cycle: How to turn conflict into collaboration when you and your patients disagree.* ACP Press.

Brodsky, D., Gupta, M., Quinn, M., Smallcomb, J., Mao, W., Koyama, N., May, V., Waldo, K., Young, S., & Pursley, D. M. (2013). Building collaborative teams in neonatal intensive care. *BMJ Quality & Safety, 22*(5), 374–382.

Brown, C., & Chitkara, M. (2014). American Academy of Pediatrics Committee on Hospital Care and Child Life Council: Policy statement child life services. *Pediatrics, 133*(5), 1471–1478.

Bush, N. R., Wakschlag, L. S., LeWinn, K. Z., Hertz-Picciotto, I., Nozadi, S. S., Pieper, S., Lewis, J., Biezonski, D., Blair, C., Deardorff, J., & Neiderhiser, J. M. (2020). Family environment, neurodevelopmental risk, and the Environmental Influences on Child Health Outcomes (ECHO) initiative: Looking back and moving forward. *Frontiers in Psychiatry, 11*, 547.

Cleland, J. A., Ross, S., Miller, S. C., & Patey, R. (2009). "There is a chain of Chinese whispers . . .": Empirical data support the call to formally teach handover to prequalification doctors. *BMJ Quality & Safety, 18*(4), 267–271.

Cole, J. C., Moldenhauer, J. S., Berger, K., Cary, M. S., Smith, H., Martino, V., Rendon, N., & Howell, L. J. (2016). Identifying expectant parents at risk for psychological distress in response to a confirmed fetal abnormality. *Archives of Women's Mental Health, 19*(3), 443–453.

Cole, J. C., Moldenhauer, J. S., Jones, T. R., Shaughnessy, E. A., Zarrin, H. E., Coursey, A. L., & Munson, D. A. (2017). A proposed model for perinatal palliative care. *Journal of Obstetric, Gynecologic & Neonatal Nursing, 46*(6), 904–911.

Forster, A. J., Murff, H. J., Peterson, J. F., Gandhi, T. K., & Bates, D. W. (2003). The incidence and severity of adverse events affecting patients after discharge from the hospital. *Annals of Internal Medicine, 138*(3), 161–167.

Hall, S. L., Cross, J., Selix, N. W., Patterson, C., Segre, L., Chuffo-Siewert, R., Geller, P., & Martin, M. L. (2015). Recommendations for enhancing psychosocial support of NICU parents through staff education and support. *Journal of Perinatology, 35*(1), S29–S36.

Hall, S. L., Famuyide, M., Saxton, S., Moore, T., Mosher, S., Sorrells, K., Milford, C., & Craig, J. (2019). Improving staff knowledge and attitudes toward providing psychosocial support to NICU parents through an online education course. *Advances in Neonatal Care, 19*(6), 490.

Hall, S., Hynan, M., & Phillips, R. (2016). Transforming NICU care to provide comprehensive family support. *Newborn and Infant Nursing Reviews, 16*, 69–73. https://doi.org/doi:10.1053/j.nainr.2016.03.008

Hallowell, S. G., Rogowski, J. A., & Lake, E. T. (2019). How nurse work environments relate to the presence of parents in neonatal intensive care. *Advances in Neonatal Care, 19*(1), 65–72.

Ho, S., & Saigal, S. (2005). Current survival and early outcomes of infants of borderline viability. *NeoReviews, 6*(3), e123–e132.

Hynan, M. T., & Hall, S. L. (2015). Psychosocial program standards for NICU parents. *Journal of Perinatology, 35*(Suppl. 1), S1.

Hynan, M. T., Mounts, K. O., & Vanderbilt, D. L. (2013). Screening parents of high-risk infants for emotional distress: Rationale and recommendations. *Journal of Perinatology, 33*(10), 748–753.

Janice-Woods Reed, D., & Sharma, J. (2016). Delivering difficult news and improving family communication: Simulation for neonatal–perinatal fellows. *MedEdPORTAL*, *12*, 10467.

Juckett, G., & Unger, K. (2014). Appropriate use of medical interpreters. *American Family Physician*, *90*(7), 476–480.

Katzenbach, R., & Douglas, K. (1993). *The wisdom of teams: Creating the high-performance organization*. Harvard Business School Press.

Moreyra, A., Dowtin, L. L., Ocampo, M., Perez, E., Borkovi, T. C., Wharton, E., Simon, S., Armer, E. G., & Shaw, R. J. (2021). Implementing a standardized screening protocol for parental depression, anxiety, and PTSD symptoms in the neonatal intensive care unit. *Early Human Development*, *154*, 105279.

National Association of Social Workers. (2005). *NASW standards for social work practice in health care settings*.

Pai, A. L., Patiño-Fernández, A. M., McSherry, M., Beele, D., Alderfer, M. A., Reilly, A. T., Hwang, W. T., & Kazak, A. E. (2008). The Psychosocial Assessment Tool (PAT2.0): Psychometric properties of a screener for psychosocial distress in families of children newly diagnosed with cancer. *Journal of Pediatric Psychology*, *33*(1), 50–62.

Pezzolesi, C., Manser, T., Schifano, F., Kostrzewski, A., Pickles, J., Harriet, N., Warren, I., & Dhillon, S. (2013). Human factors in clinical handover: Development and testing of a "handover performance tool" for doctors' shift handovers. *International Journal for Quality in Health Care*, *25*(1), 58–65.

Purdy, I. B., Craig, J. W., & Zeanah, P. (2015). NICU discharge planning and beyond: Recommendations for parent psychosocial support. *Journal of Perinatology*, *35*(1), S24–S28.

Saxton, S. N., Dempsey, A. G., Willis, T., Baughcum, A. E., Chavis, L., Hoffman, C., Fulco, C. J., Milford, C. A., & Steinberg, Z. (2020). Essential knowledge and competencies for psychologists working in neonatal intensive care units. *Journal of Clinical Psychology in Medical Settings*, *27*(4), 830–841.

Shuffler, M. L., Diazgranados, D., & Salas, E. (2011). There's science for that: Team development interventions in organizations. *Current Directions in Psychological Science*, *20*(6), 365–372.

Tuckman, B. W. (1965). Developmental sequence in small groups. *Psychological Bulletin*, *63*(6), 384.

6

TEACHING AND TRAINING DEVELOPING PROFESSIONALS IN PERINATAL AND NEONATAL SETTINGS

LATRICE L. DOWTIN, TIFFANY WILLIS,
SOUDABEH GIVRAD, AND MELISSA SCALA ■

Behavioral health clinicians (BHCs) come from a variety of disciplines and have varied levels of training experiences in prenatal, fetal, neonatal, infant, and post-natal settings. These combined subspecialty areas comprise the fields of perinatal and neonatal health and present a unique training opportunity for developing BHCs and those wishing to re-specialize. Training in perinatal and neonatal settings considers all areas of infant–parent needs for developmental, psychological, and psychiatric health. This chapter discusses those needs and makes recommendations about the essential focus of training and educating BHCs to explore and process both personal bias and bias within the perinatal and neonatal health settings.

High-risk fetuses and infants are cared for in fetal diagnostic centers, obstetrics and gynecology clinics, developmental follow-up clinics, neonatal intensive care units (NICUs), and infant/early care centers. Every infant is accompanied by at least one adult caregiver. Whether biological, adoptive, foster, or court appointed, caregivers may benefit from psychological support, which has led to a family-centered care model within these settings. In response to understanding the importance of caregiver mental health for fetal and infant development, it is important to include exposure to adult mental health support/services when training professionals to work with high-risk infants. Perinatal and neonatal settings are unique in that they can cover adult-focused (e.g., preconception and pregnancy contexts) and infant-focused (e.g., the NICU and high-risk infant follow-up clinics) environments that need family-centered care. Researchers in perinatal and neonatal health are continually developing and testing the efficacy of evidence-based practices. This includes assessments (e.g., developmental, socioemotional, and psychosocial) and interventions for infants and their caregivers. Therefore, it is imperative that BHCs are knowledgeable about adult and infant practices and examine the effectiveness of service delivery.

Discussions of training and teaching begin with understanding and assessing learners for implicit biases. The foundation of every training consideration includes opportunities for learning about and unpacking implicit biases, such as racial stereotyping, in order to serve all families and developing BHCs through equitable high-quality practice. This is vital at the outset of training because studies show that families from racially marginalized populations encounter limited access to care, discrimination by medical professionals, and higher maternal and infant mortality rates compared to White populations (Sigurdson et al., 2019). Overwhelmingly, these differences are attributed to the impact that racial implicit biases have on care practices and policies. In fact, a study in the United States showed that NICU parents of preterm infants who did not speak English or who had public insurance participated in kangaroo care (e.g., skin-to-skin holding) half as much as English-speaking and privately insured families, even after controlling for visitation (Brignoni-Pérez et al., 2021). Whereas developmental care practices delivered by parents in the NICU have been shown to have multiple positive health outcomes (e.g., greater cardio-respiratory stability, better growth, fewer infections, and possibly improved neurologic outcomes), reduced rates of parent-delivered developmental care have major implications for the outcomes of infants from racially, linguistically, and financially marginalized backgrounds. Therefore, BHCs carry the responsibility of unpacking racial implicit bias in training environments. This chapter discusses teaching considerations for developing BHCs in perinatal and neonatal settings from an anti-bias perspective.

TEACHING ACROSS DISCIPLINES

Counselors, psychologists, clinical social workers, and psychiatrists—collectively, BHCs—in perinatal and neonatal settings need to understand other fields and how those fields can impact their patients. Knowledge of related fields aids in training developing BHCs to work in perinatal and neonatal settings, which requires interactions with advanced practice providers, nurses, physicians, and ancillary staff (e.g., lactation, occupational therapists, and speech–language pathologists). Cross-disciplinary training also involves BHCs educating other disciplines about mental health services by using didactics, live practice, and supervision. For example, BHCs can teach residents, fellows, and nurses about parent–infant interactions, attachment, developmentally appropriate care, trauma, or perinatal mood and anxiety disorders (PMADs) screening. This collaborative approach will strengthen the cross-disciplinary support available for families.

Physician Training

Behavioral health clinicians have the opportunity to teach physicians and medical trainees working with women, infants, and families in fetal care centers, NICUs, and neonatal follow-up clinics to recognize signs and symptoms of psychological distress/behavioral health needs and the necessity for referrals to trained BHCs. The need for physician training in this area is supported by national agencies that have created guidelines and recommendations to impact care roles.

Training in perinatal mental health (PMH) has been slowly improving in obstetrical programs during the past decade. In 2006, 92% of obstetric residency program directors reported believing that training in PMH was minimal or suboptimal (Leigh et al., 2006). In 2015, the Council on Patient Safety in Women's Health Care established an interdisciplinary work group to develop a maternal mental health toolkit focusing on PMADs. The toolkit provides broad direction for screening, intervention, referral, and follow-up in maternity care. Similarly, in 2014, the American Board of Pediatrics (ABP) identified behavioral and mental health as the highest priority for training, after national survey data showed that up to two-thirds of pediatricians felt ill-equipped to handle parental mental health in their practices (Horwitz et al., 2015). The ABP outlined goals to promote health and resilience among patients, increase early intervention, and improve treatment, which led to the Roadmap Project (ABP, 2020). The Roadmap Project aims to educate and advocate on behavioral mental health in pediatrics, including toolkits for pediatricians.

In 2017, the ABP published guidelines with other national agencies to improve training in mental health (McMillan et al., 2017). The ABP has decided that certifying board exams will include behavioral and mental health content. Maintenance of certification activities for board-certified pediatricians will include quality improvement and learning activities in these areas. Beginning in 2019, pediatric training programs, including fellowships in neonatology and developmental behavioral pediatrics, have the following core requirements (Accreditation Council for Graduate Medical Education [ACGME], 2020):

IV.B.1.b).(1).(k) Fellows must demonstrate an understanding of the emotional impact on the family of having a child born prematurely or born with a life-threatening and/or chronic condition, and must demonstrate the communication skills necessary for encouraging dialogue.

IV.B.1.b).(1).(l) Fellows must provide care that is sensitive to the developmental stage of the patient with common behavioral and mental health issues, and the cultural context of the patient and family.

IV.B.1.b).(1).(m) Fellows must demonstrate the ability to refer and/or co-manage patients with common behavioral and mental health issues along with appropriate specialists when indicated.

Because teaching and training perinatal and infant mental health (IMH) are now required by the ACGME, program directors are creating curricula that address these new elements, and BHCs working in academic medical settings with high-risk infants and families are well-positioned to support these training initiatives.

Nurse Training

Behavioral health clinicians also have the opportunity to support nurse and nurse-trainee education related to perinatal and infant mental health. The National Association of Neonatal Nurses (NANN) has also highlighted the need for education on infant–parent mental health. NANN endorsed work by its members, in collaboration with the National Perinatal Association, to advocate for practice standards. The "Interdisciplinary Recommendations for Psychosocial Support of NICU Parents" (Hall et al., 2015) stressed the need for trauma-informed and culturally responsive approaches to NICU families. In addition to establishing recommendations for NICU nursing education, NANN created resources to support this education. Resources included a standard text regarding developmental care of newborns, learning modules, and a special neonatal developmental specialist designation program (see http://nann.org/education/neonatal-learning).

CORE COMPETENCIES FOR BEHAVIORAL HEALTH CLINICIANS

The fields of social work, psychology, and psychiatry each have a growing presence in fetal care centers, NICUs, and neonatal follow-up programs. Each specialty has its own expertise and domain of practice, although there are certainly areas of overlap across the disciplines (see Chapter 5, this volume). Thus, having universal training program may not be possible/advised, although there are certainly opportunities for interdisciplinary training among the disciplines.

Social Workers

The National Association of Perinatal Social Workers (NAPSW) has solidified guidelines, which include a code of ethics detailing nine national standards for working with patients in perinatal/neonatal settings (Box 6.1). Although not all social workers are members of NAPSW, and thus are not required to adhere to these standards, guidelines are accessible and may direct other behavioral health

Box 6.1

NATIONAL ASSOCIATION OF PERINATAL SOCIAL WORKERS' STANDARDS
FOR PERINATAL SETTINGS

STANDARDS BY TITLE
Adolescent Pregnancy
Adoptions in a Hospital Setting
Field Education in Perinatal Social Work
Patients Experiencing Postpartum Depression
Infertility Treatment Centers Offering Assisted Reproductive Technologies
    and the Use of Donor Gametes
Newborn Intensive Care Unit
Obstetrics
Perinatal Bereavement
Surrogacy in Hospitals

From the National Association of Perinatal Social Workers' (2020) Code of Ethics (https://
w.napsw.org/ethics-standards).

fields. Included in the standards are newer developing areas such as understanding the PMH needs of adolescents and complex fertility cases, such as surrogacy.

Psychologists

Training for psychologists working with families in fetal care, NICU, and neonatal follow-up settings has been limited. Saxton et al. (2020) outlined the essential six domains of psychologists preparing for and/or already practicing in these settings.

The first domain, science, includes topics related to working in a perinatal and neonatal setting, such as awareness of pregnancy complications, research and evaluation, and program development and sustainability (Saxton et al., 2020). Components from the science domain provide a foundation from which the psychologist can grow toward the second domain, systems. Many systems are involved in the care of a family in the NICU, such as developmental care, early intervention, social support services, and hospital-based support services (e.g., music therapy, child life, chaplaincy, and social work). Knowledge of the aforementioned multidisciplinary partnerships and clinical services that support families is important to ensure families have the adequate support they need.

Similarly, the third and fourth domains, professionalism and relationships, are areas of focus that encourage continued knowledge and skill development, which includes competency in professional values and attitudes, individual and cultural diversity, ethics, and decision-making, as well as reflective practice, self-assessment, and care (Saxton et al., 2020). For example, understanding the needs of both the parents and their infants, as well as navigating concerns regarding confidentiality of the parent when providing documentation in the infant's chart, is a consideration unique to settings such as the NICU. Relationships are the crux of interventions in perinatal and neonatal settings. Therefore, psychologists working in perinatal and neonatal settings should be skilled in conflict resolution; facilitating emotional identification and expression; normalizing emotional reactions; and modeling empathic, respectful engagement with families, staff, and teams (Saxton et al., 2020).

The final two domains, application and education, emphasize skills for practice management, assessment, clinical consultation, teaching, and supervision. Specifically, the application domain highlights the use of common screening and assessment tools for PMADs, trauma, and other psychological needs along with evidence-based interventions for the dyadic caregiver–infant relationship (Saxton et al., 2020). The education domain acknowledges competency needs around teaching and supervision, both for existing medical staff and for psychology and medical trainees. Psychologists working in fetal care centers, NICUs, and neonatal follow-up clinics should be regularly involved in educating all professionals across disciplines who provide care to infants and families in these settings. In a supervisory role, psychologists need to identify symptoms of vicarious trauma, compassion fatigue, and burnout in an acute trauma setting (Saxton et al., 2020).

Psychiatrists

Perinatal psychiatry is not an officially recognized subspecialty in the United States, and as of 2015, only 59% of psychiatry U.S. residencies required any level of training in reproductive psychiatry (Osborne et al., 2015). Unfortunately, many psychiatrists indicate discomfort with treating PMH, which limits referral options for obstetric, neonatal, and pediatric providers. Efforts have been made to improve training in reproductive psychiatry for general psychiatry residencies, and currently there are several reproductive psychiatry fellowships in the United States. However, the fellowships are not yet ACGME accredited, nor are they recognized by the American Board of Psychiatry and Neurology (Hudepohl et al., 2018). As a result, there is no consensus on competencies and training requirements for fellowships, resulting in interprogram variability. To partially address this lack of consensus on competencies and training requirements, the National Task Force on Women's Reproductive Mental Health was formed and developed a National Curriculum on Reproductive Psychiatry (NCRP). Psychiatrists can be trained with this curriculum by non-expert facilitators and via self-study guides. The NCRP task force identified six knowledge areas for specialists in reproductive psychiatry: (a) relationship between reproductive cycle stages and psychopathology; (b) epidemiology, pathophysiology, and phenomenology of psychiatric disorders during pregnancy and the postpartum period, including pharmacokinetic changes; (c) treatment of PMH disorders, including but not limited to psychopharmacology; (d) psychiatric symptoms related to infertility, pregnancy loss, birth trauma, and delivery of offspring with health problems; (e) premenstrual mood disorders; and (f) symptoms related to perimenopause.

In addition, psychiatrists in perinatal and neonatal settings should be knowledgeable in infant psychiatry. This adds to the complexity of the situation discussed previously because psychiatry residents often receive minimal or no training in infant and early childhood development and may not have clinical exposure to infants and their families or training in tenets of IMH. As a result, most psychiatrists are uncomfortable treating families experiencing relational disturbances or disorders of infancy and early childhood.

TRAINING BEHAVIORAL HEALTH CLINICIANS

Teaching

Behavioral health clinicians working (or training to work) in fetal care centers, NICUs, or neonatal follow-up programs typically have already received training in the core areas of their respective disciplines and are seeking advanced specialty training to work with this unique population. Teaching and training these advanced professionals include models that best suit their developmental training and career stage, which means being careful not to dismiss their prior training and knowledge as clinicians simply because they are in a learner role. It is important for training programs to facilitate intrinsic motivation in BHCs by emphasizing autonomy, competence, and a feeling of belonging. Because working with pregnant individuals, infants, and families in high-risk perinatal and neonatal settings is complicated, emotionally consuming, and at times highly stressful, it is critical to have environments in which developing BHCs can have a varied clinical caseload and adequate supervision or consultation (Taylor & Hamdy, 2013).

As noted previously, there are many domains of practice/training that need to be covered for BHCs to work with this specialty population. Thus, training programs should include education and supervision in PMH, developmental care, assessment and follow-up at post NICU discharge, IMH, and early childhood behavioral health interventions. In terms of mental health for infants and their families, long-term outpatient follow-up provides an opportunity for the developing BHCs to build deeper rapport with families and support family well-being and infant development and behavior throughout early childhood. Thus, it is important to train BHCs across fetal care, NICU, and neonatal follow-up settings. In some situations, trainees and BHCs may have opportunities to provide longer term (versus brief) interventions across settings. This can be beneficial to decreasing burnout among developing BHCs because they have the opportunity to see longer term improvements among families seen in a single integrated setting (e.g., fetal care center or NICU) who are going through an acute traumatic event.

It is also important to view developing BHCs as both learners and educators. As they increase their knowledge and skills in perinatal and neonatal services, they also serve as valuable sources of education for junior developing professionals and medical colleagues because they provide opportunities for peer consultation. There has been some progress in defining required competencies for social workers and psychologists working in the NICU and for counselors and psychiatrists working in the field of PMH; however, existing training and clinical programs in perinatal psychiatry vary in their approaches, experiences, and didactics. Because this is a developing field, further research is needed on what types of programs and collaborations would result in best patient and family outcomes. Furthermore, due to the gap between trained BHCs and the need for PMH providers, programs need a method for recruiting, training, and retaining developing BHCs. One way to decrease this gap is by increasing field experiences through practica, externships, internships, and fellowships focused on the perinatal and neonatal periods. The National Network of NICU Psychologists, via the National Perinatal Association, is developing a database of psychology training programs that outline fetal and NICU training experiences.

Box 6.2 provides a recommended list of didactic seminar topics that could be used for developing BHCs across disciplines. In addition, teaching and training

---

Box 6.2

RECOMMENDED DIDACTIC TOPICS FOR PERINATAL AND NEONATAL SETTINGS

DIDACTIC DESCRIPTION

Implicit bias training and working with historically marginalized patients and their families (i.e., race, culture, gender, ability, etc.)

Basic information on the course of pregnancy and common complications

Typical course of development during infancy and early childhood, including infant assessment

Neonatal assessment and common developmental care interventions

Typical psychological processes for parents during pregnancy, the transition to parenthood, and early parenthood

Typical social–emotional development during infancy and early childhood

PMADs and other psychiatric disorders during this period

Infant mental health (birth to five diagnoses), parent–infant relationship, and bonding

Medical and psychological matters specific to the preterm birth, medical complications in infants, and NICU admission

Trauma-informed care and psychotherapy

Grief counseling

Evidenced-based psychotherapies during perinatal period and infancy, including cognitive–behavioral therapy, interpersonal psychotherapy, dyadic and family therapy, and group psychotherapy

Risk and resiliency factors for parents and infants during this period

Collaborative, integrative, and co-located models of care with other medical teams involved in the care of parents and infants

Adolescent pregnancy and related care

Infertility care, complications, and options

Telehealth practices for in- and outpatient settings with this population for intervention and assessment

NICU, neonatal intensive care unit; PMADs, perinatal mood and anxiety disorders.

for BHCs would be incomplete without a review of quality assurance practices. Evaluations of programs, supervisors, and developing BHCs need to cover topics such as continuing education (CE) opportunities, adoption and implementation of evidence-based practices, and general self-care development and maintenance. To provide optimal behavioral health services, programs must consider how they prepare developing BHCs to work with patients, colleagues, and staff from various backgrounds (e.g., races, cultures, genders, abilities, languages, nationalities, beliefs, ages, and socioeconomic status). Perhaps two of the most critical roles that programs play is to review practices in this area of cultural responsiveness and sociodemographic equity and understand that these areas are an ongoing process that is the springboard for all interactions across settings.

Training programs are encouraged to provide BHCs knowledge and funding for CE training in the spectrum of perinatal and neonatal areas. Two urgent priorities should be covered in CE training for perinatal and neonatal settings: (a) the needs among gender-fluid and transgender people and (b) training and practice in telehealth assessments and interventions. Because few, if any, graduate programs discuss perinatal and neonatal needs, CE access may be the only way that BHCs can increase skills in these areas.

Supervision

Behavioral health clinicians work with complicated medical and psychosocial conditions and must have fluency in perinatal and IMH, integrative models of health care, and knowledge of medical complications during pregnancy, as well as within fetal, neonatal, and early childhood development. Furthermore, adherence to a specific model may be more aspirational than is actually applied in training situations. Rather than a focus on supervision models, critical components of supervision are suggested, such as cultural responsiveness, supportive feedback, and opportunities for reflective telesupervision.

Clinical supervision of developing BHCs in perinatal and neonatal settings is a critical component that may vary depending on the discipline of the learner and supervisor. Thorough supervision planning and consistent monitoring, such as evaluation of the supervisor by a peer and under a process of supervision and consultation for supervisors, are recommended. In terms of the critical component of cultural responsiveness, behavioral health fields require developing BHCs to be supervised in a manner that provides opportunities for training and discussion of culture as an active part of supervision. For example, along with other behavioral health fields, NAPSW lists both cultural responsiveness and cross-cultural supervision in its practice standards for supervision. Cultural responsiveness training includes exploration of implicit biases based on sociodemographics and identities, intersectionality within marginalized groups and among individuals, and considers the cultural backgrounds of all parties from learner to supervisor to patient and can foster a safe environment for learners to receive support and feedback while facilitating a healthy supervisory relationship.

REFLECTIVE SUPERVISION

Reflective supervision has been a critical component of the perinatal and IMH clinician's practice and is vital for self-care in perinatal and neonatal settings. A seminal work in IMH by Fraiberg et al. (1975) described reflective supervision as bringing awareness to the effects of past experiences, traumas, and early relational histories on how parents perceive and interact with their children. This process led to increasing awareness of the effects of the BHC's thoughts, feelings, and past experiences and trauma both on the clinical work and on the BHC's perceptions and perspectives toward the infant and family. Supervision should provide a safe space to build reflective functioning where the developing BHC can discuss their reactions to the infants and their families. Reflective functioning is the ability of the person to be better attuned to their thoughts, emotions, and reactions while thinking about another person's thoughts, feelings, and reactions.

Reflective supervision has three main components: reflection, collaboration, and regularity. In this model of supervision, the supervisor is ready to listen without judgment and with an open curiosity to help developing BHCs become more reflective about their work and reactions. There are guidelines about the supervisory relationship that include reflection about the infant, the infant's family, and the infant's developing early relationships, in addition to increasing the developing BHCs self-reflection (Tomlin et al., 2014). Reflective supervision has shown positive effects for BHCs, their clinical work, outcomes, and decreased rates of turnover. Without reflective supervision, BHCs may be left overwhelmed and reach burnout.

INCORPORATION OF TECHNOLOGY IN SUPERVISION

Although telesupervision (e.g., supervision conducted while the supervisor and supervisee are in separate locations using live video communication) and supervision of supervisees in their utilization of telehealth technologies have not traditionally been part of best practice in behavioral health, the global coronavirus (COVID-19) pandemic required a shift in clinical work, administrative practices, and supervision. Therefore, telesupervision is recommended to be an ongoing training initiative within perinatal and neonatal health so that future BHCs are prepared for rapid changes in access to appropriate supervision, to include live video supervision between supervisor and developing BHC, access to phone check-ins and Health Insurance Portability and Accountability Act secure messaging options for quick communications between supervision sessions. Although the technology for telehealth has existed for several decades, many perinatal and neonatal environments were underprepared and unfamiliar with training, education, practice, legalities, and privacy protection until the pandemic was well underway. Moving forward, quality assurance in perinatal and neonatal settings should include appropriate telehealth training as an integral part of supervision.

Peer Consultation to Improve Supervision

A consideration that seems to be missing in the literature and across training programs is the role of evaluation in supervision and how being evaluated holds varying levels of power that affords some developing BHCs with gains and privileges in comparison to others depending on sociodemographic dynamics. For example, the field of psychology has a disproportionate number of White psychologists in comparison to the general population demographics. According to Lin et al. (2018),

> In 2015, 86 percent of psychologists in the U.S. workforce were White, 5 percent were Asian, 5 percent were Hispanic, 4 percent were Black/African American, and 1 percent were multiracial or from other racial/ethnic groups. This is less diverse than the U.S. population as a whole, which is 62 percent White and 38 percent [racially minoritized]. (p. 19)

Without the proper training and ongoing reflection on racism and racial biases, the majority of BHCs may be unaware of the true power they hold over and within supervisory relationships when they are working with marginalized and minoritized developing BHCs. A BHC's lack of awareness or abuse of power may not allow a developing BHC to be completely open during supervisory sessions. Because a training goal for developing BHCs is to have them function as skillful, reflective BHCs who minimize harm to others, it is important that developing BHCs receive peer consultation (also referred to as peer supervision), which would allow developing BHCs to discuss cases and ideas without fear of negative impact on evaluative supervisory relationships. Peer consultation can provide a safe space where developing BHCs can increase competence and further develop as clinicians while garnering feedback from learners who are at the same training level or within a few years of their training experiences.

CONCLUSION

Educating developing BHCs as they enter perinatal and neonatal settings encompasses many considerations not limited to competencies, practice domains, didactics, supervision, and avoidance of burnout and vicarious trauma. At the core of these considerations is the necessity of building curricula and training experiences that unpack implicit biases. This creates perinatal and neonatal settings that are safe and expansive for learners, patients, and staff. When thoughtful planning and ongoing monitoring occur, training can produce BHCs who are equipped to address concerns regarding their psychological and emotional health and those of staff and families.

REFERENCES

Accreditation Council for Graduate Medical Education. (2020). *ACGME program requirements for graduate medical education in neonatal-perinatal medicine*. https://www.acgme.org/Portals/0/PFAssets/ProgramRequirements/329_NeonatalPerinatalMedicine_2020.pdf?ver=2020-06-29-162707-410

Ahlqvist-Björkroth, S., Axelin, A., Korja, R., & Lehtonen, L. (2019). An educational intervention for NICU staff decreased maternal postpartum depression. *Pediatric Research, 85*(7), 982–986. https://doi.org/10.1038/s41390-019-0306-y

American Board of Pediatrics. (2020, January). *Roadmap to resilience, emotional, and mental health*. https://www.abp.org/foundation/roadmap

Brignoni-Pérez, E., Scala, M., Marchman, V., Feldman, H. M., & Travis, K. E. (2021, October 28). Disparities in kangaroo care for premature infants in the neonatal intensive care unit. *Journal of Developmental and Behavioral Pediatrics*. Advance online publication.

Fraiberg, S., Adelson, E., & Shapiro, V. (1975). Ghosts in the nursery: A psychoanalytic approach to the problems of impaired infant–mother relationships. *Journal of the American Academy of Child Psychiatry, 14*(3), 387–421. https://doi.org/10.1016/S0002-7138(09)61442-4

Hall, S. L., Cross, J., Selix, N. W., Patterson, C., Segre, L., Chuffo-Siewert, R., Geller, P. A., & Martin, M. L. (2015). Recommendations for enhancing psychosocial support of NICU parents through staff education and support. *Journal of Perinatology, 35*(1), S29–S36. https://doi.org/10.1038/jp.2015.147

Horwitz, S. M., Storfer-Isser, A., Kerker, B. D., Szilagyi, M., Garner, A., O'Connor, K. G., Hoagwood, K. E., & Stein, R. E. (2015). Barriers to the identification and management of psychosocial problems: Changes from 2004 to 2013. *Academic Pediatrics, 15*(6), 613–620. https://doi.org/10.1016/j.acap.2015.08.006

Hudepohl, N. S., Battle, C. L., & Howard, M. (2018). Advanced training in reproductive psychiatry: The case for standardization in training and a path to sub-specialty recognition. *Archives of Women's Mental Health, 21*(1), 121–123. https://doi.org/10.1007/s00737-017-0766-1

Leigh, H., Stewart, D., & Mallios, R. (2006). Mental health and psychiatry training in primary care residency programs: Part I. Who teaches, where, when and how satisfied? *General Hospital Psychiatry, 28*(3), 189–194. https://doi.org/10.1016/j.genhosppsych.2005.10.003

Lin, L., Stamm, K., & Christidis, P. (2018, February). How diverse is the psychology workforce? *Monitor on Psychology, 49*(2). http://www.apa.org/monitor/2018/02/datapoint

McMillan, J. A., Land, M., & Leslie, L. K. (2017). Pediatric residency education and the behavioral and mental health crisis: A call to action. *Pediatrics, 139*(1), e20162141.

National Association of Perinatal Social Workers. (2020). *Code of ethics*. https://www.napsw.org/ethics-standards

Osborne, L. M., Hermann, A., Burt, V., Driscoll, K., Fitelson, E., Meltzer-Brody, S., Murphy Barzilay, E., Nagle Yang, S., & Miller, L.; National Task Force on Women's Reproductive Mental Health. (2015). Reproductive psychiatry: The gap between clinical need and education. *American Journal of Psychiatry, 172*(10), 946–948. https://doi.org/10.1176/appi.ajp.2015.15060837

Saxton, S. N., Dempsey, A. G., Willis, T., Baughcum, A. E., Chavis, L., Hoffman, C., . . . & Steinberg, Z. (2020). Essential knowledge and competencies for psychologists working in neonatal intensive care units. *Journal of Clinical Psychology in Medical Settings, 27*, 830–841. https://doi.org/10.1007/s10880-019-09682-8

Sigurdson, K., Mitchell, B., Liu, J., Morton, C., Gould, J. B., Lee, H. C., Capdarest-Arest, N., & Profit, J. (2019). Racial/ethnic disparities in neonatal intensive care: A systematic review. *Pediatrics, 144*(2), e20183114. https://doi.org/10.1542/peds.2018-3114

Taylor, D. C., & Hamdy, H. (2013). Adult learning theories: Implications for learning and teaching in medical education: AMEE Guide No. 83. *Medical Teacher, 35*(11), e1561–e1572. https://doi.org/10.3109/0142159X.2013.828153

Tomlin, A. M. M., Weatherston, D. J., & Pavkov, T. (2014). Critical components of reflective supervision: Responses from expert supervisors in the field. *Infant Mental Health Journal, 35*(1), 70–80. https://doi.org/10.1002/imhj.21420

7

OPERATIONS AND ETHICAL CONSIDERATIONS

ELIZABETH A. FISCHER, KRISTILYNN R. CEDARS,
ABBEY KRUPER, AND STEVEN R. LEUTHNER ■

As fetal and neonatal care evolves, increasing attention is brought to bear on maternal, family, and infant mental health. Psychologists and other behavioral health specialists are increasingly involved in fetal care centers and neonatal intensive care settings. These settings bring with them unique challenges to clinical care in terms of the day-to-day work of managing patient care, documentation in maternal and infant medical records, and considerations of professional and bioethical standards. This chapter provides an overview of these issues and how they impact care in fetal and neonatal settings.

ETHICAL ISSUES THAT INFORM OPERATIONS

Technical advances in fetal and neonatal medicine have brought about the development of fetal centers with pediatric subspecialty in diagnostic scanning and counseling. The development of the fetus as a patient brings the challenges of ensuring shared decision-making with families for the fetus/future child as well as the challenges of balancing fetal and maternal interests when considering a fetal intervention. As more fetal care or fetal treatment centers emerge nationally, and more pediatric subspecialists participate in the prenatal care of the fetus and woman, understanding the importance of the ethical issues that span from the prenatal to the postnatal period becomes essential (Brown et al., 2008). While there has been discussion about different medical/specialty professional ethical cultures between obstetrics and pediatrics, more centers are adding behavioral health support (Brown et al., 2012). The additional benefit of the behavioral health specialists is in providing mental health support to the pregnant woman who is dealing with her own health, as well as the grief of the loss of a normal pregnancy. The general ethical principles that apply in fetal and pediatric ethics also apply to psychology and can help direct its practice. The benefit of a multi-disciplinary approach is to enhance the pregnant woman's sense of autonomy and decision-making by ensuring she is better informed of the maternal, fetal, and infant outcomes and possible perinatal and neonatal options.

The foundation for what morality ought to be in clinical practice has been the professional obligation to protect and promote the health-related interests of a patient. Within fetal centers, the practitioners are considering the health of two patients. Perhaps the most well-developed ethical concept of the "fetus as patient" is that of Chervenak and McCullough (2003). They argue for a "dependent" moral status of the fetus when discussing the fetus as a patient. The concept of the fetus as a patient then rests on the links between the fetus and the future child it can become. The first link is when the fetus becomes viable, and the second link is previably when the woman autonomously chooses to continue the pregnancy and presents the fetus and herself for medical care. It is within this context of the woman's autonomous decision-making needs that psychologists can perhaps help because maternal/parental autonomy is enhanced with the provision of informational and emotional support.

Once the infant and, subsequently, parents transition into the neonatal intensive care unit (NICU), the ethical constructs for the family are focused on surrogate decision-making. There are three constructs of surrogate decision-making considered in pediatric ethics. The first is "best interest," which is a beneficence-based decision for a patient whose wishes are unknowable. It is considered the right and responsibility of the parent(s) to be the one(s) to make these best interest decisions on behalf of their infant (Kopelman, 1997). At the same time, there are noted limitations in parental authority, and it is not uncommon that parents and health care staff might view an infant's best interests differently, often based on their own values or interpretation of what is best (Leuthner, 2001). For example, if an infant's prognosis is poor, health care practitioners might disagree that further treatment provides enough benefit and outweighs the discomfort of life-sustaining procedures, whereas parents may still accept that outcome as tolerable. A second construct for pediatric decision-making is that of "constrained parental autonomy" (Ross, 2004). In this construct, the pediatric patient's interests are not taken in isolation but, rather, within the framework of an intimate family. If the interests of an infant conflict with the family's goals or interests, the parents may compromise the interests of the infant if doing so does not sacrifice the infant's basic needs (i.e., food and shelter). The third construct is the "harm principle," which offers families discretion up to the point of certain harms and justifies the overriding of parental decisions only when these harms are reached, such as endangerment (Diekma, 2004). Although the details of these ethical constructs are beyond the scope of this chapter, they underlie the potential importance of psychological support for parents in the NICU because all three constructs ask parents to participate in medical decision-making that is complex and uncertain. The more healthy, well-adjusted, and cared-for the parents are, the better surrogate decision-makers they can be for their infant. Parental mental health impacts neonatal and childhood health. Although the infant is biologically separated from the mother, we should consider that the child's health remains dependent on maternal mental health.

What are the professional ethical considerations for psychologists in these settings? First, who is their patient? Professionals may, at times, be working with parents directly, and therefore the infant more indirectly. This leads to issues such as maintaining confidentiality, privacy, and therefore autonomy; however, perhaps some infringement on this could be of value to help the obstetrical or neonatal team. For example, severe maternal depression could explain why a parent may seem disengaged with the team or not ready to take the infant home. Increased team integration could allow more interdisciplinary sharing to better help the parent and infant. However, there is the risk that too much sharing might limit parental comfort with disclosure of sensitive information. The ethical principle of justice could lead to the question of whether there are higher or lower risk populations that psychological services should target or whether the services should be universally screened for and/or offered. Ethically, any developing psychological service should begin with providing the support to those most in need, perhaps with a goal of developing the resources for adequate universal engagement. This clinical care leads to questions of billing for these services. Services that are proven valuable in terms of improving infant health directly, or indirectly by targeting the health of family members, provide reason to support through billing processes. Operational issues related to billing and additionally to documentation are addressed later in this chapter. Finally, appropriate ethical utilization of psychological care should include ethical research in this area to guide the appropriate screening and therapeutic measures that might help these families and infants.

TRANSITION FROM MATERNAL–FETAL CARE TO NEONATAL CARE

High-risk pregnancies with suspected or known fetal anomalies and potentially complex treatment needed in utero or in the immediate postnatal period necessitate informational and emotional support for women and their partners. Multidisciplinary support within fetal centers paired with coordinated transition of care to the pediatric/NICU setting is critical for maternal and fetal treatment decision-making and overall outcome. Special attention should be given not only to how families navigate and adjust but also to how mental health and psychosocial information is communicated. Psychology practice in fetal care centers involves direct assessment, intervention, and support for mothers as they progress through perinatal care, the details of which are outlined in Section III of this volume.

As a family transitions to the NICU and information is relayed from fetal care centers (or other medical facilities), issues of family member confidentiality, specifically maternal health history, and methods to transfer health information arise. Newborn charts are unique in that they contain personal health information for two individuals: mother and infant. This issue is complex and important, given that maternal health information may be relevant to the medical care of the infant while in the NICU. For example, maternal obstetric factors such as gestational diabetes and mental health factors such as depression, suicidal ideation, and drug use can impact the care and management of the infant. In addition, providers and other potential family members, such as fathers, may access an infant/newborn record and view sensitive health information for the mother (Scibilia, 2014). Given this, care needs to be taken to determine the clinical relevance for information to disclose and then best practices for including pertinent information in an infant chart. This raises issues of ethics, confidentiality, and documentation, described in detail in later sections of this chapter.

In the transfer of records from the fetal care center to the NICU, challenges with how information is communicated are present. Health information can be disjointed, given the presence of multiple systems, different providers, and variations in documentation models and payer source (Institute of Medicine, 2001). This impacts interoperability between systems, such as linking maternal health history to infant charts. Records transferring from adult to pediatric hospitals may not be directly linked technologically, and there may be limitations of structure within the pediatric chart for pertinent maternal health information. Best practices to include and document maternal information in the pediatric chart should be considered either through connected information technology systems or manual processes within the particular setting or system (i.e., a separate section to document maternal health history electronically or scanning maternal health information into the pediatric chart).

Multidisciplinary care and team communication are also critical to optimal maternal–fetal care. Providers and systems should consider best practice strategies to aid with collaboration and continuity of care. Teams can coordinate care through direct provider-to-provider communication, secure email, and multidisciplinary care conferences. Instant messaging applications (IMAs) have also been utilized to support efficient communication, especially across institutions. Maternal–fetal medicine specialists and fellows who utilized IMAs for education and clinical case discussion found this modality to be very beneficial for case solutions, obtaining/disseminating knowledge, and managing clinical practice (Carmona et al., 2018). All chart documentation should remain clinically appropriate, in line with patient care and billing guidelines. However, alternative forms of communication can be considered when time or distance are issues, limiting in-person, direct communication, or when there may be potential delay from methods such as email or phone. Providers may consider incorporating additional technologies such as IMA or text messages for more efficient, real-time case collaboration. Behavioral health providers may consider providing other team members with recommendations for patient care related to medical decision-making, communication needs, or mental health treatment planning. Providers should be mindful to exclude any identifying information in accordance with Health Insurance Portability and Accountability Act of 1996 (HIPAA) standards.

CARE IN THE NICU

Identifying the Target Patient in NICU Care

Once birth has occurred and the infant is transferred to an NICU setting, the focus of care ostensibly transfers from maternal and fetal care to care of the infant as the identified patient. The medical chart is set up under the infant's name, and medical providers are oriented toward assessing and treating the child.

Although the infant is the identified patient in NICU care, this can be a complex issue in a setting in which an infant is the focus of treatment but their medical status can be directly related to maternal health issues and their well-being is often evaluated and treated in the context of the family unit. In infant care, and through the lens of infant mental health, the infant–parent dyad is essential for healing and development. This holds true through the NICU course and into hospital discharge and beyond. A clinician must differentiate between direct patient care and supportive care or relationship-focused care given to family members in the process of caring for an identified pediatric patient. Once these decisions have been made, the psychologist has a responsibility to clarify relationships. According to the American Psychological Association's Code of Conduct (APA, 2017),

> When psychologists agree to provide services to several persons who have a relationship (such as spouses, significant others, or parents and children), they take reasonable steps to clarify at the outset (1) which of the individuals are clients/patients and (2) the relationship the psychologist will have with each person. This clarification includes the psychologist's role and the probable uses of the services provided or the information obtained.

Determining the psychologist's role in care will directly affect issues of consent, billing, confidentiality, and documentation.

Consent

Upon introduction of services, it is customary to obtain consent and to discuss limits of confidentiality. This is directly addressed in the APA's (2017) Code of Conduct, which directs psychologists to obtain consent when conducting research or providing assessment, therapy, counseling, and/or consulting services. A discussion about consent would include the nature of services provided and information on confidentiality, documentation, and billing. This discussion would require a clear indication of who is receiving the direct service, be it the infant, the parent, or the infant–parent dyad. Having this clear discussion with the parent at the outset of services will help the clinician and the parent establish appropriate treatment boundaries and set the standard for how treatment information is managed going forward.

Organizations and programs may differ in methods by which consent is obtained. Some organizations may recognize the consent for medical care signed upon admission as covering relevant billable psychological services when provided upon consultation from the treating medical team. In this situation, the onus is on the clinician to have an additional conversation with the parent or guardian specific to psychological services. Other organizations may require additional written consent at the time of behavioral health consultation. If the services are provided all or in part by clinicians in training, there may be state or third-party requirements for additional consent procedures. Decisions about consent procedures are best made in concert with organizational representatives and in accordance with state law and consideration of ethical principles.

Billing

Billing practices for behavioral health services in the NICU will be determined by a variety of factors, including organizational policies, third-party reimbursement and contracts, funding, legal statutes, and ethical codes. Thus, there is no one cohesive billing practice, as it will differ between organizations and from state to state. Psychologists performing consultation, assessment, and intervention for an identified patient will typically bill for their services. Such billing can support the need for psychological services in the NICU and can help psychologists advocate for additional needed positions and program expansion.

Billing is achieved through use of Current Procedural Terminology (CPT) codes. There are a variety of CPT code options, and CPT coding definitions and procedures are outlined by the American Medical Association (2020). These include assessment and testing codes, psychotherapy codes, and Health and Behavior (H&B) codes. Psychotherapy codes are commonly used in a variety of mental health settings and require a mental health diagnosis, which is not appropriate when caring for infants, although it would be potentially applicable for assessment and psychotherapy services applied to parents. H&B codes are directly relevant to treating patients in the context of medical illness. They were developed in 2002 specifically to describe psychological services applied to helping patients manage physical health conditions. These codes were updated in 2020 and are now referred to as Health Behavioral Assessment and Intervention Services, although for ease and familiarity, this discussion continues to refer to them as H&B codes. The codes can be used in the context of the NICU to bill family support or dyadic services using an infant's medical diagnosis. Similarly, in the fetal care center, pregnant individuals can receive services billed under the medical diagnosis of the fetus they are carrying.

Confidentiality

Confidentiality is governed by various codes of ethics and is written into law at the federal and state levels. The APA's (2017) Code of Conduct notes a psychologist's obligation to protect confidential information "obtained through or stored in any medium." Psychologists operating in multidisciplinary settings balance this with the ethical obligation to "cooperate with other professionals in order to serve" clients effectively (APA, 2017). State laws allow psychologists and other medical professionals to break confidentiality in certain circumstances to protect the safety of a pediatric or adult patient. When that happens, reports may be made by the psychologist, social worker, or other staff in the medical setting to Child Protective Services and/or law enforcement or another body governing involuntary hospitalization (in the case of harm to self or others).

When working in multidisciplinary teams and organizations, patient care can be facilitated through the appropriate sharing of information. The limits of confidentiality related to multidisciplinary care should be discussed with patients and guardians at the onset of treatment. Information sharing in this context is achieved by in-person conversation that might occur during patient rounding, through telephone or telefax connections, and also through use of the medical record. Initial discussions of confidentiality should include how information is accessed, maintained, and released in electronic medical records.

ELECTRONIC MEDICAL RECORD.
Increasingly, health care organizations are reliant upon use of the electronic medical record (EMR), and its evolution has changed the way in which private health information is stored, accessed, and shared. EMRs have, as benefits, easier movement and transfer of records and improved continuity of care. This, however, comes with potential risks, especially to confidentiality. Shenoy and Appel (2017) outline three ways in which access might threaten privacy: through "inside attacks" (where users inappropriately access information), security breaches from outside the system (e.g., through hacking), and/or from sharing of information between providers that is permissible but unwanted by the patient.

It is imperative that clinicians understand their organization's EMR, including privacy settings for employees; standards of access and sharing; and how information will be released to patients and guardians, outside parties, and through access regulated under treatment, payment, and operations. For example, certain note types may be designed with higher security protections, limiting which providers and staff members can see those notes. Organizational security settings will govern which providers and staff members have easy access to psychology notes and visit information.

Documentation

The issue of documentation is directly related to issues of patient identification, confidentiality, and services provided. Documentation of symptoms, background, diagnosis, and services provided is a core requirement of health care providers, including psychologists and other behavioral health clinicians (BHCs). Clear documentation can facilitate treatment; can help resolve legal and ethical questions; and is often a requirement for compliance with laws, regulations, and billing requirements.

Once a psychologist has identified the targeted patient, whether an individual or a family unit, a determination can be made regarding the type of information documented, where information is maintained, and how information is disclosed. For example, if a child is the identified patient, then documentation focuses on treatment and health care needs of the child. Health information about parents or other guardians is included only as pertinent to the health care needs of the child. Parents or other legal guardians (in the case of an infant) give consent and may receive and release records. If a parent or legal guardian is identified as the patient, their private health information is separate from that of their child and must be maintained and released as such.

The creation, contents, maintenance, and release of records kept by psychologists may be governed by a number of entities, such as the organizations for which they work, professional associations, codes of ethics, state laws and regulations, third-party contracts, and federal laws and regulations—namely HIPAA and, more recently, the 21st Century Cures Act.

EMPLOYERS/ORGANIZATIONS

Psychologists and other BHCs working in NICU settings are typically employed by hospitals or their academic partners. Such organizations have clear and detailed policies governing charting and sharing of confidential information. These policies are typically owned by departments such as Compliance, Billing, Medical Records, and Risk Management. When resolving questions about procedures related to documentation, it is important to include representatives from these departments as stakeholders in the discussion. These individuals are often experts in not only organizational policy but also the underlying state and federal laws and rules, and together with clinicians, they can help identify procedures that meet clinical needs while also maintaining compliance with the law. Medical records experts bring to the discussion an understanding of how an institution's records are accessed, kept, and released, thus helping clinicians understand how to protect patient confidentiality.

As this applies to the NICU setting, there will need to be a determination of whether and under what circumstances a parent or other family member is an identified patient and, if so, how their records will be created and maintained. Often, those in pediatric settings are unfamiliar with the idea of maintaining protected health information (PHI) for an adult family member and will need to identify methods for creating such records. If the infant is the identified patient, there will be discussions regarding what sensitive family information is appropriate for the child's chart and what to do with important sensitive collateral information that should ideally not be in the child's chart for confidentiality reasons. In some cases, this may be the rationale for creating a chart for an adult family member. Decisions about location of documentation are discussed in more detail later.

THIRD-PARTY CONTRACTS

When planning and implementing a documentation system, psychologists should be mindful of regulations attached to insurance reimbursement. Psychologists practicing in NICU settings and fetal care centers generally do not have control over the third-party contracts into which their organizations have entered. They are, however, responsible to meet the documentation standards of these entities, and they must have documentation consistent with billing codes utilized. Billing specialists and other administrators in the institution will have detailed knowledge of documentation requirements for third-party contracts.

STATE AND FEDERAL LAWS AND REGULATIONS

All psychologists and other BHCs should be familiar with the state and federal laws under which they practice. State laws governing the practice of psychology, including rules regarding documentation, can be found online and reviewed in detail. Often, demonstration of knowledge of these statutes is part of gaining initial licensure to practice in the state. Any decision regarding documentation should be made with the relevant state statutes in mind.

In the United States, HIPAA sets standards for the protection of PHI under the Privacy Rule. The Privacy Rule identifies PHI as information that is individually identifiable (or reasonably could be identifiable) and that relates to "the individual's past, present, or future physical or mental health or condition, the provision of health care to the individual, or the past, present, or future payment for the provision of health care to the individual" (U.S. Department of Health and Human Services, 2003). As such, PHI may not be released or utilized without consent of the patient (or guardian thereof). PHI may be accessed for the purposes of treatment, payment, or operations. PHI belonging to a family member (e.g., a parent or sibling) that is in an identified child patient chart could potentially be released with the child's information, which would thus be considered a violation of this rule. Related to the NICU setting, this brings into question, for example, such information as maternal and paternal perinatal/postnatal screening results and other personal information shared in the process of treating the infant or the parent–child dyad. The Office of Civil Rights documents and web page can be accessed for a thorough review of HIPAA rules and regulations.

The 21st Century Cures Act was passed by Congress in 2016 and, among other things, focuses on patient access to health information. It prohibits information blocking, which, in practical application, requires that patients have access to their electronic health records. This includes progress notes written by clinicians. Although some exceptions are allowed, these are limited. This is a significant change to patient access to health records, and clinicians will need to be aware of how their individual institutions are managing compliance with the new law.

American Psychological Association

The APA has published information relevant to this discussion of documentation in NICU settings. The APA practice directorate sets out guidelines on record-keeping and takes into account the APA ethical standards set forth in the "Ethical Principles of Psychologists and Code of Conduct" (APA, 2017). The APA also notes that documentation requirements may vary by context and by state laws, in addition to ethical considerations. When conflicts exist between APA guidelines and standards and state and/or federal laws and regulations, psychologists are expected to follow the law and to attempt to resolve conflicts in a manner consistent with the APA ethical principles (APA, 2007). APA guidelines on record-keeping include 13 separate points with examples for application. Readers are encouraged to become familiar with these by reviewing the information contained in the publication and the APA website (APA, 2007).

According to APA's record-keeping guidelines, psychologists have the responsibility to create and maintain accurate records that will inform and document treatment and that contain information relevant to the context of treatment. Psychologists further have the responsibility to maintain the security of records and the confidentiality of information contained in the records. Applied to the NICU and fetal care settings, this means ensuring that therapeutic interventions are properly recorded and available to other legitimate treatment providers and that patient confidentiality is protected. It also means ensuring that records exist to support billing and answer any potential legal or ethical questions that may arise related to treatment.

Applying these approaches to the NICU setting, the pediatric psychologist might consider the preceding issues related to documentation by first identifying the patient. Are they acting in support of the infant's care? Situations that might meet this criteria are dyadic intervention, coaching on parent attachment, or providing general family support focused on the stressors associated with the NICU setting and/or infant's illness. In this case, documentation would occur in the infant's chart with information on parent/family functioning only as it pertains to the infant's care, safety, and well-being.

At the nexus of all of these considerations is the information that is gathered about a parent or other family member when treating an infant as the identified patient. During this treatment, a clinician may encounter family members who require referral to outside providers for more significant adjustment or psychiatric disorders. They may also encounter situations that require that they document clinical information, screening, referral, and other intervention for family members in a detailed manner. Guidelines and ethical principles suggest that clinicians should strive for accurate documentation of therapeutic work for treatment and billing purposes, while ensuring that confidential family information is not inappropriately shared within the unit, the medical and nursing staff, and outside of the hospital setting (through subsequent release of the infant's records).

Unfortunately, this still leaves much gray area regarding how to handle sensitive information about parents and other collateral family members. Much is left to clinician judgment. At what point does family member information cross from relevancy to the identified patient's (infant's) care to family member PHI? For example, if a parent is expressing suicidality, does that information and resultant safety assessment belong in the infant's chart or in a separate chart dedicated to the parent? What about results of parental depression screenings?

In some medical settings, clinicians have chosen to document results of parent screening directly into patient charts. For example, postpartum depression screenings are frequently given in pediatric settings such as a pediatrician's office or in the NICU. Similarly, parents may make disclosures about individual or family psychosocial concerns. Some providers choose to place this information in the infant's chart, arguing that parent functioning is directly relevant to an infant's health, development, and safety. There are situations in which information about serious parental mental health concerns is directly relevant to the well-being of the infant and may thus be recorded in the infant's chart to facilitate care of the infant. For example, when encountering a parent who is impaired by their psychiatric symptoms and unable to provide needed care to their infant, a clinician may need to document the parent's symptoms and impairment in order to protect the infant.

However, even in situations in which parent functioning is documented as relevant to the infant's health, there is sensitive information that may not belong in an infant's chart. For example, in the case of suicidal ideation, documentation of appropriate clinical actions to mitigate risk to the parent or family member when presenting such an emergent and potentially dangerous situation is clearly required by any documentation standard. Such documentation records actions taken and also protects the clinician and the organization from any resultant legal or ethical questions. If such information is not directly relevant to an infant's medical care or needs, it could be argued that the information is parent PHI and including it in an infant's chart is a violation of parent privacy. It is not difficult to envision a scenario in which such information could become inappropriately released with the infant's records and result in harm to the parent. This could be the case, for example, in a divorce or custody proceeding. This would lead a clinician to chart in a location that guarantees parent privacy. There may be some compromise in alluding to important parent or other family member information vaguely in the infant's chart and recording any necessary detailed information in a separate parent chart. As previously noted, clinicians can involve relevant members of their administration to identify processes and procedures for opening and maintaining parent charts in their pediatric institutions. It is often helpful to have an algorithm that identifies under what circumstances a parent chart will be opened. This helps ensure consistent procedures between individual clinicians.

These are important questions, and careful consideration needs to be given to how private parent or other family member information is handled. Taking into account all of the entities involved in setting standards for documentation, and involving multiple stakeholders in the organization in decisions about documentation, will ensure appropriate documentation of assessment, impressions, and treatment and will help protect clinicians and patients and families.

INTEGRATION OF TECHNOLOGY IN SERVICES

It has often been the case that technology develops faster than the operational and ethical principles that guide practice. As discussed previously, one piece of technology that has become almost standard is the EMR. It is important to remember that an EMR can be customized by institutions, and security settings for information contained within it will differ across those institutions. The EMR provides a variety of tools that can assist the clinician with documentation, including templates to help standardize notes, flow sheets to record data in easy-to-access locations, and copy forward features. Some EMRs also have functions that allow for messages between treatment team providers that are not available for records release following discharge or are even not maintained after an inpatient admission is complete. Clinicians should familiarize themselves with all of the tools available in their organization's EMR and understand what pieces of information are released when medical records are requested. Many organizations have information available to clinicians for EMR training and continuous learning activities.

Telemedicine

In the spring of 2020, the 2019 novel coronavirus (COVID-19) was declared a pandemic, changing the landscape of health care significantly. One of the major changes seen in health care was the widespread adoption of telehealth. For many years, institutions have attempted to adopt telehealth procedures and have encountered a variety of difficulties related to clinician licensing, patient safety, and confidentiality. Perhaps the major hurdle in telehealth had been reimbursement for services. However, with pandemic-era recommendations for physical distancing and protection of vulnerable populations, telemedicine has become widely accepted and reimbursed. As each institution adopted telehealth services, rigorous processes were put into place to ensure patient confidentiality, including use of secure platforms on which to provide telephone or video services. Clinicians who are new to telemedicine should become familiar with the APA's (2013) guidelines for the practice of telepsychology.

In NICUs and fetal care centers, the ability to provide services via phone or video conferencing during the pandemic allowed psychologists to protect some of the most vulnerable patients by limiting exposure to in-person contact. Although direct contact with parents was limited, telehealth opportunities increased clinician access to some parents, who, for a variety of reasons, were unable to be at their child's bedside during typical work hours. In the past, these parents or caregivers might have been excluded from benefiting from psychological services. It could be the case that these families are the most in need of psychological support given the stressors that prevent them from being at bedside with their infant. Telehealth services may reduce barriers and allow for a more equitable provision of services. The literature on psychological telemedicine services (prior to COVID-19) across the life span shows that there is consistent feasibility of telehealth models, and telehealth interventions are highly acceptable from both a patient and provider point of view (Bashshur et al., 2016). Research focused on efficacy, cost, and cost:benefit ratios of telehealth during this unique time in health care will help determine future uses and may help advocate for ongoing reimbursement of these services in a consistent manner.

Social Media

Many hospitals have specific policies around the use of social media for their staff. Psychologists have a duty to protect the confidentiality of their patients and therefore should refrain from informal (unofficial) connections with patients and families on social media platforms. Such relationships violate the accepted boundaries between patients and clinicians, and they raise ethical concerns about inappropriate information sharing. It is best to have clear communication early in the treatment relationship with patients and families about policies related to social media. This may include communicating about policies prohibiting social media connections between clinicians and patients. Such communication can prevent ethical dilemmas, awkward social situations, and/or hurt feelings.

One potential benefit of social media is the ability for families with unique circumstances to connect through disease-specific or NICU-specific support groups. Some families find these groups very helpful in reducing isolation and obtaining social support. It is, however, important that families understand that these groups are largely unmonitored and the information/advice presented in them may not be accurate or generalizable to their child. For some families, online groups can increase distress through inaccurate, misleading, or incomplete information.

Other Novel Technologies

WEB-BASED VIDEO TECHNOLOGY

In recent years, many NICUs have added web-based video camera services (e.g., AngelEye camera) to their care environments. These cameras allow parents to view their infant remotely and can help them feel more connected to their infant when separated. This technology involves a camera available at bedside, pointed toward the infant, which then transmits a picture via secure internet connection. Families can be given the option to create an account on the internet-based user platform and then can log in and observe their child. Hacking and resultant breach of confidentiality are possible risks related to use of this technology.

From an operations standpoint, the adoption of this technology requires clear policies and procedures around its use. Consideration should be given to when the cameras are activated and deactivated. For example, some hospitals direct that cameras are turned off during staff care or handling of the infant. Many institutions have policies against filming or photographing staff, which would be violated by staff appearing on camera during care of the infant. When developing a policy regarding web-based camera use, there are a number of issues to consider. These include having a process for consenting families regarding the purpose and the agreed-upon guidelines for use of the technology. In addition, consideration should be given to whether the hospital will revoke a family's access and under what circumstances this might occur. Families should have a clear understanding of whether screenshots (if possible) and recording (if possible) are allowed.

Data on how the use of web-based cameras at the bedside affects families are very limited. Guttmann and colleagues (2020) at Children's Hospital of Philadelphia recently completed a study of the impact of AngelEye cameras on NICU-specific parental stress using the Parental Stress Scale–NICU, a validated tool. In general, they found that parents reported high levels of stress related to being separated from their infants, their infants appearing in pain, and feeling helpless to protect or help their infants. Parents who reported using the AngelEye cameras reported lower levels of stress related to the sights/sounds of the NICU, the appearance of the infant, and their relationship with the infant and parental role. Specifically, camera use was associated with significantly less distress about being separated from their infants. Guttmann et al. did not find an association between bedside camera use and reported levels of stress with staff behaviors and communication.

Additional research needs to be conducted on the positive and negative impacts of this technology on families coping and adjustment to the NICU. Anecdotally, the authors have seen these cameras have some unintended consequences. Some families appear to experience increased anxiety and interruptions to sleep related to constant attention to the bedside camera. Parent anxiety can be exacerbated by watching events but being unable to respond directly (e.g., seeing their infant cry) or by having the camera turned off during care tasks. Such anxiety can contribute to distrust and communication difficulties, giving rise to conflict with staff and medical teams, and can also increase stress for bedside staff.

Parental Support and Information Applications

A variety of free applications (apps) on both the Apple and Android platforms are available specifically for families of premature infants, such as What to Expect, Pregnancy Tracker, March of Dimes' My NICU Baby (available in English and Spanish), and MyPreemie. It may be helpful to provide families with a list of vetted apps as an informational resource (see apps listed in Box 7.1 and Box 7.2). One of the advantages of having a list of vetted apps is the ability to guide families to accurate and reliable sources of information. In addition, providing families

---

Box 7.1

APPLICATIONS TO TRACK INFANT PROGRESS

MyPreemie
   Available in English or Spanish, depending on the language settings on
      one's phone
   Has trackers, a diary, education, and suggested questions

My NICU Baby
   Developed by the March of Dimes and includes their educational content
   Allows one to track feedings, weight, pumping, and kangaroo care time
   Available in both English and Spanish (Mi Bebe en NICU)

Box 7.2

APPLICATIONS FOR RELAXATION AND STRESS MANAGEMENT

   Insight Timer—app for meditation, sleep, anxiety, and mindfulness
   Breathe2Relax—tools for learning deep breathing for stress management
   Sanvello for Anxiety and Depression (formerly Pacifica)—tools for
      depression, anxiety, and post-traumatic stress disorder
   Yoga Studio—beginner yoga app that includes a yoga for mental health
      collection
   HeadSpace—mindfulness app
   Liberate—relaxation strategies developed for people of color by people of
      color

---

with apps to help with anxiety management, relaxation, and mindfulness may help them cope with the stress and anxiety.

Some institutions have created unique interactive NICU apps to help families stay involved in care. For example, Geisinger Medical Center's "My NICU Newborn" allows parents to track weight and feedings and even to offer feedback to the institution. Depending on the information available in this type of app, there may be significant measures that must be taken during application development to protect privacy and confidentiality. This is particularly important if information available in the app (e.g., weight and height) is connected to and uploaded from the EMR. When the infant's information is parent-entered, there are fewer concerns about privacy and confidentiality because the family is choosing what information to put in the app. When developing an app specific to an institution or hospital, it is necessary to gather a multidisciplinary team that includes experts from health information management, app development, and direct care providers.

CONCLUSION

The increasing inclusion of psychological services into fetal care center and NICU settings allows for more comprehensive behavioral health and developmental care for families and infants. It does, however, bring accompanying challenges for clinicians regarding application of ethical and legal issues related to patient identification, consent, documentation, confidentiality, and billing. Careful attention to these concerns is important in developing programs of care in these settings.

REFERENCES

American Medical Association. (2020). *CPT professional edition.*

American Psychological Association. (2007). Record keeping guidelines. *American Psychologist*, *62*(9), 993–1004. https://www.apa.org/practice/guidelines/record-keeping

American Psychological Association. (2013). *Guidelines for the practice of telepsychology.* *American Psychologist*, *68*(9), 791–800. https://www.apa.org/practice/guidelines/tel epsychology

American Psychological Association. (2017). *Ethical principles of psychologists and code of conduct, including 2010 and 2017 amendments.* https://www.apa.org/ethics/code

Bashshur, R. L., Shannon, G. W., Bashshur, N., & Yellowlees, P. M. (2016). The empirical evidence for telemedicine interventions in mental disorders. *Telemedicine Journal and E-Health*, *22*, 87–113.

Brown, S. D., Donelan, K., Martins, Y., Burmeister, K., Buchmiller, T. L., Sayeed, S. A., Mitchell, C., & Ecker, J. L. (2012). Differing attitudes toward fetal care by pediatric and maternal–fetal medicine specialists. *Pediatrics*, *130*, e1534. doi:10.1542/peds.2012-1352

Brown, S. D., Lyerly, A. D., Little, M. O., & Lantos, J. D. (2008). Paediatrics-based fetal care: Unanswered ethical questions. *Acta Pædiatrica*, *97*, 1617–1619.

Carmona, S., Alayed, N., Al-Ibrahim, A., & D'Souza, R. (2018). Realizing the potential of real-time clinical collaboration in maternal–fetal and obstetric medicine through WhatsApp. *Obstetric Medicine*, *11*(2), 83–89. https://doi.org/10.1177/1753495x1 8754457

Chervenak, F. A., & McCullough, L. B. (2003). The fetus as a patient: An essential concept for the ethics of perinatal medicine. *American Journal of Perinatology*, *20*, 399–404.

Diekma, D. S. (2004). Parental refusals of medical treatment: The harm principle as threshold for state intervention. *Theoretical Medicine and Bioethics*, *25*, 243–264. doi:10.1007/s11017-004-3146-6

Guttmann, K., Patterson, C., Haines, T., Hoffman, C., Masten, M., Lorch, S., & Chuo, J. (2020). Parent stress in relation to use of bedside telehealth, an initiative to improve family-centeredness of care in the neonatal intensive care unit. *Journal of Patient Experience*, *7*, 1378–1383.

Institute of Medicine, Committee on Quality of Health Care in America. (2001). *Crossing the quality chasm: A new health system for the 21st century.* National Academies Press.

Kopelman, L. M. (1997). The best-interests standard as threshold, ideal, and standard of reasonableness. *Journal of Medicine and Philosophy*, *22*, 271–289.

Leuthner, S. R. (2001). Decisions regarding resuscitation of the extremely premature infant and models of best interest. *Journal of Perinatology*, *21*, 193–198.

Ross, L. F. (2004). *Children, families, and health care decision making*. Oxford University Press.

Scibilia, J. (2014). How to protect maternal health information in a newborn's medical record. *AAP News*, *35*(12), 4.

Shenoy, A., & Appel, J. M. (2017). Safeguarding confidentiality in electronic health records. *Cambridge Quarterly of Healthcare Ethics*, *26*, 337–341. https://doi.org/10.1017/S0963180116000931

U.S. Department of Health and Human Services, Office of Civil Rights. (2003). *Summary of the HIPAA Privacy Rule: HIPAA compliance assistance*. https://www.hhs.gov/hipaa/for-professionals/privacy/laws-regulations/index.html

Cross-Cutting Mental Health Issues and Approaches

8

INFANT MENTAL HEALTH FOR HIGH-RISK INFANTS ACROSS THE CONTINUUM OF CARE

MILLER SHIVERS, ANNELISE CUNNINGHAM, NATALIA HENNER, AND KERRI MACHUT ∎

CASE EXAMPLE

Yessenia is a 32-year-old married Hispanic woman with a history of depression, anxiety, and infertility challenges. During a prenatal ultrasound at 20 weeks of gestation, her baby, Aiden, was noted to have intrauterine growth restriction with double-outlet right ventricle, transposition of the great arteries, and aortic coarctation. Aiden was born preterm at 32 weeks of gestation and was also found to have several areas of intestinal atresias. He required help with breathing and was placed on a ventilator. Aiden underwent many surgeries, and his heart defect was deemed too complex to repair, significantly limiting his chances of surviving past 1 year of age. Aiden spent the next 9 months of his life in the neonatal intensive care unit (NICU), where teams of doctors and nurses attempted to stabilize him enough to reach the next surgery. He spent many months sedated in order to tolerate a ventilator and was often too agitated to be held by anyone other than Yessenia.

Yessenia remained at Aiden's bedside every day while her partner, Jose, worked. The staff quickly noticed how progressively withdrawn, quiet, and thin Yessenia became, and many raised concerns about her mental health. Behavioral health and care coordinators spent many hours attempting to help, but Yessenia was reluctant to seek any professional support, as she preferred to use her deep religious faith as comfort and guidance. She noted feeling dissatisfied and limited in her parenting, especially with breastfeeding. At the time of transfer from the NICU to a rehabilitation facility at 10 months of life, Aiden was somewhat withdrawn, often frowning or with a blank facial expression, which greatly worried his medical team. The most remarkable moments for the behavioral health and medical teams to observe were when Yessenia and her son would interact. Even when deeply sedated, Aiden's heart rate would stabilize with Yessenia's presence, and his mood would seemingly lift. This remarkable connection between mother's and baby's moods remained through his illness and slow recovery.

Infants and their parents simultaneously cue one another over and over again, creating the foundational/core choreography of their relationship. Cries, proximity, touch, eye contact, and words are the steps of the delicate dance that ultimately build attachment. For all parent–infant relationships, responsiveness and attunement to these cues can be impacted by both infant and parent factors, such as anxiety and depression, physical health complications, environmental stress, temperament, and exposure to trauma. Parents of high-risk infants hospitalized in the NICU enter into the parent–infant relationship with additional challenges, including adjustment to medical complications and diagnoses, establishing trusted relationships with medical providers, making critical care decisions for their infants, and facing financial and employment stress. Parents of high-risk infants face these mentioned obstacles while getting to know and building their relationship with their infants. Behavioral health clinicians (BHCs) working with parents and infants in the NICU setting are encouraged to approach assessment and intervention within the context of the parent–infant relationship. This chapter provides an overview of common issues and transition points encountered by families in the NICU, followed by suggestions for assessment and intervention.

COMMON ISSUES PERTAINING TO HIGH-RISK INFANTS

Much of how parents perceive their infant and their personality starts during the early stages of pregnancy. When there are deviations from the "norm" during pregnancy or soon after birth, such as genetic conditions, unexpected surgical complications, or premature birth, parents begin to reframe their own narrative, and that of their infant, as part of coping. Many factors influence parental perceptions of their infant in the NICU setting, which has a major impact on parent and infant mental health and the parenting relationship.

Behavioral health in the setting of fetal or neonatal anomalies often focuses on explanation of each specific condition, anticipated NICU course, short- and long-term medical and developmental outcomes, and resources to aid with decision-making. Behavioral health services should ideally include discussions of disrupted bonding, ways to support parenting in the NICU environment, information processing, and coping skills.

There is significant variability in how expectant parents interact with the health care system, which impacts future interactions with their infant and the NICU medical team. Parents may choose a very "hands-on" approach and may view themselves as part of the health care team. These parents will often educate themselves in-depth about their infant's condition, join support groups, seek additional opinions, and remain highly engaged in all nuances of their infant's medical care. Their coping is aided by being prepared, and they believe that having some control impacts their infant's outcome. Other parents may cope by avoiding in-depth medical interactions because they believe predictions about their unborn or newly born infant are irrelevant and/or that outcomes are predetermined by fate or religious beliefs. As in the case of Aiden, Yessenia's faith served as her primary source of coping and guidance, and she perceived she had little choice in his care. Parents' affect when interacting with providers is very different among these two groups of parents and may lead providers to make incorrect assumptions about level of investment and attachment. Yessenia became withdrawn in response to discussions of surgeries and extended hospitalization with health care providers, but she remained very much invested in her faith in achieving a healthy outcome for Aiden.

Cultural considerations, as well as past experiences with health care, are often a part of these differences. African American mothers often voice distrust of prenatal diagnostics (especially when their prenatal care has been limited or dispersed through several hospitals) and believe the health care system has been devaluing their experience and their infants (Peters et al., 2014). It is difficult to argue with this viewpoint because many statistics indicate great racial disparities in maternal and infant outcomes. As such, some African American mothers feel a need to protect their infants not only against the ongoing invasiveness of an NICU but also against the societal injustices that make them more vulnerable. There is also a prevailing sense of ongoing community and individual trauma, making mothers adapt a stance of "making it" despite the odds, while relying on their families, communities, and faith. This may lead to further distancing between families and providers, with families' mistrust shaping how they process information. Ongoing "bad news" may cause the family to feel like providers are no longer advocating for their infant, which often leads to increased anger and reduced presence at the bedside, with obvious negative impact on bonding and mood.

Non-English-speaking families face unique challenges in perinatal interactions with health care providers. When a language barrier is present, not all providers are consistent in their utilization of interpreters, leading to increased familial isolation and confusion about directions of care. In some cultures, it may be common for mothers to defer some of the decision-making to their partners and to their broader families, leading providers to incorrectly conclude that these mothers are passive and/or indifferent in their approach to the infant's care (Galanti, 2003; Ilowite et al., 2017). Such assumptions may lead to physicians being overly paternalistic, which may further alienate the mothers and disrupt their parenting, with negative impact on infant health and parent–infant attachment (Chertok et al., 2014).

All parents, irrespective of race, age, and/or cultural backgrounds, assign characteristics to their infants based on their own perceptions. Those who have struggled with infertility challenges, for example, may view this long-awaited infant who now has medical issues as more vulnerable and more prone to complications. Alternatively, such an infant may be seen as a "miracle" or one who is "meant to be." Parents who have overcome many personal or health care odds themselves may view their infants with congenital anomalies as "fighters" who will prove the medical providers wrong. These parentally predetermined infant characteristics may not reflect reality, but it is obvious they shape that family's narrative, coping, and interactions with their infant well beyond the NICU.

TRANSITIONS FROM PREGNANCY TO NICU DISCHARGE

Pregnancy

All families undergo many important transitions across the prenatal, labor and delivery, newborn, and infant periods. In the NICU, these experiences are especially challenging, and parents face many difficult decision points that impact them as well as their infants. While navigating the NICU stay, parents risk the development or exacerbation of mental health disorders. Access to infant mental health–informed social work and/or psychological services is critical to support parents and their infants throughout each transition during the NICU stay.

The initial parenthood transition all families encounter is the realization of pregnancy, which carries a multitude of emotions and accompanying thoughts. Although pregnancy may be a time of joy for many families, the news may also be a source of distress. The point at which a pregnancy becomes high risk ranges from as early as the first trimester to as late as the day of birth, depending on a variety of maternal and fetal clinical conditions. There may be maternal health conditions that increase risk for fetuses and infants, such as lupus and diabetes. Some families experience infertility challenges, require assisted reproductive technologies, and/ or face higher rates of preterm birth and congenital anomalies. Pregnancies with preterm labor, conditions leading to preterm delivery, and congenital anomalies may require decision-making regarding termination of pregnancy, perinatal palliative care planning, fetal intervention, or immediate postnatal intervention. Each of these decisions can be complex and difficult for families to navigate. In the case of Aiden, several of the mentioned factors were present for the family's transition to pregnancy. Yessenia and Jose experienced multiple years of infertility challenges, learned of Aiden's compromised development at 20 weeks of gestation, and experienced preterm birth at 32 weeks. These factors influence not only the experience of pregnancy but also the parents' perceptions of their infant and the parent–infant relationship.

In addition, families with high-risk pregnancies have heightened stress, worry, or fear of a poor neonatal outcome. Families may need to grieve the loss of a "normal" pregnancy or face feelings of guilt that they caused or exacerbated their infant's condition in some way (Janvier et al., 2016). Parents often experience isolation and believe their friends, family members, and even partners do not fully understand their clinical scenario and feelings. In addition, parents may have family members who actively disagree with decisions they are making for themselves and their infants.

Parenthood

All parents face numerous adjustments transitioning into parenthood, including navigating postpartum recovery, managing changes in stress and hormones, and establishing new sleep and feeding routines (often breastfeeding in particular)—all while balancing many other life factors. Family factors, being a first-time parent, and parental health conditions all influence the adjustment to parenthood. Families with single, adoptive, and/or teenage parents, as well as parents with their own health conditions and postpartum maternal complications, may face added challenges (Lean et al., 2018; Russell et al., 2014). Parents may feel more or less efficacious in tackling this transition depending on whether this is their first child. For most parents, these adjustments are made in the comfort of their own home; in contrast, parents of high-risk infants face the transition to parenthood while in a foreign and unfamiliar environment.

As mentioned previously, parents of a high-risk infant in a NICU environment may experience a wide range of emotions, including increased anxiety and depression (Garfield et al., 2021). Some enter the transition to parenthood aware of a high-risk health condition (e.g., congenital anomaly diagnosed in pregnancy) that necessitates NICU admission and intervention after birth. These parents may have had time to process and plan for their infant's condition, but they may also carry significant worry and fear over the clinical scenario as it begins to unfold. For other parents, the NICU admission may be completely unexpected, bringing about its own set of challenges. The admission may be indicated immediately after birth (e.g., following a placental abruption), following a clinical deterioration after a period of apparent health and "normalcy" in the normal newborn nursery, or even following initial discharge home (e.g., late-onset sepsis). Families may have limited baseline knowledge of their infant's condition and understanding of the NICU environment and interventions. High-risk infants may also require transfer to a regional NICU (sometimes hours away) and be separated from their parents. For many high-risk infants, their condition, diagnosis, and treatment plans may be unknown and/or change frequently and acutely through the infant's hospitalization course.

The NICU environment itself is challenging for most parents, despite the effort of the NICU team to address such issues. Often, it is a foreign environment in which most parents have no or limited exposure prior to their infant's admission. For many, seeing their infant in the NICU environment for the first time, often with monitoring wires and medical equipment, can be very stressful. Parents may be unfamiliar with the policies and procedures of a NICU. Managing visitation can be a difficult task with limitations for when and who can be on the unit. Families additionally may have to juggle work demands and organizing care for their other children. As in the case of Aiden, Yessenia drove 2 hours daily to the hospital while Jose worked overtime due to financial strain.

When parents visit the hospital, privacy and space may be limited in some open-bay NICUs, whereas isolation may be a concern in private-room NICUs. Many

NICU environments do not have space for fatigued parents to comfortably eat meals, nap, and/or stay the night. The physical environment can often be loud with conversations and frequent alarms. While trying to familiarize themselves with the new surroundings, parents are also acclimating to numerous health care providers. Because shift schedules change frequently, parents are continuously meeting new nurses, doctors, trainees, consultants, and staff; as a result, establishing long-term relationships can be challenging. At times, parents' ideas and preferences regarding their infant's care, or simply their personality, may differ from those of their child's health care providers and may lead to conflict and distrust. Some parents have additional burdens of limited health literacy, language barriers, and level of acculturation (Barragan et al., 2011). Navigating the road of parenthood within the fetal care and NICU landscape may be especially difficult for these families.

Given the constraints of the NICU environment and their infant's high-risk condition, bonding with their infant can be difficult. Many conditions preclude the infant being held for days up to weeks, and parents may be fearful of touching their high-risk infant. Maternal (potentially induced by stress) or infant health contraindications can result in parents being unable to deliver basic personal care, breastfeed, or provide expressed breast milk. Even when mothers can provide breast milk, infants are sometimes too sick to receive any feedings. This occurred often for Aiden, and as a result, Yessenia confided to the NICU team how little satisfaction she received from pumping. Not having these parental roles and connection to their infant can often be very difficult and disappointing for parents.

Parents may have barriers to visiting regularly (e.g., other children, work, distance from the hospital, and transportation issues) during the sometimes-prolonged hospitalization. Aiden's father, although heavily invested in his son's recovery, was limited in his visiting the NICU due to his work schedule. Parents can face challenges maintaining optimal relationships with others in their life, including with their other children and partners. Traveling back and forth between the NICU and home, they have limited time to balance between these important family members and their own self-care. Due to these complex factors, many struggle with a loss of control and parental identity during their NICU stay (Janvier et al., 2016). Although some parents may demand involvement in shared decision-making, others may feel uncomfortable or inadequate in participating. Parents may believe they cede their role to the medical team and have limited importance to their infant. These crucial issues need to be addressed and rectified to re-establish the central role of the parent, for both infant and parental mental health in the NICU and after discharge (Hynan et al., 2015). In the case of Yessenia, the NICU team noticed her progressively losing weight and becoming more withdrawn and quiet over the course of Aiden's hospitalization.

Discharge from NICU to Home

The transition from NICU to discharge home is an important milestone for all NICU families. Nearly all parents eagerly await this day, and frustration mounts if it is delayed. From a medical standpoint, an infant's clinical condition can change abruptly and lead to discharge delays. Some infants have ongoing complex care needs, necessitating an abundance of discharge education and coordination of outpatient care, including medical equipment, home nursing, and appointments. Because infants have not been home before, they may not yet have a primary care provider or medical home established.

Parents often are again confronted with a mix and range of emotions. Feelings of anxiety about the transition may build as the anticipated discharge date approaches. Parents may carry concerns about their adequacy as a parent, fears of having primary responsibility for their infant's health at home, and/or worry something may happen to their infant's health under their watch (Soghier et al., 2020). There may be feelings of panic and uncertainty because their infant will no longer be on continuous monitors, have the safety of emergency equipment, and/ or providers will no longer by immediately and continuously present. Parents may grieve the loss of relationships with providers they have built during the NICU stay. Thoughts and feelings of distress may arise in anticipation of facing personal relationships with partners and family members that were strained during hospitalization (Boykova, 2016; Boykova & Kenner, 2012). Parents can feel they have missed out on a "normal" homecoming at a more natural newborn time point. NICU parents also may gain a perception of their infant as more vulnerable due to the infant's medical history, which can impact parents' confidence in feeling ready for discharge. These emotions are all exacerbated by the fatigue that quickly builds when caring for an infant 24/7 at home, especially one that may have additional medical needs.

Infant

Of great importance is the experience of the infant in the NICU. Infants in the NICU are receiving and processing sensory stimuli from their environment with each change and transition (Thompson et al., 2019). As infants develop and increase their state of awareness and bonding to medical parents, they utilize their own affect and behavior to signal notification of change. The transition from the NICU to home, changes in medical staff, and the awareness of the presence of caregivers bedside are all events for infants to regulate. Each of these stressors may impact subsequent functioning in the central nervous system (D'Agata et al., 2017), highlighting the importance of infants' early interactions with their environments. Observation of infants during transitions provides a multitude of information regarding their affective state and medical and behavioral health providers. In the case of Aiden, after spending 10 months in the NICU, he was transferred to a rehabilitation facility. Aiden displayed affective cues of withdrawal during this transition, including frowning at times and, at other times, showing a blank expression. It is critical for the well-being of the infant that health care professionals be mindful of the infant's experience throughout hospitalization(s) in an effort to support the infant's mental health and regulation during the many transitions.

INFANT MENTAL HEALTH ASSESSMENT TECHNIQUES IN THE NICU

What Is Infant Mental Health?

An accepted explanation of infant mental health (IMH; Zero to Three, 2001) is

> the young child's capacity to experience, regulate, and express emotions, form close and secure relationships, and explore the environment and learn. All of these capacities will be best accomplished within the context of the caregiving environment that includes family, community, and cultural expectations for young children. Developing these capacities is synonymous with healthy social and emotional development.

Thus, infant–parent relationships are the primary focus of assessment and are especially important with high-risk infants and their families. Infants are dependent on their caregiving contexts, and infants in NICU settings are even more so dependent on their parents and on the medical staff who intervene with them. In the case of Aiden, his extended stay in the NICU for 10 months included a range of relationships among health care providers. The majority of the first year of his life depended on care from a multitude of different relationships.

IMH focuses on infant behavior and parent behavior to change or improve the relationship between the two. IMH work is a constant dyadic balance, with a simultaneous focus on assessing the concerns and issues of the parents along with the developmental and well-being concerns of the infant. IMH is a strengths-based discipline, and the focus of assessment should aim to create ways to support and improve the infant–parent relationship as it impacts the development of high-risk infants.

Parental Factors and Internalized Representations

It is important to assess the parent's cultural context and internalizations of the parenting role when evaluating the parent–infant relationship. In order to do this, the clinician must have an understanding of the parent's perceptions of parenting, their role as a parent, their cultural beliefs in parenting, and their feelings of how they themselves were parented. Equally important are the parent's perceptions, beliefs, and representations of their infant. These internal representations of the infant and their parenting have been shown to predict parent and young child behavior, infant attachment classifications, and infant and young child symptomatic behavior (Vreeswijk et al., 2012). Because high-risk infants have additional medical needs, it is paramount to gain an understanding of all of these factors in addition to the parent's perceptions, beliefs, and understanding of the medical complexities of the infant. It was critical in the case of Aiden to understand his parents' strong religious beliefs and how religion impacted perceptions of Aiden and his health.

The Working Model of the Child Interview (WMCI; Zeanah et al., 1994) has been used to assess internal representations of an infant. The WMCI takes approximately 1 hour to complete and is meant to be administered in the context of a supportive conversation. The WMCI provides a rapport-building exercise for the clinician and the parent. It is also easily administered via telephone or video conferencing, which is useful for parents who are not able to physically be in the NICU to be interviewed and/or for those who cannot spend an hour of time in person. A shorter version of the interview is available and may be used when there is limited time. The interview asks about parents' experiences during pregnancy and birth, parent's perception of their infant's personality and their relationship with their infant, infant's difficult behaviors and their responses to them, and hopes and fears parents have for their infant in the future. Based on the parent's responses, a typology of their internal representation is assigned as balanced, disengaged, or distorted. Parents whose interviews are balanced describe both strengths and weaknesses, and they speak about empathy for their infant's experience. Parents with disengaged representations have vague information and lack an emotional connection with their infant. Parents whose interviews are distorted show dissatisfaction with their infant. Parents with distorted interviews can be confused about their infant, have unrealistic expectations, and can be preoccupied with themselves or a particular aspect of their infant. In the NICU and other high-risk infant settings, parents may have a disengaged or distorted view of their infant because they often feel little control over decisions being made, have limited understanding of the medical terminology, and have difficulty forming a relationship with their infant.

Parental Adverse Experiences

Because contextual factors play a significant role in how parents perceive their role as parents, it is useful to assess experiences and cultural contexts of the parents. The Adverse Childhood Experiences Study in 1995–1997 (Felitti et al., 1998) found that adverse childhood experiences (ACEs) are linked to poor health outcomes, mental illness, substance misuse, among others, but that ACEs can also be prevented. The Adverse Childhood Experiences Scale assesses childhood traumatic experiences of the parents (have mother and father complete separately), which can be useful in determining internal representations. ACEs are linked to chronic health problems, negative educational experiences, and can increase parental and child health problems, in addition to many other negative effects. An associated condition, toxic stress, can change brain development and affect attention, decision-making, learning, and responses to stress. These negative conditions can be passed to children, so it is critical to intervene with parents to prevent the transmission to their fragile infants, and the first step in intervention is a thorough assessment.

Factors in the NICU Environment

Creating safe, stable, and nurturing caregiving relationships and environments is key to prevention in fragile infants. NICU BHCs must work to develop a rapport with families and reduce the stigma of asking for and accepting help from a BHC so that they can establish an optimal trajectory for infant health and development. This starts with warm and receptive relationship building during the assessment process. An assessment of a parent–infant relationship cannot be complete without observation of the interaction between the two (Table 8.1). The quality of the parent–infant interaction is critical for the infant's development into early childhood—their attachment, social–emotional development, and cognitive development (Evans & Porter, 2009). Although there are many observational measures for infant–parent interactions, no tool is considered the "gold standard."

Observing the Parent–Infant Relationship in the NICU

Observational measures vary in the constructs they aim to measure, availability of the measure, and training to administer and score. In addition, core constructs are believed to be relevant across cultures, and this universalist approach to assessment is problematic (Bernstein et al., 2005). Generally, tools measure some form of parent behavior, infant behavior, and the dyadic interaction. Salient parent behaviors include those that are considered positive, such as responsive caregiving, sensitivity, contingent responsiveness, and emotional availability; and those that interfere with development, such as intrusiveness, control, and hostility (Beebe et al., 2010). Infant behaviors assessed by observational measures of parent–infant interaction often include infant responsiveness, engagement, and involvement. In addition, infant's positive and negative affect are evaluated. Measures also address the coordination of the parent and their infant's interaction by assessing their behaviors in terms of synchrony, reciprocity, and mutuality.

Many factors can impact parent–infant interaction quality, particularly for families of high-risk infants. The NICU environment, physical constraints with medical equipment and devices, and the simple fact that the infant is hospitalized

Table 8.1 KEY CONSTRUCTS TO OBSERVE PARENT–INFANT INTERACTIONS

Parent	Infant	Parent–Infant Interaction
Encouragement	Engagement	Synchrony
Responsiveness	Responsiveness	Reciprocity
Affection	Involvement	Mutuality
Physical proximity	Physical proximity	
Warmth	Curiosity	
Expression/affect	Expression/affect	
Support	Exploration	

and fragile influence interactions and parent–infant relationships. It may be difficult for the BHC to observe meaningful interactions due to medical constraints or a family's limitations in being physically present with their infant at the bedside. The high-risk environment taxes parents, and there is a higher prevalence of stress, anxiety, depression, and trauma symptoms in parents of infants in the NICU, which affects their ability to interact and form meaningful relationships with their infant (Hawes et al., 2016). During Aiden's lengthy admission, he and his family faced a variety of challenging obstacles; however, the family's religious values steadily influenced their perceptions and experiences. Cultural considerations and contexts of the family must be taken into consideration and discussed with each family during a thorough assessment of the parent–infant relationship. Understanding the cultural norms of a family and the family's cultural context is essential for gaining an understanding of the quality of their interactions and relationship (Box 8.1).

IMH INTERVENTIONS IN THE NICU

Transitioning into the intervention phase requires consideration of the unique factors of the family obtained through assessment. Formulating an appropriate treatment plan rests on inclusion of what has been learned about the culture of the family and their identified needs. At the same time, BHCs need to be mindful of the culture of the health care staff and environment. Factors such as identities, roles, expressions, behaviors, values, and beliefs all shape the views and understanding of what "healthy," "safety," and "security" mean. At times, the values of the family

---

Box 8.1

Suggested Probes for a Culturally Informed Assessment

1. What does the parent see as the problem? And, what is the parent's understanding of the problem(s)?
2. What are the parent's expectations with regard to treatment? (Medically, developmentally, and socioemotionally)
3. How does the NICU stay affect the infant, parents, and other family members?
4. What does the parent see as the optimal outcome for their infant?
5. What are the parent's beliefs about infant development, medical interventions, and social–emotional supports?
6. How have community members connected with the infant and parents while in the NICU?
7. What is the predominant attitude regarding help seeking in the parent's community?
8. How do the community members see the hospital in which the infant is hospitalized?

and medical staff may align or differ. BHCs in the NICU often serve as a liaison between families and staff. It is essential for providers to gain an appreciation and respect for individuals' cultural variables in order to best support the relationships between families and providers. Individualized family-based interventions during NICU hospitalization, as well as during the transition home, have been associated with improved infant–parent interactions, lower levels of depression and stress, and increased parental self-esteem (Muller-Nix & Ansermet, 2009).

Targets of Intervention in the NICU

In 2015, the *Journal of Perinatology* listed IMH training as a recommendation for mental health professionals in the NICU (Hynan et al., 2015). As previously mentioned, while in the NICU, infants are in relationships not only with their family but also with their medical providers. IMH-focused intervention efforts in the NICU strive to incorporate all of the different individuals who have relationships with the infant. Throughout various time points in the hospitalization, individuals involved in interventions may change and can include infants, parents, other family members, and health care staff. Treatment efforts can target a variety of needs for the family, including psychoeducation, parental factors, sibling stress, trauma responses, parental self-efficacy, response to infant needs, development, parental psychopathology, and attachment.

Specific parental concerns may play a role in overall adjustment for the family in the NICU, including parental stress, personality, mental health, social support, and pregnancy variables (J. Carter et al., 2007). Recent recommendations for parental services in the NICU advocate for a universal-care-for-all approach that includes systematic support and education focused on developmental needs and peer-to-peer support provided by trained volunteers (Hynan et al., 2015). In addition to universal care, Hynan and colleagues (2015) also explain the need for psychologists, psychiatrists, social workers, NICU staff, and pastoral care for parents with increased risk factors or acute stress symptoms. Taking an IMH approach, when working exclusively with the parents (either individually or in group format), BHCs aim to model secure attachment behaviors within their relationship.

In traditional outpatient care, IMH treatment largely focuses on the infant–parent relationship. Often, this takes course by targeting attachment behaviors to strengthen the security of the relationship to foster regulation and exploration. Traditional attachment theory includes specific behaviors that occur between the infant and the parent to signal safety and facilitate regulation such as following, clinging, crying, and holding. During hospitalization, behaviors that facilitate soothing, proximity, and communication may be compromised. It is the challenge for IMH providers in the NICU setting to identify, foster, and support the mechanisms of attachment occurring within the context of medical complications. The interventions discussed next serve to enhance infants' mental health through increasing both support for parents and attachment behaviors in the NICU.

Existing IMH NICU Interventions

Emotional bonding between parents and their infants in the NICU has been encouraged through the use of kangaroo care. Kangaroo care includes the practice of skin-to-skin contact between the parent and the infant and has been linked to beneficial outcomes for infants across both high- and low-income countries (Jefferies, 2012). The practice of skin-to-skin contact not only provides physical benefits for infants, including sleep organization, improved neurodevelopmental outcomes, breastfeeding, and cardiorespiratory and temperature stability, but also serves as a behavior in which the parent can respond to the needs of the infant and foster attachment security. Despite being too agitated to be held by others, Aiden consistently responded to being held by his mother. While engaged in kangaroo care, Yessenia sang to Aiden in Spanish, and daily he responded with a small smile or light squeeze of her hand. Her mere presence in the room, even when deeply sedated, regulated Aiden's heart rate and his mood would seemingly lift.

The use of technology has more recently served as a source of intervention among NICU populations in efforts to target parental stress and attachment. Applications have included web-based videoconferencing and webcam systems, including NICView (Joshi et al., 2016) and AngelEye (Rhoads et al., 2015). Such interventions aim to provide opportunities for parents to access alternative methods of communication with health care providers and interactions with their infants when there are barriers to being physically present in the NICU. Parent outcomes with regard to the use of technology are mixed, with reports of increased stress and decreased anxiety. The qualitative data provide more details regarding the impact of stress and anxiety on parents, including being able to see their infant when not on the unit, if the camera was turned on or off, and/or seeing their infant without being able to behaviorally provide comfort (Epstein et al., 2017).

Outpatient Adaptations for Intervention in the NICU

Two existing outpatient-based programs, Circle of Security (Cooper et al., 2009) and Speaking for the Baby (S. Carter et al., 1991), can be applied in the NICU setting to support parent–infant relationships. Circle of Security–Parenting (COS-P) is a video-based program that aims to increase parents' capacity to identify and respond to the emotional needs of their child to strengthen attachment. The program focuses on encouraging the parent to reflect on their own developmental history and how that plays into their emotional and behavioral responses with their child (Cooper et al., 2009). COS-P can be delivered individually or in a group format. Speaking for the Baby, a therapeutic intervention that has been used with parents and their infants, is based on the seminal work of Selma Fraiberg. Speaking for the Baby aims to encourage parents to express their own emotions while also interpreting infant cues within the parent–infant relationship (S. Carter et al., 1991). Both COS-P and Speaking for the Baby involve working with parents to increase not only reflection on their own emotions but also the cues offered by their infants within the relationship.

IDEAS WORTH SHARING

- Application of IMH requires establishing a trusted relationship with the parents in order to understand their perceptions of their infant's medical, emotional, and behavioral states.
- Providing IMH in the NICU is not limited to direct work with parents; rather, it is critical to involve all the active relationships for the parent(s) and infant, including health care providers.
- Parents may go through states of change with regard to involvement with BHCs. IMH providers are encouraged to meet families where they are and continue to foster a relationship at a level that is comforting to the family.

CONCLUSION

Yessenia was faithfully at Aiden's side daily even when she became more withdrawn and distant from the medical staff. Yessenia was ultimately uninterested in receiving behavioral health support and persisted that her source of comfort and coping was her faith. As Aiden's hospitalization continued, Yessenia became familiar with the behavioral health team and her engagement in casual conversations increased over time. Yessenia eventually shared details of her past, including struggling with depression and anxiety since adolescence and experiencing past trauma. Although she did not engage in formalized assessment or intervention, the BHCs were able to serve as a liaison to the other health care providers (e.g., the chaplain) to build context to better understand Yessenia's culture, values, and beliefs.

Whether serving as a liaison between providers and families, working exclusively with parents, or supporting the infant–parent dyad, providing IMH services in the NICU requires investment in relationships. The needs and goals for each family may differ, and individualized treatment plans are recommended in addition to overall systematic universal services. The use of recommended assessment approaches described previously positions providers to know the intimate and valued unique factors of each family that are impacting their perspectives of themselves, their infant, the medical staff, and their overall NICU experience.

REFERENCES

Barragan, D. I., Ormond, K. E., Strecker, M. N., & Weil, J. (2011). Concurrent use of cultural health practices and Western medicine during pregnancy: Exploring the

Mexican experience in the United States. *Journal of Genetic Counseling*, 20(6), 609–624.

Beebe, B., Jaffe, J., Markese, S., Buck, K., Chen, H., Cohen, P., Bahrick, L., Andrews, H., & Feldstein, S. (2010). The origins of 12-month attachment: A microanalysis of 4-month mother–infant interaction. *Attachment & Human Development*, 12(1–2), 3–141.

Bernstein, V. J., Harris, E. J., Long, C. W., Iida, E., & Hans, S. L. (2005). Issues in the multi-cultural assessment of parent–child interaction: An exploratory study from the Starting Early Starting Smart Collaboration. *Journal of Applied Developmental Psychology*, 26(3), 241–275.

Boykova, M. (2016). Transition from hospital to home in parents of preterm infants: A literature review. *Journal of Perinatal & Neonatal Nursing*, 30(4), 327–348.

Boykova, M., & Kenner, C. (2012). Transition from hospital to home for parents of preterm infants. *Journal of Perinatal & Neonatal Nursing*, 26(1), 81–89.

Carter, J. D., Mulder, R. T., & Darlow, B. A. (2007). Parental stress in the NICU: The influence of personality, psychological, pregnancy and family factors. *Personality and Mental Health*, 1(1), 40–50.

Carter, S. L., Osofsky, J. D., & Hann, D. M. (1991). Speaking for the baby: A therapeutic intervention with adolescent mothers and their infants. *Infant Mental Health Journal*, 12(4), 291–301.

Chertok, I. R. A., McCrone, S., Parker, D., Leslie, N., & Catlin, A. (2014). Review of interventions to reduce stress among mothers of infants in the NICU. *Advances in Neonatal Care*, 14(1), 30–37.

Cooper, G., Hoffman, K., & Powell, B. (2009). *Circle of Security parenting: A relationship based DVD parenting program*. Marycliff Institute.

D'Agata, A. L., Sanders, M. R., Grasso, D. J., Young, E. E., Cong, X., & McGrath, J. M. (2017). Unpacking the burden of care for infants in the NICU. *Infant Mental Health Journal*, 38(2), 306–317.

Epstein, E. G., Arechiga, J., Dancy, M., Simon, J., Wilson, D., & Alhusen, J. L. (2017). Integrative review of technology to support communication with parents of infants in the NICU. *Journal of Obstetric, Gynecologic & Neonatal Nursing*, 46(3), 357–366.

Evans, C. A., & Porter, C. L. (2009). The emergence of mother–infant co-regulation during the first year: Links to infants' developmental status and attachment. *Infant Behavior and Development*, 32(2), 147–158.

Felitti, V. J., Anda, R. F., Nordenberg, D., Williamson, D. F., Spitz, A. M., Edwards, M. P., & Marks, J. S. (1998). Relationship of childhood abuse and household dysfunction to many of the leading causes of death in adults: The Adverse Childhood Experiences (ACEs) Study. *American Journal of Preventive Medicine*, 14(4), 245–258.

Felitti, V. J., Anda, R. F., Nordenberg, D., Williamson, D. F., Spitz, A. M., Edwards, V., & Marks, J. S. (1998). Relationship of childhood abuse and household dysfunction to many of the leading causes of death in adults: The Adverse Childhood Experiences (ACE) Study. *American Journal of Preventive Medicine*, 14(4), 245–258.

Galanti, G.-A. (2003). The Hispanic family and male–female relationships: An overview. *Journal of Transcultural Nursing*, 14(3), 180–185.

Garfield, C. F., Lee, Y. S., Warner-Shifflett, L., Christie, R., Jackson, K. L., & Miller, E. (2021). Maternal and paternal depressive symptoms during NICU stay and transition home. *Pediatrics*, 148(2), e2020042747.

Hawes, K., McGowan, E., O'Donnell, M., Tucker, R., & Vohr, B. (2016). Social emotional factors increase risk of postpartum depression in mothers of preterm infants. *Journal of Pediatrics*, *179*, 61–67.

Hynan, M. T., Steinberg, Z., Baker, L., Cicco, R., Geller, P. A., Lassen, S., Milford, C., Mounts, K. O., Patterson, C., Saxton, S., Segre, L., & Stuebe, A. (2015). Recommendations for mental health professionals in the NICU. *Journal of Perinatology*, *35*(1), S14–S18.

Ilowite, M. F., Cronin, A. M., Kang, T. I., & Mack, J. W. (2017). Disparities in prognosis communication among parents of children with cancer: The impact of race and ethnicity. *Cancer*, *123*(20), 3995–4003.

Janvier, A., Lantos, J., Aschner, J., Barrington, K., Batton, B., Batton, D., Berg, S. F., Carter, B., Campbell, D., Cohn, F., Drapkin Lyerly, A., Ellsbury, D., Fanaroff, A., Fanaroff, K., Gravel, S., Haward, M., Kutzsche, S., Marlow, N., Montello, M., . . . Lyerly, A. D. (2016). Stronger and more vulnerable: A balanced view of the impacts of the NICU experience on parents. *Pediatrics*, *138*(3), e20160655.

Jefferies, A. L.; Canadian Paediatric Society & Fetus and Newborn Committee. (2012). Kangaroo care for the preterm infant and family. *Paediatrics & Child Health*, *17*(3), 141–143.

Joshi, A., Chyou, P. H., Tirmizi, Z., & Gross, J. (2016). Web camera use in the neonatal intensive care unit: Impact on nursing workflow. *Clinical Medicine & Research*, *14*(1), 1–6.

Lean, R. E., Rogers, C. E., Paul, R. A., & Gerstein, E. D. (2018). NICU hospitalization: Long-term implications on parenting and child behaviors. *Current Treatment Options in Pediatrics*, *4*, 49–69.

Muller-Nix, C., & Ansermet, F. (2009). Prematurity, risk factors, and protective factors. In C. Z. Zeanah, Jr. (Ed.), *Handbook of infant mental health* (3rd ed., pp. 180–196). Guilford.

Peters, R. M., Benkert, R., Templin, T. N., & Cassidy-Bushrow, A. E. (2014). Measuring African American women's trust in provider during pregnancy. *Research in Nursing & Health*, *372*(2), 144–154.

Rhoads, S. J., Green, A., Gauss, C. H., Mitchell, A., Pate, B., & Dowling, D. (2015). Web camera use of mothers and fathers when viewing their hospitalized neonate. *Advances in Neonatal Care*, *15*(6), 440–446.

Russell, G., Sawyer, A., Rabe, H., Abbott, J., Gyte, G., Duley, L., & Ayers, S. (2014). Very Preterm Birth Qualitative Collaborative Group: Parents' views on care of their very premature babies in neonatal intensive care units: a qualitative study. *BMC Pediatrics*, *14*, 440.

Soghier, L. M., Kritikos, K. I., Carty, C. L., Glass, P., Tuchman, L. K., Streisand, R., & Fratantoni, K. R. (2020). Parental depression symptoms at neonatal intensive care unit discharge and associated risk factors. *Pediatrics*, *227*, 163–169.

Thompson, S. F., Kiff, C. J., & McLaughlin, K. A. (2019). The neurobiology of stress and adversity in infancy. In C. Z. Zeanah, Jr. (Ed.), *Handbook of infant mental health* (4th ed., pp. 81–94). Guilford.

Vreeswijk, C. M., Maas, A. J. B., & van Bakel, H. J. (2012). Parental representations: A systematic review of the working model of the child interview. *Infant Mental Health Journal*, *33*(3), 314–328.

Zeanah, C. H., Benoit, D., Hirshberg, L., Barton, M. L., & Regan, C. (1994). Mothers' representations of their infants are concordant with infant attachment classifications. *Developmental Issues in Psychiatry and Psychology, 1*(1), 1–14.

Zero to Three Infant Mental Health Task Force Steering Committee. (2001). *Definition of infant mental health.* National Center for Clinical Infant Programs.

9

PERINATAL MOOD AND ANXIETY DISORDERS AMONG PARENTS OF HIGH-RISK FETUSES AND INFANTS

BIRDIE G. MEYER, BRENDA PAPIERNIAK, AND CHRISTENA B. RAINES ■

Perinatal mood and anxiety disorders (PMADs) represent a common and serious risk for all pregnant and postpartum women, with a prevalence rate close to 21% in the postpartum period. A landmark study regarding the onset and timing of PMADs that included 10,000 women (Wisner et al., 2013) revealed that 1 in 7 women developed depression or anxiety during pregnancy or within the first 3 months postpartum and 1 in 5 women developed depression and/or anxiety in the first year postpartum. The study also reported 19% of the population endorsed self-harm ideation and a prevalence of 22.6% for bipolar disorder diagnosis (Wisner et al., 2013). New fathers can also be affected by PMADs. A meta-analysis of 43 studies over a 29-year span (Paulson & Bazemore, 2010) found a prevalence of PMADs in 10% of men. A moderate positive correlation between maternal depression and paternal depression was also found. There is an increased risk for PMADs in parents who experience high-risk pregnancy or when an infant is admitted to the neonatal intensive care unit (NICU). As parents deal with the stress and uncertainty involved with a high-risk pregnancy and possible NICU admission, it is vital for staff who work with both infants and their families to understand the risks for PMADs and learn how to recognize symptoms in these parents.

PMADs is an umbrella term that encompasses a set of disorders occurring during pregnancy and the first year postpartum. These disorders include major depression, generalized anxiety, panic disorder, obsessive–compulsive disorder, post-traumatic stress disorder, psychosis, and bipolar disorder. Although these disorders can occur at any time in life, some parents demonstrate an increase in reactivity during the perinatal period. Women often describe the changes in mood as "this feels different than my usual depression" or "I do not really feel depressed but more anxious," making it difficult to distinguish between typical stress, worry, and more clinically significant emotional distress.

PERINATAL MOOD AND ANXIETY DISORDERS

Perinatal Depression

The diagnostic criteria specified in the fifth edition of the *Diagnostic and Statistical Manual of Mental Disorders* (DSM-5; American Psychiatric Association [APA], 2013) for major depressive disorder (MDD) with peripartum onset states that this diagnosis can be made even without full criteria for MDD if it occurs during pregnancy or within the first 4 weeks postpartum. The symptoms that are often observed and reported by parents are sadness, tearfulness, and feeling that nothing is ever going to be the same again. Mothers are often withdrawn and have difficulty caring for themselves and their infant. Fathers with depression can appear withdrawn or uncaring because many often physically retreat or isolate. These behaviors can be perceived as feeling negative toward their partner or infant and can precipitate poor communication within the couple. Anger, irritability, and rage are often seen in both parents and may be a result of decreased sleep and increased stress, or they may be a sign of worsening mood (Fairbrother et al., 2016). Parents also need to be assessed for safety concerns including suicidal ideation, support systems, possible targeted therapy, and medication management.

CASE EXAMPLE 1

Kim was hospitalized for several weeks on the antepartum unit due to increased blood pressure and need for monitoring. She required a preterm, emergent cesarean section being diagnosed with pre-eclampsia. Kim's baby was admitted to the NICU at 32 weeks of gestation, and she was unable to see him for the first 48 hours after birth. Kim is noted to be sad and tearful. Her partner, John, appears quiet and withdrawn. These might be perceived as "typical" behaviors given the circumstances. Their infant had an uncomplicated course of treatment and at 4 weeks the staff and parents have begun discharge planning. As the parents are in the NICU, staff notice they do not talk much with each other or staff. John stands back and lets Kim ask questions; he just nods. After the team rounds on the infant, John leaves to get some coffee and Kim bursts into tears and states, "He never talks about the baby and I don't know how I am going to be able to do all of this." Kim is crying, does not want to help with her infant's care, and removes herself to sit in the corner of the room. She feels embarrassed by her outburst and states, "I never should have gotten pregnant, I can't do this, it is too hard and now I am losing my relationship too."

What is going on in this example? Is this perinatal depression, normal reactivity with lack of sleep, or the "baby blues"? Baby blues is regularly talked about but is not a mood disorder. It is the normal fluctuation of mood after birth brought on by significant hormonal adjustments and decreased sleep. It has been reported that up to 80% of all women may have some form of baby blues after birth. It is time limited and often resolves within the first 2 weeks postpartum. The predominant mood is happiness with periods of tearfulness and feeling overwhelmed (Bennett & Indman, 2019). Women with infants in the NICU may experience increased stress resulting in fluctuation in mood, worry, changes in sleep, changes in appetite, feelings of guilt, and possible feelings of detachment from their infant; however, these symptoms are generally short-lived.

In this vignette, the infant is more than 2 weeks old and the parents' symptoms no longer meet criteria for baby blues and may now meet criteria for major mood disorder with peripartum onset. Both parents are exhibiting symptoms of depression and may need further assessment and additional supports as they transition home with baby. Areas of needed support may include skills in communication, psychoeducation about sleep and diet, discussion about healthy coping skills, and self-care. Such support can be an important step in the treatment plan for the infant and discharge planning. As part of the discharge planning for this family, a referral should be made to perinatal trained providers to assess for the needs for therapy and medication management.

Generalized Anxiety Disorders

Generalized anxiety disorders that occur during the perinatal period are often overlooked and have not been studied as rigorously as perinatal depression. In Fairbrother et al.'s (2016) study of 310 women, perinatal anxiety was more prevalent than perinatal depression. Farr et al. (2013) found among 4,451 postpartum women that the prevalence of perinatal anxiety was 18%, with overall symptoms of perinatal depression at 6.3%.

Symptoms most often associated with perinatal anxiety are excessive worry and fears, difficulty falling and/or staying asleep, racing heart rate, and feelings of restlessness with ruminating thoughts (Fairbrother et al., 2016). Ruminating thoughts may include intrusive thoughts of harm to the infant that frighten parents. Examples include fear of dropping the infant down the stairs, sexual thoughts involving the infant, fear of stabbing the infant with a sharp object, thoughts about seeing the infant turn blue, and fear of drowning the infant in the bath. Although these thoughts are common for new parents, actual harm to the infant is rare. It is recommended to refer to a perinatal mental health professional for further assessment and to better understand the risk for safety. Providing psychoeducation regarding intrusive thoughts can help parents understand these are intrusive thoughts and not intentions.

CASE EXAMPLE 2

Jabina and her partner, Mark, were excited when they found out they were pregnant after trying for several years without success. Jabina had several early trimester losses, and now that she was moving into the third trimester, she had her hopes up. Then she began to experience leaking of her amniotic fluid and was admitted to the antepartum unit at the hospital. She began experiencing heightened worry and anxiety. She developed a fever and had an emergent cesarean section at 30 weeks of gestation. Her son was stabilized in the delivery room and transported to the NICU. When Jabina and Mark saw their son, he was intubated and monitoring was in place. It was a difficult sight, and Jabina began to cry. When the physician came to the bedside to tell the parents that their son had a heart defect, Jabina began to breathe rapidly, she felt dizzy, and she began to have chest pain with a rapid heart rate and profuse sweating.

What is happening? Is this a panic attack? In order to determine what Jabina is experiencing, medical conditions must first be ruled out. A diagnosis of a panic attack is made as an exclusion of any medical condition or substance use that could better explain the symptoms (APA, 2013). NICU staff can help decrease anxiety levels for parents by providing difficult news in a safe place; using calm, sensitive, validating language; and allowing parents to express their emotions without restraint. Being emotionally present for the parents as they process difficult news can decrease their stress and help establish a caring and trusting relationship with the staff.

Perinatal panic disorder is a type of perinatal anxiety disorder and is specified by recurrent panic attacks. A panic attack is described as a sudden feeling of intense fear or discomfort that peaks within minutes (APA, 2013). A panic attack can include symptoms of heart palpitations, sweating, shortness of breath, nausea, chest pain, paresthesia, and the fear of "losing control" or dying. A panic attack might be precipitated by new parents being told that their infant has a life-threatening condition or when an unexpected NICU admission occurs. Upon hearing this news, parents may feel a rush of fear and can have a sense of derealization or depersonalization preventing them from hearing what is said. Parents may experience symptoms of panic with specific triggers, such as when holding the baby or from the heightened smells or sounds in the NICU. They may also experience anxiety/panic attacks when away from the hospital, such as when they are driving or sleeping.

Perinatal Obsessive–Compulsive Disorder

The DSM-5 defines obsessions as recurrent and persistent thoughts with images that are disturbing, intrusive, and unwanted (APA, 2013). Compulsions are repetitive behaviors that the individual feels driven to perform in order to decrease levels of anxiety. There is no specifier for pregnancy or postpartum, but what has commonly been seen in the perinatal period is the need for cleaning/cleanliness, checking and rechecking, and a sense of order. These behaviors can manifest with either parent, and they often intensively focus on their infant and their environment being clean and safe. There may be a compulsion to check and recheck to determine if their sleeping infant is breathing and whether the house is locked. A preoccupation with death and dying of their infant or other family members is often seen with perinatal obsessive–compulsive disorder (OCD) and can lead to intrusive or "scary" thoughts or images (Collardeau et al., 2019). When an infant is in the NICU, these tendencies can increase greatly. The worry about germs and their infant becoming ill and/or dying increases, and thoughts can become intrusive.

Intrusive thoughts experienced with OCD are the most misunderstood symptoms of all the disorders. Intrusive thoughts are ego-dystonic, meaning that they are not in line with the parent's thoughts of "normal" behavior (Collardeau et al., 2019). Parents, particularly mothers, will "see" their infant in a scary or compromised position and will become extremely frightened, believing that if they think the thought, then it must mean it will come true. These images or thoughts involve harm coming to their infant or even of the parent harming the infant. A thought such as "What if I drop the baby?" can become a mental image of actually throwing the baby to the floor or down the stairs. Parents are often quite upset by these thoughts and need encouragement that the thoughts are just thoughts and are not an intent to harm. This can be an effective way to help parents normalize these thoughts and help them understand that being scared of the thoughts is the "normal" reaction to fear. It is helpful to normalize these thoughts and to educate parents that having these thoughts does not mean they have perinatal psychosis, as long as the thoughts remain ego-dystonic, but that they are a common symptom of postpartum OCD. Some common ways that parents may experience OCD symptoms include fear of contamination with germs, excessive hand washing, repeatedly checking the infant's breathing, fear of others touching and getting the baby sick, and the need to keep a schedule for the baby with feeding/sleep/diapers in order to control the parents' anxiety and worry. Unfortunately, sometimes these symptoms are misunderstood, and mothers are misdiagnosed as having postpartum depression with psychotic ideations or even postpartum psychosis and do not receive the appropriate treatment. Other times, if providers do not understand the nature of a parent's behavior or intrusive thoughts, they may assume that the infant is in danger and involve the Department of Child and Family Services, increasing parents' stress and worry.

Perinatal Bipolar Disorder

Bipolar disorder (BD) represents a complex set of symptoms when experienced in pregnancy and postpartum. BD is defined by the DSM-5 as distinct periods of depression (2 weeks) and either mania (1 week) or hypomania (4 days) that are required in order to meet diagnostic criteria (APA, 2013). The lifetime prevalence of BD, including bipolar spectrum disorder, is 3–6.5% in the general population, with equal and similar incidence in both men and women (Clark & Wisner, 2018). The average onset of BD is late adolescence (Wisner et al., 2019) when people are moving into the reproductive years, making women particularly vulnerable during pregnancy and postpartum for new onset or recurrence of BD (Clark & Wisner, 2018). In a study of women with diagnosed unipolar depression or BD, the women with BD had a 50% increased risk of relapse and were seven times more likely to be admitted to the hospital for the first time related to their mental health. In addition, women with a diagnosed history of BD had a 25–50% increased risk for developing perinatal psychosis (Sit & Wisner, 2009).

Risk factors for BD include a prior history of depression or a family history of BD. The mainstay of treatment is medication for stabilization and to prevent relapse. Unfortunately, many women on medications prior to pregnancy often discontinue them for fear of harm to their infant and can be supported in this by providers unfamiliar with the current research on the use of medications in pregnancy and lactation (Wisner et al., 2019). Untreated BD has been associated with preterm birth; low birth weight; intrauterine growth restriction; fetal distress; adverse neurodevelopmental outcomes in the infant; and maternal risk-taking behaviors, which are a hallmark of BD. Risky behaviors can include decreased prenatal care, poor nutrition, participating in high-risk sexualized behavior, impulsive shopping/spending of money, and/or substance abuse. Behaviors that mothers with untreated BD might present in the NICU setting could include irritability, high energy, impulsivity, combativeness, inability to process information, and waxing and waning mood. These symptoms may also be indicative of untreated PMADs in general, so further assessment is necessary.

Balancing the risk of untreated BD complications with risks to the fetus of using medication is imperative to benefit mother and infant and ensure a stable and engaged parental attachment. A second and equally important aspect of both treated and untreated BD during pregnancy and postpartum is the increased incidence of perinatal psychosis (Wisner et al., 2019).

Perinatal Psychosis

The prevalence of perinatal psychosis is 1–2% per 1,000, and it is considered a medical emergency (Osborne, 2018). Perinatal psychosis is perhaps the most dangerous and misunderstood illness associated with PMADs. Onset is usually sudden and often within the first 2 weeks postpartum. With clinical features of "delirium-like waxing and waning of consciousness, disorganization and confusion, depersonalization, and bizarre delusions [often concerning the child or childbirth]," perinatal psychosis poses a threat to both mother and infant (Osborne, 2018, p. 456). Early warning signs and symptoms include insomnia, anxiety, irritability, paranoia, and mood fluctuations. Recognizing these early symptoms can help the provider be proactive with treatment and may help decrease the severity and longevity of the illness.

The differential diagnosis of perinatal psychosis from perinatal OCD with intrusive thoughts can be complex. Intrusive thoughts (obsessions) are common with OCD and are characterized as frightening and unwanted thoughts. Delusions in perinatal psychosis are a fixed belief, and although they might seem frightening to mothers, mothers are often not disturbed by them and feel compelled to act upon these beliefs (Osborne, 2018).

An inpatient psychiatric hospitalization for medical stabilization and ongoing medication management is commonly needed for perinatal psychosis. Assessing risk versus benefits of treatment is part of the provider's responsibly because untreated perinatal psychosis can create a dangerous condition, with maternal suicide rates at 5% and infanticide rates at 4% (Spinelli, 2009). Having a multidisciplinary treatment team is vital to the care of the mother, her infant, and the family unit. Stabilization of BD with a mood stabilizer and possible antipsychotics has been found to decrease risk. Continuing pre-pregnancy medication and reviewing risks versus benefits of these medications, as well as risks of untreated illness, are an integral part of informed consent (Spinelli, 2009). Providing evidence-based information is necessary for helping mothers make the best decisions for themselves and their infants. Finally, psychoeducation and involvement of the family in the mother's care provide for better outcomes post hospitalization.

Risk and Protective Factors

Developing a PMAD is one of the most common complications in the perinatal period. Multiple factors can predispose an individual to this risk. A biological family history of mood disorders or having a previous maternal mood disorder are two of the most common risk factors. Prior sensitivity to hormonal changes during menstrual cycles and with the use of birth control can also be a risk factor. For a subset of women with PMAD symptoms, they are triggered by the rapid, hormonal changes of pregnancy and placental delivery, as well as the hormonal changes that accompany lactation. Additional medical conditions including thyroid imbalance and other endocrine-related illnesses have been reported as risk factors during the perinatal period.

Epigenetic/Biological Factors

Epigenetics has been shown to play an important role in one's predisposition to PMADs. Elwood et al. (2019) reported in their systematic review that a subset of women who had a predisposition to postnatal depressive disorder because of hereditary factors had a heightened sensitivity to the psychological changes during childbirth. That is, the stress of childbirth often triggered or set into motion the epigenetic changes that were genetically present. An international group of researchers formed a consortium—Postpartum Depression: Action Towards Causes and Treatment (PACT)—to better understand how genetic markers interact with environmental stressors, which will improve understanding of the etiology of postpartum depression. The PACT consortium has developed a telephone application for data collection to better understand how genetics play a role in maternal mental health (Guintivano et al., 2018). This application screens women who have a lifetime history of PMADs and collects a salivary sample for analysis in the hope of finding a genetic connection leading to early or proactive identification of women who are genetically susceptible to PMADs.

The area of epigenetics that has been most studied involves the methylation of DNA. Methylation is a process in which an additional methyl is added to DNA. This modifies the gene expression by turning off or repressing the gene expression. Environmental exposures can alter methylation, as can inherited changes in DNA. These changes have been implicated in mental health disorders (Lin & Tsai, 2019).

Oxytocin is also a key regulator in stress and anxiety, and the epigenetic variability in the oxytocin receptors has been linked to postnatal depression (McEvoy et al., 2017), making the postpartum period especially sensitive to these changes. The rapid decrease in estrogen and progesterone at birth is often the trigger for these changes. Several studies have shown that the effects of epigenetics on mood happen within four weeks of birth (Elwood et al., 2019; McEvoy et al., 2017). Combining the stress of birth with an infant admitted to the NICU can then become a "perfect storm" for parents who are potentially susceptible to these genetic and epigenetic changes.

COMORBID MATERNAL MEDICAL COMPLICATIONS

In the holistic model of care and treatment, it is important to understand what pre-existing medical conditions parents may have experienced and how co-occurring medical conditions can affect moods. Research shows that chronic medical conditions such as diabetes, epilepsy, or hypertension may increase the risk for depression and anxiety (Fisher et al., 2016). When adding a chronic medical condition to the stress of a high-risk pregnancy or having a preterm infant or an infant who requires the specialized care in the NICU, it is important to consider how this scenario might complicate an already fragile family.

Fertility Challenges

Parents who experience fertility challenges may encounter higher levels of stress throughout the pregnancy and postpartum period. Lynch and Prasad (2014) did not find a correlation between depression and fertility treatments. Likewise, in a cross-sectional study including 40,337 women using data from the Centers for Disease Control and Prevention's (CDC) Pregnancy Risk Assessment Monitoring

System, 12.9% of mothers reported feelings of depression and 6% reported feeling hopeless. The study did not find a correlation between depression and fertility after adjusting for confounder effects. However, when combined with complications such as preterm delivery, fetal loss of a singleton in a multiple gestation, and/or admission to the NICU, there was an increased risk of postpartum mental health symptoms (Lynch & Prasad, 2014).

Diabetes

Managing a chronic illness such as type I diabetes mellitus (DM) can also lead to emotional stress (Fisher, 2016). In a prospective study, Hinkle et al. (2016) found a moderate association between depression in pregnancy and the incidence of gestational DM. This study highlighted the increased susceptibility, during this time frame, for the interplay of depression and glucose intolerance phenotypes (Hinkle et al., 2016). It is common for infants to be admitted to the NICU for glucose stabilization. This can increase a stress response from parents and possibly be the trigger for postpartum anxiety and depression. Parents with type I/type II DM express concern for themselves and fear that their infant will have long-term sequelae from their chronic conditions, which adds to the parents' stress.

Hypertension

Both chronic and new-onset hypertension are another subset of medical and co-occurring disorders that can affect the mood of the mother during pregnancy and the postpartum period. It is well known that chronic hypertension and depression are often seen together (Li et al., 2015). Determining the exact prevalence is difficult secondary to variance in depression rating scales, but it is estimated that one in three people with hypertension also have a co-occurring diagnosis of depression, which increases the risk in the perinatal population. Pre-eclampsia, both mild and severe, has also been shown to trigger a depressive episode in mothers. In one of the first studies examining the impact of pre-eclampsia on the mood of the mother, Hoedjes et al. (2011) found that although severe pre-eclampsia was associated with depression, the consequences of the illness (e.g., prolonged maternal hospital admission, emergency delivery, admission to the NICU, and/or prenatal death) dictated the severity of the depression.

Chronic Pain

The prevalence of chronic pain and depression as comorbid conditions is becoming increasingly recognized, and these conditions seem to occur at higher rates together than either alone (Darakhshan, 2019). In a meta-analysis, Darakhshan (2019) found roughly 65% of the study subjects with clinical symptoms of depression also had chronic pain. Treatment for chronic pain is often with opioid medications that increase the risk of a NICU admission at birth (Ray-Griffith et al., 2018). Chronic pain and the presence of opioid medications can be a double stressor for parents, along with the realization that their treatment for pain may be one of the medical reasons for the NICU admission. Nonjudgmental attitudes are most effective when helping families cope with the stress of a dual diagnosis of chronic pain and opioid addiction. A mother who is in treatment for an opioid use disorder because of chronic pain, a medical illness, or self-medicating needs to be supported in her ongoing treatment while she is also caring for her new infant. Helping mothers and their partners see the benefit of treatment even with the difficulty of seeing their infant in withdrawal is part of the support needed to prevent added trauma during this already difficult time.

Effects of Adverse Childhood Events

Adverse childhood experiences (ACEs) are distressing events that occur during the first 18 years of life, such as emotional, physical, and sexual abuse, as well as a variety of different forms of dysfunction in the home, including parental separation, violence, and mental illness (Angerud et al., 2018). Studies have shown that experiencing a high number of ACEs can increase the risk for poor psychosocial outcomes and result in higher rates of mental health and medical concerns over the course of a person's lifetime. Research with pregnant and postpartum mothers has indicated that ACEs may increase the risk for mental health concerns for both mothers and their infants. McDonald and colleagues (2019) found that mothers who reported three or more ACEs were more likely to struggle with PMADs. These mothers were seen to be at a higher risk for experiencing difficulties with parenting and may choose maladaptive coping strategies in times of high stress. Women with higher levels of childhood maltreatment may also be at increased risk for higher levels of depressive symptoms that can persist for long periods of time (McDonnell & Valentino, 2016). Danese and McEwen (2012) hypothesized that ACEs may lead to perinatal depression through a process of biological embedding because the endocrine, immune, and nervous systems are altered due to the repeated and high levels of stress exposure. It is important for health care providers to assess for ACEs in parents. It is crucial for providers to understand how past experiences might impact new parents and may influence how they cope with the heightened stress of medical complications or a NICU admission.

Teen Pregnancy

According to the CDC, in 2017, the birth rate for women aged 15–19 years was 18.8 per 1,000. Although the numbers continue to be near record lows, the teen pregnancy rate is substantially higher in the United States than in other Western industrialized nations, and racial/ethnic and geographic disparities in teen birth rates persist (CDC, 2019). The rate of depression identified for pregnant teens is higher than that for their nonpregnant peers, varying between 25% and 42% (Corocoran, 2016). It is widely acknowledged that teen pregnancy and early motherhood can be associated with increased risk for mental and physical health problems, social isolation, poor educational outcomes, poverty, and other related social factors. Many of these psychosocial factors may be the cause for teen pregnancy, as well as a long-term consequence of teen pregnancy. Teen mothers must find ways to integrate their life roles as an adolescent, student, daughter, and partner with their role as a new mother. When a teen becomes pregnant, a number of these developmental tasks may be impacted. The constant demands and responsibilities associated with being a parent can impact the opportunity to develop these important developmental skills, putting these teen mothers at an increased risk for PMADs.

According to Corcoran (2016), teen mothers who are depressed may be emotionally unavailable to attend to their infant's emotional needs. They may feel a sense of helplessness while learning how to parent and deal with everyday parenting challenges. Having a baby in the NICU with multiple medical needs can prove challenging for teen mothers as they learn how significant these needs may be for their infant or the risk for potential long-term effects. According to Boss and colleagues (2009), teens often believed that NICU nursing staff offered useful information in day-to-day interactions. However, many teens did not believe their infant's physicians provided them with understandable information, and they often struggled with asking questions to better understand medical information. Health care providers have a duty to assess what questions teen parents might have and provide them with clear information so they can make appropriate health care decisions for their infants.

Teen mothers may also struggle with attachment to their infants. Long-term adverse consequences can be seen in cognitive, adaptive, and behavioral domains in infants with poor attachment to their primary caregiver (Flaherty & Sadler, 2011). According to Flaherty and Sadler, "Adolescent mothers may not intuitively be able to assume these characteristics that foster secure attachment because of their own developmental stage" (p. 114). It is essential for health care providers working with teen mothers of hospitalized infants to assess for and identify the signs of poor attachment. Providing encouragement and modeling of appropriate parenting skills can assist with fostering a healthy attachment, which is an important building block for healthy long-term outcomes for these infants.

PROTECTIVE FACTORS

Although it is not possible to prevent PMADs, there are things that can be done to help reduce symptom severity. Medical providers (obstetricians and pediatricians) who provide ongoing care should conduct regular screenings to identify patients experiencing possible PMADs. Ongoing psychoeducation about risks and symptoms should occur during pregnancy and in the postpartum period, and discussing ways to cope if PMADs occur can help lessen symptoms. self-care including sleep hygiene, good nutrition, exercise and utilizing a support network are a few of the tools individuals can utilize to help reduce symptoms. Providing education regarding PMADs to mothers, families, and their health care providers demystifies the illness and can reduce the fear and anxiety associated with reaching out for help.

Health care providers can help support women and their families by exploring their own thoughts and biases regarding PMADs. Understanding beliefs about mental health illness can make their care and support more genuine and compassionate, which can assist in preventing additional stress and trauma. Having a mood disorder or anxiety, whether it is a chronic illness or triggered by the birth of an infant, often leaves families emotionally raw, irritable, and sometimes angry. Health care providers may also be impacted by the difficult emotions and stories of others, touching places that are tender and may reflect areas of unhealed trauma.

IDEAS WORTH SHARING

What can health care providers do to help parents on antepartum units and in the NICU?

- Support parents in a nonjudgmental way by encouraging them to "tell their birth story." Trauma is often experienced differently by each parent. By allowing them to tell their story, they can begin the healing process. Validate their feelings of sadness, fear, and inadequacy as parents with compassion and understanding.
- Encourage parents to talk about their feelings related to their pregnancy, birth, and NICU experience. This gives parents courage, and talking about their feelings can help them process difficulties and also see the positives. Allowing for this discussion provides an opportunity to process and cope with the variety of emotions they may be experiencing.
- Reinforce that they are the parents and they know their infant better than anyone else does. Provide supportive feedback when parents are caring for and bonding with their infant. Allow parents to help with the first bath or put on the first outfit. This encourages them to bond with their infant and helps them feel they have a role as parents. This can help them to not retreat inward emotionally.
- Ask parents what cultural or religious traditions they might like to integrate into caring for their infant while in the NICU. Integrating the family's cultural and religious traditions acknowledges the importance of these traditions and will allow the family to begin building positive memories despite being in the NICU environment.
- Assess for symptoms of worsening moods and anxiety that may impact parents' ability to bond with their infant or other symptoms that develop

that may indicate a worsening condition, and refer to a mental health provider if necessary. Provide psychoeducation regarding postpartum depression and anxiety and risk factors due to having an infant in the NICU. Provide information on resources that are available to support antepartum families or new NICU parents. Educate on the critical importance of self-care, sleep, proper nutrition, and utilizing family and social supports during this time. Psychoeducation regarding postpartum depression and anxiety provides an opportunity for the mother and her partner to ask questions and to help them understand any emotions and reactions they may be experiencing. Having this discussion also allows for parents to feel more comfortable asking for further resources or support. New parents, particularly NICU parents, often need reminders of the importance of managing their own needs and well-being during times of stress.

- Prepare new parents for what the transition from the NICU to home with their infant might look like, and remind them that they continue to be at risk for new onset of PMADs after that time. Discuss the mix of feelings that parents may feel as they get close to discharge and the fears that they may feel about their ability to manage once they are home. NICU staff can help parents identify community resources that might be available to them once they are home if they find they are in need of additional support.

CONCLUSION

When parents experience the stress and trauma of a high-risk pregnancy or having their infant in the NICU, they are at increased risk for experiencing PMADs. Although sadness and worry may be a normal reaction to this experience, it can be difficult to determine whether challenges with mood and anxiety precipitate or are the sequelae of stress and the intensity of a NICU stay. Parents often find themselves in a world of unknowns and much uncertainty, having to learn about medical illness and rare neonatal conditions during what should be one of the happiest times of their lives. Parents may not understand their own risk factors or be able to identify symptoms of depression and anxiety, which puts antepartum and NICU staff in an important position to provide necessary support and resources for new parents. Interventions that validate the difficulties these families are facing may be an important buffer and lessen the intensity of their grief and trauma response. This can also provide an opportunity to educate new parents about PMADs and to help them identify symptoms they may be struggling with prior to their infant going home. Encouraging these discussions will help destigmatize PMADs and dispel any myths that may fuel reluctance to seek support. Finally, there is still much work to do to continue increasing support available in all hospitals and providing new parents with the resources needed while their infant remains in NICU care.

REFERENCES

American Psychiatric Association. (2013). *Diagnostic and statistical manual of mental disorders* (5th ed.).

Angerud, K., Annerback, E.-M., Tyden, T., Boddeti, S., & Kristiansson, P. (2018). Adverse childhood experiences and depressive symptomatology among pregnant women. *Acta Obstetricia et Gynecologica Scandinavica, 97*(6), 701–708.

Bennett, S. S., & Indman, P. (2019). *Beyond the blues: Understanding and treating prenatal and postpartum depression and anxiety.* Untreed Reads.

Boss, R. D., Donohue, P. K., & Arnold, R. M. (2009). Adolescent mothers in the NICU: How much do they understand? *Journal of Perinatology, 30,* 286–290.

Centers for Disease Control and Prevention. (2019). *Reproductive health: Teen pregnancy.* https://www.cdc.gov/teenpregnancy/about/index.htm

Clark, C., & Wisner, K. L. (2018). Treatment of peripartum bipolar disorder. *Obstetrics and Gynecology Clinics of North America, 45*(3), 403–417. https://doi.org/10.1016/j.ogc.2018.05.002

Collardeau, F., Corbyn, B., Abramowitz, J., Janssen, P., Woody, S., & Fairbrother, N. (2019). Maternal unwanted and intrusive thoughts of infant-related harm, obsessive–compulsive disorder and depression in the perinatal period: Study protocol. *BMC Psychiatry, 19,* Article 94. https://doi.org/10.1186/s12888-019-2067-x

Corocoran, J. (2016). Teenage pregnancy and mental health. *Societies, 6*(3), 21. https://doi.org/10.3390/soc6030021

Danese, A., & McEwen, B. S. (2012). Adverse childhood experiences, allostasis, all static load, and age-related disease. *Physiological Behavior, 106,* 29–39. https://doi.org/10.1016/j.physbeh.2011.08.019

Darakhshan, J. H. (2019). Targeting serotonin 1A receptors for treating chronic pain and depression. *Current Neuropharmacology, 7*(12), 1098–1108. https://doi.org/10.2174/1570159X17666190811161807

Elwood, J., Murray, E., Bell, A., Sinclair, M., Kernohan, W. G., & Stockdale, J. (2019). A systematic review investigating if genetic or epigenetic markers are associated with postnatal depression. *Journal of Affective Disorders, 253*(15), 51–62. https://doi.org/10.1016/j.jad.2019.04.059

Fairbrother, N., Janssen, P., Antony, M. M., Tucker, E., & Young, A. H. (2016). Perinatal anxiety disorder prevalence and incidence. *Journal of Affective Disorders, 200,* 148–155. https://doi.org/10.1016/j.jad.2015.12.082

Farr, S. L., Dietz, P. M., O'Hara, M. W., Burley, K., & Ko, J. Y. (2013). Postpartum anxiety and comorbid depression in a population-based sample of women. *Journal of Women's Health, 23*(2), 120–128. https://doi.org/10.1089/jwh.2013.4438

Fisher, L., Hessler, D. M., Masharani, U., Peters, A. L., Blumer, I., & Strycker, L. A. (2016). Prevalence of depression in type I diabetes and the problem of over-diagnosis. *Diabetic Medicine, 33*(11), 1590–1597. https://doi.org/10.1111/dme.12973

Flaherty, S. C., & Sadler, L. S. (2011). A review of attachment theory in the context of adolescent parenting. *Journal of Pediatric Health Care, 25*(2), 114–121.

Guintivano, J., Krohn, H., Lewis, C., Byrne, E. M., Henders, A. K., Sullivan, P., & Meltzer-Brody, S. (2018). PPD ACT: An app-based genetic study of postpartum depression. *Translational Psychiatry, 8,* 260.

Hinkle, S. N., Buck Louis, G. M., Rawal, S., Zhu, Y., Albert, P. S., & Zhang, C. (2016). A longitudinal study of depression and gestational diabetes in pregnancy and the postpartum period. *Diabetologia, 59,* 2594–2602. https://doi.org/10.1007/s00 125-016-4086-1

Hoedjes, M., Berks, D., Vogel, I., & Franx, A. (2011). Postpartum depression after mild and severe preeclampsia. *Journal of Women's Health, 20*(10), 1535–1542.

Li, Z., Li, Y., Chen, L., Chen, P., & Hu, Y. (2015). Prevalence of depression in patients with hypertension: A systematic review and meta-analysis. *Medicine, 94*(31), 1317.

Lin, E., & Tsai, S.-J. (2019). Epigenetics and depression: An update. *Psychiatry Investigation, 16*(9), 654-661. https://doi.org/10.30773/pi.2019.07.17.2

Lynch, C. D., & Prasad, M. R. (2014). Association between infertility treatment and symptoms of postpartum depression. *Fertility and Sterility, 102*(5), 1416–1421.

McDonald, S. W., Madigan, S., Racine, N., Benzies, K., Tomfohr, L., & Tough, S. (2019). Maternal adverse childhood experiences, mental health, and child behaviour at age 3: The All Our Families Community Cohort Study. *Preventive Medicine, 118,* 286–294.

McDonnell, C. G., & Valentino, K. (2016). Intergenerational effects of childhood trauma: Evaluating pathways among maternal ACESs, perinatal depressive symptoms, and infant outcomes. *Child Maltreatment, 21*(4), 317–326.

McEvoy, K., Osborne, L. M., Nanavati, J., & Payne, J. L. (2017). Reproductive affective disorders: A review of the evidence for premenstrual dysphoric disorder and post-partum depression. *Reproductive Psychiatry and Women's Health, 19,* Article 94. https://doi.org/10.1007/s11920-017-0852-0

Osborne, L. M. (2018). Recognizing and managing postpartum psychosis: A clinical guide for obstetric providers. *Obstetrics and Gynecology Clinics of North America, 45*(3), 455–468. https://doi.org/10.1016/j.ogc.2018.04.005

Paulson, J. F., & Bazemore, S. (2010). Prenatal and postpartum depression in fathers and its association with maternal depression: A meta-analysis. *JAMA Network, 303*(19), 1961–1969. https://doi.org/10.1001/jama.2010.605

Ray-Griffith, S., Wendel, M. P., Stowe, Z. N., & Magann, E. F. (2018). Chronic pain during pregnancy: A review of the literature. *International Journal of Women's Health, 10,* 153–164.

Sit, D. K. Y., & Wisner, K. L. (2009). Identification of postpartum depression. *Clinical Obstetrics and Gynecology, 52*(3), 456–468. https://doi.org/10.1097/GRF.0b013e318 1b5a57c

Spinelli, M. G. (2009). Postpartum psychosis: Detection of risk and management. *American Journal of Psychiatry, 166*(4), 405–408. https://doi.org/10.1176/appi. ajp.2008.08121899

Wisner, K. L., Sit, D. K. Y., & McShea, M. C. (2013). Onset timing, thoughts of self-harm, and diagnoses in postpartum women with screen-positive depression findings. *JAMA Network, 70*(5), 490–498. https://doi.org/10.1001/jamapsychiatry.2013.87

Wisner, K. L., Sit, D. K. Y., O'Shea, K., Bogen, D. L., Clark, C., Pinheiro, E., Yang, A., & Ciolino, J. D. (2019). Bipolar disorder and psychotropic medication: Impact on pregnancy and neonatal outcomes. *Journal of Affective Disorders, 243*(15), 220–225. https://doi.org/10.1016/j.jad.2018.09.045

10

SCREENING FOR PERINATAL MOOD AND ANXIETY DISORDERS ACROSS SETTINGS

AMY E. BAUGHCUM, OLIVIA E. CLARK, SHANNON L. GILLESPIE, AND JEANNE DECKER ■

The prevalence rate of postpartum depression (PPD) is approximately 13–19% (O'Hara & McCabe, 2013), and postpartum anxiety estimates range from 11% to 17% of new mothers within this general population (Fairbrother et al., 2015; McCabe-Beane et al., 2018). Parents of high-risk infants experience perinatal mood and anxiety disorders (PMADs) at even higher rates due to the unique stress of complicated pregnancy and hospitalization in the neonatal intensive care unit (NICU) (Hynan et al., 2013). Research has shown that PMADs are associated with poorer outcomes for parents and infants alike (Gaynes et al., 2005; Hall et al., 2017). Maternal depression is well known to negatively impact the dyadic relationship between parent and child, including decreased warmth and responsiveness (Rogers et al., 2020). This can subsequently impact infant neurodevelopment longer term, which is especially important to consider in the context of infants who are already at increased neurodevelopmental risk due to prematurity and/or other medical diagnoses.

There are inherent risks for all new parents, and experiences in the NICU may exacerbate mood symptoms. In particular, the NICU course may increase significant emotional distress due to fluctuating infant medical status; altered sleep, eating, and self-care patterns; disruptions to planned transition to parenthood; concerns about other children and responsibilities; and stressors of the hospital environment (Hoffman et al., 2021). NICU admission may also distance parents and families from culturally relevant coping mechanisms and social supports. Some stress reactions may be adaptive because they may lead to re-prioritizing values, mobilizing resources, and utilizing social support; however, distinguishing between adaptive and problematic stress responses may be challenging for providers in the NICU. Furthermore, heightened situational stress for families in the NICU is quite common and does not represent pathology but, rather, highlights the need to promote parental adjustment and coping during the NICU admission to prevent clinical levels of emotional disturbance (Hynan et al., 2013). Most often, screening for emotional distress is conducted via in-person or phone interview by a social worker integrated into that particular setting. However, this type of service may not be readily available, and using a screening tool may help alert staff to parental distress. Therefore, efficient screening for PMADs, particularly use of brief questionnaires, has been recommended as an important element of triaging appropriate support for parents in the NICU (Hynan et al., 2013).

GUIDELINES

The U.S. Preventive Services Task Force revised the recommendation to screen all adults for depression by adding a specification for pregnant and postpartum women (Siu et al., 2016). This helped spur subsequent legislation and states' efforts to address this issue (Rhodes & Segre, 2013). Although this was a major step in improving clinical care, implementation has been a challenge, and only four states currently mandate PPD screening (Illinois, Massachusetts, New Jersey, and West Virginia; Rowan et al., 2015). Multidisciplinary work groups (e.g., American Academy of Pediatrics [AAP], American College of Obstetrics and Gynecology [ACOG], March of Dimes [MOD], National Perinatal Association [NPA], and Postpartum Support International) recommend consideration of universal postpartum screening for new parents, particularly those within the NICU, to not only assess for mood disorders but also screen for post-traumatic stress symptoms (Earls, 2010; Kendig et al., 2017; O'Connor et al., 2016; Willis et al., 2018). ACOG recommends obstetric care providers screen patients at least once during the prenatal period for depression and anxiety symptoms as well as perform a full assessment during the comprehensive postpartum visit. The NPA advocates for extensive and routine screening for depression throughout pregnancy, following the birth, and throughout a NICU admission. The NPA also recognizes the importance of training NICU staff and other health care providers involved in peripartum care to recognize signs and symptoms of perinatal mood and anxiety disorders, with specific attention to the effects of race, class, culture, and ethnicity on clinical presentations (Willis et al., 2018). This research, however, is lacking, and culturally responsive evaluation and treatment approaches are underdeveloped.

Similarly, the AAP urges implementation of screening for maternal depression into prenatal visits and well-child visits following the birth. However, given that infants admitted to the NICU are not yet attending well-child visits, the onus falls to health care providers in the NICU (Earls, 2010). MOD offers that universal, routine screening for PPD and post-traumatic stress disorder (PTSD) in conjunction with management and treatment efforts (i.e., counseling and collaboration among health care providers) should be incorporated into postpartum care (Berns, 2010).

Specifically, MOD recommends women be screened for PPD at minimum once between 2 and 12 weeks postpartum. Routine screening earlier than 2 weeks after giving birth may result in false positives because women often experience "maternity blues" (i.e., transient anxiety, tearfulness, or mood changes) during this time. If a mother screens negative for PPD during these first few weeks, then she may need to be screened again later because onset of PMADs can occur any time from pregnancy through the first year postpartum.

These valuable screening guidelines and efforts are primarily concerned with PPD symptoms; there is a notable lack of screening guidelines pertaining specifically to anxiety disorders (McCabe-Beane et al., 2018). Significant comorbidity across depression and anxiety disorders should be recognized; however, mandated screening that focuses primarily on depression may allow parents with maladaptive anxiety symptoms to go undetected, which may have significant implications for these families in the postpartum period, both in the NICU and following discharge. Research indicates a need for further validation of anxiety measures for this population to better determine screening and clinical cutoff guidelines (McCabe-Beane et al., 2018).

In general, benefits offered by screening in the NICU include early identification of mood disorder risk factors, linkage to support services and resources, and raising awareness of potential vulnerabilities for the care team. However, there is limited evidence to suggest that widespread screening leads to better treatment outcomes within the general population. Critics argue screening could lead to overdiagnosis and inappropriate prescription of antidepressant medication (Mojtabai, 2017; Rhodes & Segre, 2013). This argument may be relevant for general population screening, but parents of high-risk infants represent a higher risk group and potentially derive greater benefit from early identification and access to treatment. In both cases, antidepressants and nonpharmacological treatments (including psychotherapy and support groups) may be potential effective treatment options and should be encouraged on an individual basis.

Following screening and follow-up evaluation from a positive screen, mental health interventions for parents in the NICU may focus on managing stress, improving family function, and/or cultivating parent–infant bonding, while working to manage PPD, anxiety, and PTSD symptoms (Hoffman et al., 2021). These services may be provided within the NICU or fetal medicine clinic and/ or later post-discharge through follow-up clinics. Parents may be able to receive mental health support within the health care setting itself through use of embedded providers or through referral to community providers. Importantly, experts recommend that screening be carried out only if and when support and treatment options are readily available (Hoffman et al., 2021).

SCREENING MEASURES

For a description of commonly used screening tools in perinatal settings, see Table 10.1. Most tools are designed for the general population, but some are specific

Table 10.1 MENTAL HEALTH SCREENING INSTRUMENTS COMMONLY USED FOR PARENTS OF INFANTS

Screening Tool	Domain Assessed	No. of Items	Public Domain	Notes
Edinburgh Perinatal Depression Scale (EPDS)[a]	Perinatal depression	10	Yes	Available in several languages; contains suicidal ideation question
Postpartum Depression Screening Scale (PDSS)[b]	Postpartum depression	35	No	Contains suicidal ideation question; has total score and seven subscale scores
Public Health Questionnaire (PHQ-2, PHQ-9)[c]	Depression in the general population; validated in perinatal population	2, 9	Yes	PHQ-2 uses the first two items of the PHQ-9; lower specificity than others; available in several languages
Center for Epidemiological Studies Depression Scale (CES-D)[d]	Depression in the general population	20	Yes	Original does not have suicidal ideation question, but revised version does
Columbia Suicide Severity Rating Scale (CSSRS) Lifetime/Recent[e]	Suicide risk assessment	2–6, structured interview	Yes	Spanish versions available; full-scale version also available for those who are trained
Impact of Events Scale–Revised (IES-R)[f]	Post-traumatic stress	22	Yes	Four symptom clusters
Davidson Trauma Scale[g]	Post-traumatic stress	17	No	Three symptom clusters
PTSD Checklist for DSM-5 (PCL-5)[h]	Post-traumatic stress	20	Yes	Items map onto DSM-5 diagnostic criteria
Modified Perinatal Post-Traumatic Stress Disorder Questionnaire (modified PPQ)[i]	Perinatal specific post-traumatic stress	14	Yes	Maps onto three symptom clusters
General Anxiety Disorder (GAD-7)[j]	Anxiety	7	Yes	Has item examining functional impact

[a] Cox, J. L., Holden, J. M., & Sagovsky, R. (1987). *Edinburgh Postnatal Depression Scale* [Measurement instrument]. https://med.stanford.edu/content/dam/sm/ppc/documents/DBP/EDPS_text_added.pdf

[b] Beck, C. T., & Gable, R. K. (2002). (PDSS) *Postpartum Depression Screening Scale* [Measurement instrument]. https://www.wpspublish.com/pdss-postpartum-depression-screening-scale

[c] Spitzer, R. L., Williams, J. B., & Kroenke, K. (1999). *Patient Health Questionnaire-9* [Measurement instrument]. https://www.phqscreeners.com

[d] Radloff, L. S. (1977). *Center for Epidemiologic Studies Depression Scale (CES-D)* [Measurement instrument]. http://www.chcr.brown.edu/pcoc/cesdscale.pdf

[e] The Columbia Lighthouse Project. (2007). *Columbia-Suicide Severity Rating Scale (C-SSRS)* [Measurement instrument]. http://cssrs.columbia.edu/the-columbia-scale-c-ssrs/about-the-scale

[f] Weiss, D. S., & Marmar, C. R. (1996). *The Impact of Event Scale–Revised (IES-R)* [Measurement instrument]. https://www.ptsd.va.gov/professional/assessment/adult-sr/ies-r.asp

[g] Davidson, J. R. T., Book, S. W., Colket, J. T., Tupler, L. A., Roth, S., David, D., Hertzberg, M., Mellman, T., Beckham, J. C., Smith, R., Davison, R. M., Katz, R., & Feldman, M. (1997). *Davidson Trauma Scale (DTS) for DSM-IV* [Measurement instrument]. https://www.ptsd.va.gov/professional/assessment/adult-sr/dts.asp

[h] Weathers, F. W., Litz, B. T., Keane, T. M., Palmieri, P. A., Marx, B. P., & Schnurr, P. P. (2013). *The PTSD Checklist for DSM-5 (PCL-5)* [Measurement instrument]. https://www.ptsd.va.gov/professional/assessment/adult-sr/ptsd-checklist.asp

[i] Callahan, J. L., Borja, S. E., & Hynan, M. T. (2006). *Modified Perinatal Post-Traumatic Stress Disorder Questionnaire (modified PPQ)* [Measurement instrument]. https://www.nature.com/articles/7211562/tables/6

[j] Spitzer, R. L., Kroenke, K., Williams, J. B. W., & Lowe, B. (2006). *General Anxiety Disorder (GAD-7)* [Measurement instrument]. https://jamanetwork.com/journals/jamainternalmedicine/fullarticle/410326

to postpartum individuals. Regardless, these questionnaires can be applied to perinatal settings. However, not all questionnaire items may seem applicable to parents within these settings, and the measures are not normed for these settings. For example, the Edinburgh Perinatal Depression Scale (EPDS) contains items that start with "I have been anxious or worried" or "I have felt scared or panicky" and conclude with "for no good reason." This can be confusing because parents in the fetal care and the NICU settings may experience these feelings as normative reactions to parenting a child with a medical condition. Parents may be unsure how to most accurately respond to these items. Therefore, caution should be used in interpreting results because there is potential for confusion and underreporting for certain individuals, including fathers and parents who culturally may be reluctant to share about their true emotional status.

General Screening

Parents with an infant admitted to the NICU may experience high levels of distress. Distress may manifest in many ways, including symptoms of depression, traumatic stress, and anxiety; therefore, more broad screeners for general distress may prove useful as well. The Brief Symptom Inventory (BSI-18) and the Symptom Checklist-90–Revised (SCL-90-R) are valuable in assessing distress in this population, although they are broad. The Clinical Interview for High-Risk Parents of Premature Infants (CLIP) is a semistructured interview designed for parents of infants in the NICU for evaluation of distress beyond particular diagnoses (Hynan et al., 2013). The Psychosocial Assessment Tool (PAT) has been recently revised (PAT-NICU/CICU) and piloted within a large NICU population and found to be a helpful screener for overall family psychosocial risk across several key domains, including caregiver problems, caregiver support, stress reactions, family structure/resources, and family beliefs (Pai et al., 2008).

These more general measures tend to be more extensive and thus time-intensive than those pertaining to a specific mood issue, but they may provide greater insight into what parents are experiencing beyond mood symptomatology. It is important to note, as well, that measures of PMADs may not take into account adverse childhood experiences, other sources of stress and vulnerability (e.g., food insecurity), or culturally specific expressions of PMADs. However, this type of general evaluation can help triage parents who require minimal resources (universal); those who require more significant intervention (targeted); and those who require intensive psychosocial care and support (clinical), which is particularly beneficial for NICUs with limited psychosocial staff (Kazak, 2006).

Postpartum Depression

Most research on PPD has focused on mothers, although fathers/partners may also experience PPD symptoms, with greater prevalence among fathers in the

NICU (Hynan et al., 2013). From research on mothers, screening programs with or without additional treatment-related support have been demonstrated to reduce depression prevalence in pregnant and postpartum women, and they have increased rates of remission and/or treatment response (O'Connor et al., 2016). Note that most research in this area has focused on heterosexual couples, so little is known about postpartum adaptation within other types of familial structures.

Studies note that depression screening is largely acceptable to parents (Hynan et al., 2013). Several PPD-specific measures are available, although there are sizable differences in terms of number of questions, time to completion, sensitivity, and specificity (see Table 10.1). Many hospitals and professional groups recommend a brief verbal screen prior to more in-depth screening if a positive screen occurs, although staff availability to conduct and respond to the screening must be taken into account. One example of such a screener is the Public Health Questionnaire-2 (PHQ-2), recommended by the U.S. Preventive Task Force Screen, which asks "1) In the past two weeks have you ever felt down, depressed or hopeless?" and "2) In the past two weeks have you had little interest or little pleasure in doing things?" (Siu et al., 2016).

Post-Traumatic Stress Disorder

Research indicates that parents of infants in the NICU experience heightened rates of post-traumatic stress symptoms (PTSS), identifying the NICU experience as a source of potential trauma and acute stress for both mothers and fathers/partners (Hynan et al., 2013). PTSS can lead to diagnosis of acute stress disorder and even PTSD, depending on duration and severity of symptoms. PTSS prior to birth may also contribute to worse infant outcomes and lead to greater vulnerability post-birth (Hynan et al., 2013). PTSS are readily identifiable with appropriate screening measures examining stress responses and risk factors (Berns, 2010). Again, recommendations regarding when screening for PTSS should take place vary, although many recommend maternal screening prior to childbirth to begin linkage to resources and support to prevent development of PTSD (Berns, 2010).

Similar to screening for PPD, some recommend a brief, verbal screen prior to more in-depth, pen-and-paper PTSS diagnostic evaluations (see Table 10.1 for PTSS screening measures). The Primary Care PTSD Screen (PC-PTSD) is an example of such a four-question screener. It asks,

In your life, have you ever had any experience that was so frightening, horrible or upsetting that in the past month you . . . 1) have had nightmares about it or thought about it when you did not want to? 2) tried hard not to think about it or went out of your way to avoid situations that remind you of it? 3) were constantly on guard, watchful or easily startled? 4) felt numb or detached from others, activities or in your surroundings?

Three "yes" responses constitute a positive screen and recommend a more extensive follow-up evaluation (Berns, 2010).

Several PTSS pen-and-paper screening tools, including the Davidson Trauma Scale, Impact of Events Scale–Revised (IES-R), and PTSD Checklist (PCL-5), are available. However, only one, the modified Perinatal Post-Traumatic Stress Disorder Questionnaire (PPQ2), is specific to perinatal settings and designed specifically for parents of high-risk infants.

Anxiety Disorders

The NICU environment is highly stressful, potentially resulting in both normative and clinically concerning anxiety responses for parents (Hoffman et al., 2021; McCabe-Beane et al., 2018). Similar to depression, clinical levels of anxiety may contribute to reduced ability to care for the infant and other children during the postpartum period, challenges with self-care and management of responsibilities, and more (Hoffman et al., 2021). Measures specifically designed for evaluating anxiety symptoms during the postpartum period and during a NICU admission are extremely limited, and existing screening measures fail to adequately distinguish anxiety symptoms from depressive symptoms.

Balancing benefits of additional screening for anxiety disorders and demands on parent time is paramount. This has resulted in the identification of a three-item anxiety subscale on the Edinburgh Postnatal Depression Scale (EPDS-A) as well as the three-item Pregnancy Risk Assessment Monitoring System–Anxiety Items (PRAMS-A), both of which have cutoff scores validated in postpartum women (McCabe-Beane et al., 2018). Other approaches utilizing measures such as the Beck Anxiety Inventory and the SCL-90-R anxiety scale () have demonstrated some incremental identification of anxiety disorders in postpartum women (McCabe-Beane et al., 2018). Both of these, however, are longer and more time-consuming to complete, and neither one has specific clinical thresholds pertaining to peripartum parents and/or the NICU experience specifically.

OBSTETRICAL CARE AND FETAL MEDICINE CENTERS

In addition to screening parents following the birth of their child, it is recommended that screening be conducted throughout pregnancy, but only if treatment options are available immediately for those who score in the clinical range. This is especially important for parents who are experiencing fetal complications because these are often accompanied by uncertainty, loss, disruption in routines, and complex decision-making (Dempsey et al., 2021). Although there is limited literature for fetal care centers, Cole et al. (2016) found higher rates of traumatic stress symptoms and clinically significant depression symptoms. Dempsey et al. (2021) advocate for screening in fetal care centers and for provision for follow-up mental health services such as counseling that includes problem-solving skills training, behavioral exposure, and biofeedback. This may also help build resiliency and better prepare families for potential NICU admissions if PMADs were assessed and treated earlier in their journey (Cole et al., 2016).

Developing a well-designed, detailed protocol for screening administration is of paramount importance, and many factors must be considered. Again, medical care providers who identify symptoms of a PMAD through screening have an ethical responsibility to further assess and connect the caregiver(s) to appropriate support services. If there is no access to support services for parents at risk, then screening should not be conducted. Given the sensitive nature of this type of assessment, informed consent should be obtained prior to screening and include transparency regarding purpose and related procedures. Protocols must be applied consistently and universally through incorporation into the setting's standard of care to maintain fairness and avoid causing harm.

The first consideration involves the "who": Who will complete the screening tool and who will administer it? There is compelling evidence that in addition to mothers, fathers/partners should complete the screening tool because they also experience mood changes during transition to new parenthood and, like mothers, are at increased risk of emotional difficulties during NICU admission (Hynan et al., 2013). This may be difficult within the NICU or clinic setting because both parents may not be available, but reasonable attempts to screen both parents should be made whenever feasible. Who administers the screening tools may depend on the complexity of the measures used. In some NICU settings, parents may be provided with screening instruments at bedside by a nurse or unit clerk. Similarly, clinic settings might have the front desk staff provide questionnaires to parents in the waiting room prior to their office visit. Scoring may take place immediately or once delivered to a psychosocial care team member before the person completing the screening measure leaves the facility. Ultimately, the screening data will eventually need to be conveyed to a psychosocial staff member for interpretation and further assessment. However, it is not uncommon for social workers or psychologists to also serve as the administrators and incorporate screening into their initial consult.

The second consideration involves which screening instrument(s) to utilize. Perinatal depression is screened most commonly, but as described previously, it may be helpful to also screen for anxiety and/or traumatic stress given the higher prevalence in this population. In selecting instruments, ease of administration, length of time for completion, parent literacy, and language should be considered. Fortunately, several of the more frequently used screening tools are published in languages other than English (e.g., EPDS and PHQ-9), but providers need to be mindful of other language and cultural barriers (Willis et al., 2018). For some families, questionnaires may need to be read aloud or an interpreter may be required, which can be more time-intensive. Most measures are brief and may be used in combination if screening for more than one PMAD is advisable.

Inclusion of an item assessing suicidal ideation and/or thoughts of self-harm could be potentially upsetting or aversive to parents, causing hesitation from some clinicians. However, not asking these questions could have harmful outcomes that might have been prevented had they been asked. Avoiding these difficult questions contributes to the silence and stigma associated with mental health issues and possibly delays treatment for severe symptoms.

There has been some variability in recommendations pertaining to the timeline of evaluation, with some research indicating early screening, other research recommending screening further into a NICU admission, and still other research advocating for repeated screenings, including pre- and post-discharge (Willis et al., 2018). Each strategy offers some benefits and drawbacks; whereas early screening increases the potential for false positives, it also offers the opportunity for prolonged and continuous resource provision and relationship building and minimizes overlooking parents with short NICU stays (Hynan et al., 2013). However, adjustment and symptoms often vary through the course of a NICU admission, and repeated screenings may be beneficial for tracking symptoms over time.

The most important consideration is how staff respond when a parent is found to have an elevated score or endorses suicidal ideation. A perinatal setting must have access to services for parents identified as at increased risk, preferably onsite or through referral to community partners with priority access of within 2 weeks. Networking with community providers and hospital-based mental health providers, such as social workers, counselors, and/or psychologists, is critical in determining workflow. Also, within the protocol design, one must consider the scheduling of screening and provision of timely follow-up as key. For example, leaving questionnaires at bedside to be completed overnight is inappropriate because hypothetically a parent could endorse significant suicidal ideation and staff are likely not available at that time to conduct further assessment. It is recommended that completion of measures take place during the day when psychosocial staff are more available, particularly when using a measure that contains an item assessing suicidality. There must be clearly identified providers who will follow up with families and potentially an on-call system in case of emergency. It is important that the NICU or clinic have the appropriately trained staff to provide parents with feedback regarding their screening results and suggest appropriate resources. It is recommended that all screening protocols be reviewed by the institution's legal and/or compliance teams prior to implementation to ensure consistency with policies.

One example of a hypothetical workflow process for screening within the NICU setting highlights many of these factors and is displayed in Figure 10.1.

DOCUMENTATION

Documentation of screening results poses an ethical dilemma in the NICU because the medical patient is technically the infant, and therefore documentation would typically be placed within the infant's chart. An argument can successfully be made for the importance of screening caregivers for mood difficulties; however, it can be difficult to know how and where to document these results.

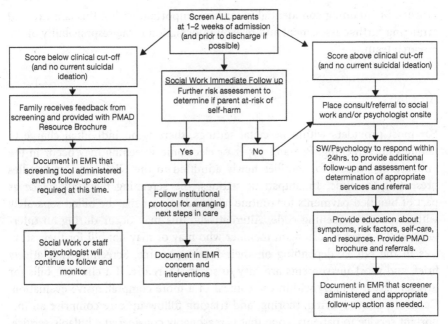

Figure 10.1. Sample workflow for screening protocol. EMR, electronic medical record; PMAD, perinatal mood and anxiety disorder; SW, social work.

Documenting results risks compromising parents' privacy and potentially upsetting parents by including this type of information in their child's chart. Medical charts are subject to release for legal proceedings, and there is potential that they could be included in child custody, parental competence, or child protection cases. For these reasons, most providers who use pen-and-paper screening for parents do not scan in the actual test forms and instead describe scores in a broad manner with use of descriptive risk categories or clinical significance, rather than a raw score. Typically, this type of documentation may be part of a larger parent–infant evaluation report or note. In addition, some settings may use a specially designed flowsheet within the medical chart for entering scores. Furthermore, to address privacy concerns, some providers may create a new chart for the patient's parent to document further assessment and follow-up care in a more confidential manner, separate from their infant's chart. Due to these privacy concerns, review of the screening protocol by the institution's legal and compliances teams is highly recommended prior to implementation.

Screening may also be part of research studies, in which case the data are not part of the official medical record but, rather, maintained by the principal investigator(s). However, even in the context of research, there must be a protocol for addressing parents found to be at increased risk of mood disorder and/or suicidal ideation/thoughts/risk via screening. This may or may not involve disclosure to and utilization of clinical staff, but this should be clear in the informed consent process. Maintaining confidentiality remains important within this context, and arranging further assessment and referral information is the responsibility of the research team.

BILLING

For most providers within neonatal settings, there is no individual charge to families for screening. Pen-and-paper or electronic screening may occur in the onboarding process for families newly admitted to the NICU and/or families presenting to clinic. In outpatient settings, the screening may take place as part of bundled payments for routine health checks or may be billed separately with a specific screening code. Alternatively, this may occur during an interview with a psychosocial team member who may or may not bill for their services in the NICU, depending on their funding source. Screening is relatively brief, and most instruments are easy to score. Therefore, if a clinician bills for this service, it is likely within the context of a more comprehensive evaluation. Certainly, administering, scoring, and triaging follow-up care comprise an important service to patients—one that is reasonably considered a billable service. A CPT code, "Caregiver-focused health risk assessment" (96161), was developed specifically for this type of screening and labeled as follows: "Administration of caregiver-focused health risk assessment instrument (e.g., depression inventory) for the benefit of the patient, with scoring and documentation, per standardized instrument." The requirements to report 96161 are as follows: "Practice expense is incurred to administer the instrument (such as nurse time or for purchase of the screening instrument), the instrument is standardized and scorable, and results are documented in the medical record." This code would apply to parental screening in the NICU, but to our knowledge, this may be underutilized due to concerns for reimbursement and/or limitations related to the type of setting (inpatient versus ambulatory/outpatient) or provider type that can bill for the code. In addition, state-specific billing considerations should be taken into account by providers, and clinicians working in hospitals and clinic settings are urged to consult with their billing compliance and revenue cycle managers to discuss whether billing for screening is appropriate.

RESPONSE

Despite recommendations, currently there is no standard protocol for screening parents in perinatal settings. However, many hospitals have started implementing their own protocols to assess for parental mood concerns. A brief informal interview survey was designed by the authors of this chapter to explore the use of screening within NICU and outpatient follow-up clinic settings. The authors sent out an invitation email to members of a professional U.S. network of NICU psychologists to complete the survey. The authors recognize this is a limited sample and only included psychologists, resulting in a convenience sample of seven respondents who are currently utilizing a screening protocol within their settings. Generally, screening appears more common in NICU settings, but some fetal medicine (Cole et al., 2018; Dempsey et al., 2021) and outpatient follow-up clinics are also screening parents (Zerden et al., 2017). This is consistent with our respondents, four of whom screen within NICU, three within outpatient clinics, and/or two within fetal health centers. The results of this convenience survey are consistent with research literature because mothers tend to be the focus, but screening with fathers/partners is receiving more attention—two of the respondents also screen fathers. Team members conducting the screening vary across sites, often relying on a psychologist, social worker, or nurse to administer screening tools to parents. Nurse administration is less common due to the many other demands on nurses' time and perhaps less familiarity or comfort with PMADs. Most sites use pen-and-paper questionnaires because they are less expensive and require little technology to administer. However, use of electronic tablets/iPads in the clinical setting is becoming more common and could be helpful for tracking and scoring. The EPDS is the most commonly used measure, but several sites also screen for anxiety or traumatic stress using the Generalized Anxiety Disorder-7 (GAD-7) or IES-R. Each respondent reported different procedures to follow up with the family when concerns were identified, but each respondent emphasized the importance of linking parents with appropriate resources. Screening results are often used as a trigger for referral to the NICU psychologist or increased involvement from social work. Some follow-up programs include an on-site psychologist, and other programs created a direct referral line with nearby outpatient providers. Most respondents utilize screening tools, which included an item regarding suicidal ideation, and all had a plan for immediate safety assessment and follow-up care if this type of concern was identified.

Advocates for screening argue this helps identify those at risk earlier than may otherwise be possible, which may help expedite professional intervention for parents. Designing a screening program requires enthusiastic support from health care administration because staff time and effort are required not only for administration but also for scoring, tracking, and follow-up care. This requires staff education about the purpose of screening and follow-up plans. Some of the psychologists surveyed believed the medical teams were very appreciative of the screening and follow-up processes and that these processes deepened staff's empathy for the families. Some found their team members reached out more often to psychosocial providers when they had concerns about a family because they had greater firsthand recognition of the need and benefits of their services.

A majority of respondents reported parents reacted favorably to screening and appreciated the staff's attention to their emotional needs. According to several respondents, even when no concerns were identified, parents expressed appreciation for the psychoeducation about perinatal mood disorders provided during the screening process, which increased their awareness of signs to look for and resources available. However, inevitably there will be some parents who, due to cultural concerns, stigma, or personal circumstances, may not appreciate completing more paperwork or view it as an invasion of privacy. Parents may also fear their responses could lead to staff judgment and subsequently affect their infant's care. On a practical level, finding parents at bedside can be challenging given competing demands for their time and desire to focus on their infant during visits. This may lead to some parents with limited or no opportunity for screening. Guidelines advocate for serial screenings throughout pregnancy, NICU, and follow-up clinics, but most sites have focused on the early weeks of NICU admission or the first clinic visit because multiple screenings may not be feasible and too many parents are lost to follow-up.

IDEAS WORTH SHARING

- It is crucial to have support of administration and staff in developing and executing a screening program. This includes prioritizing training, allocating staff time, and providing resources.
- Screening programs require mechanisms for follow-up assessment and referral. This highlights the critical need of having mental health providers embedded in multidisciplinary teams in fetal care, obstetric, NICU, and follow-up settings.
- Protocols for screening should be well designed to expeditiously address parents identified as higher risk. This includes considerations for readily available referral resources, time of day, and staffing in emergent situations.
- To facilitate outreach to more families, clinicians should consider screening measures that are translated into other languages and work with referral agencies to help best serve non-English-speaking parents.
- Screening is not only important at the beginning of a NICU admission but also may be useful in fetal medicine programs, prior to NICU discharge, and again at developmental follow-up clinic visits because the transition to home can be emotionally challenging for families given multiple new responsibilities and parenting a child with possible behavioral and developmental challenges.

CONCLUSION

Perinatal mood and anxiety disorders are more prevalent among parents in medical settings due to their unique stress related to situational demands of new parenthood coupled with the complexity of having a medically high-risk infant. Many professional organizations advocate for screening for PMADs within perinatal settings, and validated screening tools are readily available. Screening allows for earlier identification of clinically significant distress and also allows for better triage of limited support services. Screening protocols can be challenging to develop and implement due to practical barriers, including staffing, tracking, and documentation. Screening programs must include procedures for addressing emergencies and provide timely access to further mental health evaluation and professional treatment resources, highlighting the need for integration of mental health professionals within perinatal care teams. Further research is needed to evaluate the impact of screening on treatment of mood disorders for families within the perinatal setting as well as to develop more specific measures that examine the unique stress of caring for a medically complex infant.

REFERENCES

Berns, S. D. (Ed.). (2010, December). *Toward improving the outcome of pregnancy III*. March of Dimes. https://www.marchofdimes.org/toward-improving-the-outcome-of-pregnancy-iii.pdf

Cole, J. C. M., Moldenhauer, J. S., Berger, K., Cary, M. S., Smith, H., Martino, V., Rendon, N., & Howell, L. J. (2016). Identifying expectant parents at risk for psychological distress in response to a confirmed fetal abnormality. *Archives of Women's Mental Health, 19*(3), 443–453. https://doi.org/10.1007/s00737-015-0580-6

Cole, J. C. M., Olkkola, M., Zarrin, H. E., Berger, K., & Moldenhauer, J. S. (2018). Universal postpartum mental health screening for parents of newborns with prenatally diagnosed birth defects. *Journal of Obstetric, Gynecologic, & Neonatal Nursing, 47*(1), 84–93. doi:10.1016/j.jogn.2017.04.131

Dempsey, A. G., Chavis, L., Willis, T., Zuk, J., & Cole, J. C. M. (2021). Addressing perinatal mental health risk within a fetal care center. *Journal of Clinical Psychology in Medical Settings, 28*(1), 125–136. https://doi.org/10.1007/s10880-020-09728-2

Earls, M. F. (2010). Incorporating recognition and management of perinatal and postpartum depression into pediatric practice. *Pediatrics, 126*(5), 1032–1039. doi:10.1542/peds.2010-2348

Fairbrother, N., Young, A. H., Janssen, P., Antony, M. M., & Tucker, E. (2015). Depression and anxiety during the perinatal period. *BMC Psychiatry, 15*, 206. doi:10.1186/s12888-015-0526-6

Gaynes, B. N., Gavin, N., Meltzer-Brody, S., Lohr, K. N., Swinson, T., Gartlehner, G., Brody, S., &Miller, W. C. (2005, February). Perinatal depression: Prevalence, screening accuracy, and screening outcomes. *Evidence Report/Technology Assessment (Summary)* (119), 1–8. doi:10.1037/e439372005-001

Hall, S. L., Hynan, M. T., Phillips, R., Lassen, S., Craig, J. W., Goyer, E., Hatfield, R. F., & Cohen, H. (2017). The neonatal intensive parenting unit: An introduction. *Journal of Perinatology, 37*(12), 1259–1264. doi:10.1038/jp.2017.108

Hoffman, C., Greene, M., & Baughcum, A. E. (2021). Neonatal intensive care. In B. Carter & K. Kullgren (Eds.), *Clinical handbook of psychological consultation in pediatric medical settings* (pp. 277–293). Oxford University Press.

Hynan, M. T., Mounts, K. O., & Vanderbilt, D. L. (2013). Screening parents of high-risk infants for emotional distress: Rationale and recommendations. *Journal of Perinatology, 33*(10), 748–753. doi:10.1038/jp.2013.72

Kazak, A. E. (2006). Pediatric Psychosocial Preventative Health Model (PPPHM): Research, practice, and collaboration in pediatric family systems medicine. *Families, Systems, & Health, 24*(4), 381–395. doi:10.1037/1091-7527.24.4.381

Kendig, S., Keats, J. P., Hoffman, M. C., Kay, L. B., Miller, E. S., Moore Simas, T. A., Frieder, A., Hackley, B., Indman, P., Raines, C., Semenuk, K., Wisner, K. L.,& Lemieux, L. A. (2017). Consensus bundle on maternal mental health: Perinatal depression and anxiety. *Obstetrics & Gynecology, 129*(3), 422–430. doi:10.1097/aog.0000000000001902

McCabe-Beane, J. E., Stasik-O'Brien, S. M., & Segre, L. S. (2018). Anxiety screening during assessment of emotional distress in mothers of hospitalized newborns. *Journal of Obstetric, Gynecologic, & Neonatal Nursing, 47*(1), 105–113. doi:10.1016/j.jogn.2017.01.013

Mojtabai, R. (2017). Universal depression screening to improve depression outcomes in primary care: Sounds good, but where is the evidence? *Psychiatric Services, 68*(7), 724–726. doi:10.1176/appi.ps.201600320

O'Connor, E., Rossom, R. C., Henninger, M., Groom, H. C., & Burda, B. U. (2016). Primary care screening for and treatment of depression in pregnant and postpartum women: Evidence report and systematic review for the US Preventive Services Task Force. *JAMA, 315*(4), 388–406. doi:10.1001/jama.2015.18948

O'Hara, M. W., & McCabe, J. E. (2013). Postpartum depression: Current status and future directions. *Annual Review of Clinical Psychology, 9*, 379–407. doi:10.1146/annurev-clinpsy-050212-185612

Pai, A. L. H., Patiño-Fernández, A. M., McSherry, M., Beele, D., Alderfer, M. A., Reilly, A. T., Hwang, W.-T., & Kazak, A. E. (2008). The Psychosocial Assessment Tool (PAT2.0): Psychometric properties of a screener for psychosocial distress in families of children newly diagnosed with cancer. *Journal of Pediatric Psychology, 33*(1), 50–62. doi:10.1093/jpepsy/jsm053

Rhodes, A. M., & Segre, L. S. (2013). Perinatal depression: A review of US legislation and law. *Archives of Women's Mental Health, 16*(4), 259–270. doi:10.1007/s00737-013-0359-6

Rogers, A., Obst, S., Teague, S. J., Rossen, L., Spry, E. A., Macdonald, J. A., Sunderland, M., Olsson, C. A., Youssef, G., & Hutchinson, D. (2020). Association between maternal perinatal depression and anxiety and child and adolescent development: A meta-analysis. *JAMA Pediatrics, 174*(11), 1082–1092. doi:10.1001/jamapediatrics.2020.2910

Rowan, P. J., Duckett, S. A., & Wang, J. E. (2015). State mandates regarding postpartum depression. *Psychiatric Services, 66*(3), 324–328. https://doi.org/10.1176/appi.ps.201300505

Siu, A. L., Bibbins-Domingo, K., Grossman, D. C., Baumann, L. C., Davidson, K. W., Ebell, M., Garcia, F. A. R., Gillman, M., Herzstein, J., Kemper, A. R., Krist, A. H., Kurth, A. E., Owens, D. K., Phillips, W. R., Phipps, M. G., & Pignone, M. P. (2016). Screening for depression in adults: US Preventive Services Task Force recommendation statement. *JAMA, 315*(4), 380–387. doi:10.1001/jama.2015.18392

Willis, T., Chavis, L., Saxton, S., Insoft, A. N., Lassen, S., & Milford, C. (2018). *National Perinatal Association position statement on perinatal mood and anxiety disorders.* http://www.nationalperinatal.org/resources/Documents/Position%20Papers/2018%20Position%20Statement%20PMADs_NPA.pdf

Zerden, M. L., Falkovich, A., McClain, E. K., Verbiest, S., Warner, D. D., Wereszczak, J. K., & Stuebe, A. (2017). Addressing unmet maternal health needs at a pediatric specialty infant care clinic. *Women's Health Issues, 27*(5), 559–564. doi:10.1016/j.whi.2017.03.005

11

PSYCHOTHERAPY AND MEDICATION INTERVENTIONS FOR PERINATAL MOOD AND ANXIETY DISORDERS ACROSS SETTINGS

TENI DAVOUDIAN, JACQUELYN M. KNAPP, LANA S. WEBER, AND NICOLE CIRINO ∎

Mothers of medically fragile infants are at higher risk of developing perinatal mood and anxiety disorders (PMADs) compared to the general perinatal population. Untreated or undertreated depression and anxiety disorders experienced during pregnancy and/or postpartum can adversely impact the psychological well-being of mothers and their infants. Evidence-based psychotherapies, such as cognitive–behavioral therapy (CBT) and interpersonal psychotherapy (IPT), are effective in treating PMADs among women with high-risk infants. For moderate to severe illness, psychotropic medications should be considered as a treatment option.

For most perinatal psychiatric illness, medications are considered compatible during pregnancy and breastfeeding because the risk of untreated psychiatric illness exceeds the risk of medication exposure. Antidepressants are the mainstay of treatment of perinatal depression and anxiety disorders and are well-studied to support that they do not increase any significant risk to mother or infant. Sedative hypnotic medications may be used adjunctively with close monitoring to target acute anxiety and insomnia. Antipsychotics and mood-stabilizer agents, which carry a higher risk profile during the perinatal period, are used to treat severe or refractory depression and anxiety, perinatal bipolar disorder, and postpartum psychosis. Risk–benefit analysis, informed consent, and shared decision-making should be used when considering treatment with medications.

INDIVIDUAL VERSUS GROUP PSYCHOTHERAPY

Perinatal mental health disorders can lead to multigenerational mental health issues. Impaired maternal–fetal bonding, marital discord, and neuro-affective development issues in children are associated with untreated and undertreated PMADs (e.g., depression, anxiety disorders, post-traumatic stress disorder [PTSD], and bipolar disorder that occur during pregnancy and/or within 1 year following birth of child). Given the vast impact that untreated mental health conditions can have on both mother and child, effective treatments during pregnancy and postpartum are imperative (Nillni et al., 2018).

Greater than 63% of perinatal women prefer psychotherapy as first-line treatment of their psychological symptoms (Alvidrez & Azocar, 1999; Sockol, 2018). While pregnant and breastfeeding, some mothers worry that taking medications to treat their mental health symptoms will adversely impact their infant. Therefore, many women perceive psychotherapy as a safer option during the perinatal period. The U.S. Preventative Services Task Force, the American College of Obstetricians and Gynecologists (ACOG), and the American Psychiatric Association (APA) recommend evidence-based psychotherapies, such as CBT and IPT, for the prevention and treatment of perinatal depression.

Interpersonal Therapy

Interpersonal psychotherapy is a semistructured, time-limited treatment that addresses life transitions, interpersonal challenges, and grief (Sockol, 2018). Focusing on interpersonal functioning during the perinatal period is particularly important given that low social support and marital discord are associated with depression and anxiety among pregnant and postpartum women (Nillni et al., 2018; Sockol, 2015, 2018). IPT's emphasis on role transitions and grief is also relevant when considering the identity and lifestyle modifications that occur during the transition to parenthood (Nillni et al., 2018). For example, grieving the loss of a healthy or "perfect" child is common among parents with high-risk infants. Caring for a medically fragile infant often requires clear, effective communication between caregivers. IPT can help parents of high-risk infants identify and emotionally process the losses associated with having an infant with medical conditions as well as improve their communication skills related to child care.

CASE EXAMPLE

Amy is a 29-year-old female who presents to individual psychotherapy for major depressive symptoms at 7 months postpartum. Her son was born at 29 weeks, weighed 3.2 pounds, and spent 64 days in the neonatal intensive care unit (NICU). Her son's physical health stabilized at 5 months of age. Amy reports feeling "emotionally stuck" when she thinks about her son's birth and first few months of his life. After engaging in IPT, Amy comes to the realization that some aspects of her postpartum depression are due to her unprocessed grief related to her son's birth. Her expectations of labor, delivery, and postpartum were nothing like what she actually experienced. Amy had not previously examined and verbalized the losses she endured because her wife, in a sincere attempt to be supportive, encouraged Amy to focus on their son's improving health and bright future. Amy's psychotherapist encourages her to process her grief and role disputes by asking Amy to do the following:

- Identify sources of anger (e.g., her medical team, family, herself, and others)
- Process underlying emotions related to the significant losses she endured (e.g., not being able to hold her baby right after birth and not being able to breastfeed)
- Reconnect with some pre-pregnancy activities/hobbies to help balance Amy's life roles as a wife and friend in addition to being a mother
- Practice clear, assertive, and respectful communication with her wife regarding her emotional experiences and needs

IPT is effective in the prevention and treatment of perinatal depression and anxiety disorders (Nillni et al., 2018; Sockol, 2018). In addition to experiencing reduction of symptoms, perinatal women treated with IPT report increased relationship satisfaction, improved social adjustment, and decreased worrying (Sockol, 2018). IPT is also effective in treating perinatal depression among mothers from low socioeconomic and ethnic minority backgrounds (Nillni et al., 2018). These mothers often experience several stressors in addition to caring for a high-risk infant, such as difficulties accessing transportation to the hospital for their infant's many medical appointments and having limited or no health insurance. Stigma surrounding mental illness and participation in mental health treatment can be particularly potent in some cultures and possibly act as another barrier to receiving psychological care during the perinatal period.

Cognitive–Behavioral Therapy

Cognitive–behavioral therapy is a manualized, time-limited treatment focused on the connections between one's thoughts, emotions, and behaviors. The goals of CBT include (a) recognition and modification of incorrect/unhelpful thought patterns, (b) calibration of unrealistic expectations, (c) cultivation of relaxation skills, (d) development of problem-solving skills, and (e) increased engagement in enjoyable activities. CBT's focus on generating practical solutions to present-day issues is compatible with the psychotherapeutic needs of the perinatal population.

Given its efficacy and safety, CBT is often recommended as a first-line approach for the prevention and treatment of PMADs (Marchesi et al., 2016; Sockol, 2015). In addition to treating antenatal and postpartum depression, CBT is also effective in reducing symptoms of perinatal PTSD, obsessive–compulsive disorder, specific phobias (e.g., fear of injections or blood), panic disorder, and generalized anxiety (Marchesi et al., 2016).

CASE EXAMPLE

Maria is a 39-year-old single mother by choice. She is 1 month postpartum following a cesarean section birth at 32 weeks. Her twin daughters have been in the NICU since birth. Maria was referred to individual psychotherapy by a NICU social worker. Maria has a history of chronic but mild generalized anxiety disorder. Her symptoms, which include difficulties controlling her worries, irritability, and sleep disturbances due to anxious thoughts, increased in frequency and severity postpartum. Maria had initially planned on having one child. She states, "I worry about every single parenting decision that I make. I feel like I'm going to permanently damage my girls if I make one little mistake." Despite feeling physically exhausted, she has difficulties falling and staying asleep due to her anxious thoughts. Maria's psychotherapist utilizes the following CBT interventions in order to help reduce her generalized anxiety:

- Psychoeducation is provided regarding the connections between sleep deprivation and increased anxiety. Relaxation skills, such as diaphragmatic breathing and progressive muscle relaxation, are practiced in session.
- Maria is asked to bring awareness to her anxiety- or stress-provoking thoughts by identifying and documenting such thoughts. Amy discovers that she is often overestimating danger ("An earthquake will happen tonight and we will all die"), personalizing the behaviors of her daughters ("Lisa pushed me away when I tried to comfort her. That means I'm a bad mom and she doesn't like me"), and mind-reading ("My friend has offered to help babysit but I can tell that she doesn't really want to").
- Maria is reminded that thoughts are not facts and is asked to challenge her unhelpful/inaccurate thoughts. For example, Maria's psychotherapist asks, "What is the evidence for and against each of those thoughts? What are the benefits and drawbacks of holding on to those thoughts?"
- Maria's expectations of motherhood and herself as a mother are examined in the context of her cultural background. Expectations that appear to be unrealistic are placed in the context of her current life and challenged ("You work full-time but are comparing yourself to your mother, who was a stay-at-home parent. We can't equate those two circumstances").

The administration of CBT can occur in various contexts and is modifiable to address the needs of diverse patient populations (Nillni et al., 2018; Sockol, 2015). Within the NICU setting, CBT is effective in reducing maternal depression, anxiety, and PTSD (Nillni et al., 2018; Shaw et al., 2014).

Group Psychotherapy

Cognitive–behavioral therapy, IPT, and peer support can be delivered in group psychotherapy formats, during which one or more therapists meet with several patients simultaneously. Providing mental health treatment in a group setting can help increase access to care. Each psychotherapy session typically focuses on one or two topics that are relevant to the group of patients. If conducted effectively, patients participating in group psychotherapy feel supported by their therapist(s) as well as one or more of their peers in the group. The therapeutic advantages of group psychotherapy include reduced social isolation and increased normalization of difficult experiences. These advantages can be particularly relevant given that many women experience loneliness and isolation postpartum.

The complexities associated with caring for a medically fragile infant can further exacerbate the sense of social disconnection felt by parents. Some parents may not be able to recruit child care from their support networks because their infant requires advanced care that only the infant's parents are trained to provide. Some mothers of medically high-risk infants may feel emotionally disconnected from mothers with healthy infants and thus reduce the overall amount of contact they have with others. As a result of these isolating stressors, group psychotherapy may be particularly helpful for parents with high-risk infants. It is important to note, however, that parents of high-risk infants may prefer to participate in group psychotherapy that specifically addresses the unique challenges associated with parenting a medically fragile infant. Some hospitals, clinics, and organizations, such as Postpartum Support International and Hand to Hold, offer group psychotherapy specifically for NICU parents.

Although there are no known studies examining structured, evidence-based group psychotherapy for parents of high-risk infants, research suggests that group psychotherapy can be beneficial for the general perinatal population. IPT administered in a group setting does prevent and decrease perinatal depression among women of various ages and social/ethnic backgrounds (Field et al., 2013; Lieberman et al., 2014). CBT delivered in a group format reduces depression, generalized anxiety, and phobias in pregnant and postpartum women (Lieberman, 2014). Among the general perinatal population, peer support groups, which are led by individuals with relevant lived experiences rather than formalized psychological training, are perceived as being acceptable forms of treatment and are sought-out options (Sockol, 2015).

Despite the advantages of group psychotherapy, most new mothers prefer individual treatment over group psychotherapy (Goodman, 2009). Women are more likely to participate in groups that are described as being "psychoeducational" rather than group psychotherapy. Psychoeducational groups are likely more familiar (especially in the context of parenting) and provide an environment that is perceived as being less emotionally vulnerable. Peer support groups are perceived as being acceptable forms of treatment among the perinatal population and are as effective as IPT groups in reducing perinatal depression (Field et al., 2013; Sockol, 2015).

Parents of high-risk infants may experience particular challenges with regard to participating in group psychotherapy given the uncertainties and demands of caring for a medically fragile infant. The lack of flexibility associated with the date, time, and frequency of group psychotherapy can lead to nonattendance among parents with high-risk infants (Kraljevic & Warnock, 2013). If psychotherapy is implemented while parents of high-risk infants are experiencing severe distress, those parents may not be able to fully engage in treatment and thus do not reap the benefits of group or individual psychotherapy. Therefore, psychological treatments, whether administered in a group or individual format, should be made available for parents of high-risk infants during hospitalization and following discharge (Hynan et al., 2015). During the COVID-19 pandemic, most psychotherapy groups have converted to virtual formats to enable ongoing support in a safe manner.

INTRODUCTION TO PSYCHOTROPIC MEDICATIONS USED IN THE PERINATAL PERIOD

Psychotropic medications are generally well-studied and effective treatments for women who experience a mental health condition during pregnancy or the postpartum period. Many resources are available to help the patient and the clinician decide the best intervention. Psychotropic medication can improve cognition, negative emotions, and behavior, and it is used in approximately 8% of pregnancies (Frayne et al., 2017). Antidepressants, a broad class named by their mechanism of action, are the mainstay treatment of perinatal depression and anxiety disorders, used in treating approximately 70% of perinatal depression cases (Molenaar et al., 2018). Selective serotonin reuptake inhibitors (SSRIs) and serotonin norepinephrine reuptake inhibitors (SNRIs) are the most commonly used antidepressants during the perinatal period. Effects on neurotransmitter modulation—specifically serotonin, norepinephrine, and dopamine neurotransmitters—are the primary targets of antidepressants. Yet, the unique physiology of the perinatal period has given rise to a myriad of additional hypotheses to explain depression in this vulnerable stage of a woman's life, apart from aberrations in the neurotransmitter system. These include, but are not limited to, abnormalities in the hypothalamic–pituitary–adrenal axis (i.e., the endocrine system), the immune system, thyroid function, genetics, and sex hormones (Yonkers et al., 2011). Given the interplay among these systems, in addition to emotional stress and environmental factors, a multimodal approach is utilized and medications alone may not be the only therapeutic option. Examining lifestyle factors, such as a healthy diet, sleep, exercise, and other biopsychosocial considerations, is essential to the prevention and on-going management of psychiatric conditions. For many women, treatment may involve both medications and psychotherapy.

In the perinatal period, most psychotropic medications are considered compatible with pregnancy and breastfeeding, with the exception of some mood stabilizers (e.g., valproic acid) that may have teratogenic effects during gestation. The American Academy of Pediatrics recommends breastfeeding be continued if the mother is taking psychiatric medication (Sachs et al., 2013). Age and comorbidities of the infant are always considered and inform the decision to continue certain medications. Case series and case reports have been published reporting infant side effects, but these are rare. Sertraline is often regarded as the safest choice for pregnant and breastfeeding women for the de novo treatment of postpartum depression and/or anxiety; it is found in relatively low amounts in infant serum and breast milk (Table 11.1). Generally, less exposure occurs during lactation than during pregnancy, so medications taken in pregnancy are typically continued during lactation and a change is not recommended. Fact sheets on medication exposures during pregnancy and lactation are available online at https://mothertobaby.org. For prescribers, the Reprotox and LactMed mobile applications are widely used for medication management during pregnancy and breastfeeding, respectively.

Psychiatric Illnesses with Antidepressant Indications

Antidepressants are indicated for moderate to severe depression. These may also be initiated for generalized anxiety disorder, social anxiety disorder, specific phobias, agoraphobia, and obsessive–compulsive disorder. Anxiety, sleep disturbances, and panic attacks may require benzodiazepines or other antianxiety medications or hypnotics. Antidepressants are also used to target the negative cognitions, anxiety, and low mood associated with perinatal PTSD.

Initiation of antidepressants in women with bipolar disorder may increase the risk of inducing a manic or hypomanic episode. Screening for bipolar disorder in women presenting with depression is recommended, utilizing the Mood Disorder Questionnaire (Osborne & Payne, 2017). Severe illnesses such as postpartum psychosis or acute mania may require antipsychotic medications and may likely require inpatient psychiatric hospitalization.

Clinical Practice Guidelines

Managing antidepressant medications in the perinatal population is informed by practice guidelines from the ACOG and the APA. A review of international clinical practice guidelines of perinatal depression by Molenaar et al. (2018), in conjunction with ACOG's 2008 guidelines (reaffirmed in 2018), is discussed in this section. Nuances from when to initiate, switch, or discontinue any psychotropic

Table 11.1 ANTIDEPRESSANT CONSIDERATIONS FOR BREASTFEEDING

Medication	Percentage of Maternal Dose to Breastfeeding Infant	Reported Side Effects to Breastfeeding Infants[a]
Bupropion	2.0–5.1	Possible seizures
Citalopram	2.5–9.4	Uneasy sleep, drowsiness, irritability, weight loss, restlessness
Desipramine	1.0	None
Desvenlafaxine	5.5–8.1	None
Duloxetine	0.14–0.82	None
Escitalopram	3.9–7.9	Enterocolitis
Fluoxetine	1.1–12.0	Excessive crying, irritability, vomiting, watery stools, difficulty sleeping, tremor, somnolence, hypotonia, decreased weight gain, hyperglycemia, hyperactivity, reduced rooting, reduced nursing, grunting, moaning
Mirtazapine	0.6–3.5	More rapid weight gain, sleeping through the night earlier
Nortriptyline	1.3	None
Paroxetine	0.1–4.3	Agitation, difficulty feeding, irritability, sleepiness, constipation, syndrome of inappropriate antidiuretic hormone
Sertraline	0.4–2.3	Benign sleep myoclonus, transient agitation
Venlafaxine	3.0–11.8	None

[a]Based on case reports or case series of exposure as monotherapy during breastfeeding; no causal relationship is established in most cases.

Used with permission from Laura Miller, MD.

medications vary case-by-case and should be made in collaboration with the patient, weighing the risks and benefits.

Most guidelines suggest treating mild to moderate depression with psychotherapy and other environmental and behavioral interventions, reserving medications (with or without therapy) for moderate to severe depression. Typically, antidepressants are continued during pregnancy, especially if efficacious pre-pregnancy, to prevent relapse of depressive symptoms. To decrease the potential risk of numerous exposures to the fetus or neonate, prescribing a single medication at a higher dose is preferred over multiple medications. There are no U.S. guidelines on switching antidepressants that are effective during pregnancy, and several other countries discourage this. It is widely accepted to start antidepressant medication in the setting of newly diagnosed moderate to severe depression during pregnancy regardless of gestational age. Hospital delivery is recommended by most guidelines with postpartum observation of the neonate for a variable length of time, ranging from 12 hours to 3 days (Molenaar, 2018).

Review of Pharmacotherapy by Class

SELECTIVE SEROTONIN REUPTAKE INHIBITORS (E.G., Escitalopram [Lexapro], Fluoxetine [Prozac], and Sertraline [Zoloft])

With the largest volume of data about their use in pregnant and postpartum women, SSRIs are the most commonly prescribed and well-tolerated medications for the treatment of mood and anxiety disorders both outside of and within the perinatal period. SSRIs are initiated at a low dose to establish tolerability, with eventual dose increase to therapeutic levels and clinical effect over 2–8 weeks. Side effects most often occur in the first week following initiation of the medication and typically include gastrointestinal upset (e.g., nausea or diarrhea); headaches, drowsiness, or jitteriness may also occur. Over the longer term, changes in appetite, sleep, weight gain, and sexual side effects (e.g., anorgasmia) may result.

Data reviewed jointly by ACOG and the APA demonstrate that SSRIs likely have little independent effect on birth outcomes, such as spontaneous abortion, stillbirth, neonatal death, fetal growth, preterm labor and gestational age, as well as cognitive and behavioral outcomes in children later in life. With regard to structural malformations, current data demonstrate no consistent evidence to support specific teratogenic risks. The possible exception to this is first-trimester use of paroxetine, which was found in a linked analysis to demonstrate increased risk of cardiac malformations. For this reason, paroxetine is generally not started prior to the first trimester; for women already on paroxetine, the risks of continuation versus switching to an alternative should be considered. Although some studies have shown associations with SSRI use and low birth weight, it is also recognized that untreated major depressive disorder shares this association and may confound outcomes.

Antidepressants (SSRIs, SNRIs, and tricyclic antidepressants [TCAs]) have been associated with a 15–30% increased risk of developing neonatal abstinence syndrome, also termed poor neonatal adaptation syndrome, after birth when exposed to the medication in the third trimester (ACOG, 2008). Symptoms have been reported to include irritability, a weak or absent cry, hypoglycemia, temperature instability, tachypnea, and seizure. Symptoms resolve within hours to 2 weeks after birth. It is estimated that less than 5% of infants with this condition require additional medical intervention, and no long-term sequelae have been found. Several hypotheses have been posited to explain this syndrome, including genetic factors, a transient withdrawal or discontinuation phenomena, and neonatal toxicity at higher drug levels. SSRI use in late pregnancy is also associated with an increased risk (absolute risk elevation from 0.05–0.2% to 0.3–0.6%) of persistent pulmonary hypertension of the newborn, which can result in respiratory distress and NICU level of care (ACOG, 2008). These risks are always balanced against the risk of untreated depression. For instance, neonates born to mothers with depression have increased risk of irritability, less activity and attentiveness, and diminished facial expression compared to infants born to mothers without depression (Thorsness et al., 2018).

SEROTONIN NOREPINEPHRINE REUPTAKE INHIBITORS (E.G., Duloxetine [Cymbalta], Venlafaxine [Effexor], and Desfenlafaxine [Pristiq])

Whereas SSRIs are typically used as the first-line treatment, SNRIs are common medications for depression and anxiety with similar initiation schedules and side effect profiles. These medications may be used if one or two SSRIs have failed to be effective. Contrary to SSRIs, SNRIs are more likely to be associated with an unpleasant maternal discontinuation syndrome (e.g., headache, anxiety, insomnia, nausea, and electric shock sensations) following abrupt cessation of the medication. Venlafaxine may increase hypertension and should be avoided in preeclampsia; duloxetine should be avoided in severe maternal renal or hepatic disease (Thorsness et al., 2018). Acting on the noradrenergic and serotonergic systems, SNRIs are also used for the treatment of chronic pain and migraines. Based on the limited amount of data on pregnant women taking SNRIs, there is no evidence of increased risks of teratogenic effects or stillbirths. In a review of the Swedish Birth Registry, 732 pregnant women with exposure to SNRIs or norepinephrine–dopamine reuptake inhibitors (NDRIs; e.g., bupropion) in early pregnancy showed increased risk of preterm birth and neonatal symptoms akin to SSRIs (ACOG, 2008).

TRICYCLIC ANTIDEPRESSANTS (E.G., Amitriptyline [Elavil], Desipramine [Norpramin], and Nortriptyline [Pamelor])

Tricyclic antidepressants were more commonly used before the development of SSRIs and SNRIs and may be trialed in patients who have not responded to these newer classes of medications. They also have an indication for use in daily migraine prophylaxis (e.g., amitriptyline). One benefit of TCAs is the ability to check serum drug levels. The side effect profile of TCAs often hinders their use because they have anticholinergic activity and are associated with dry mouth, constipation, and sedation. Sedating properties can be used as an advantage in agitated depression. Toxic in overdose, they are not indicated for patients with a history of suicide attempts or safety concerns (ACOG, 2008). In terms of safety data, there is no association with TCAs and congenital malformations; TCAs have been associated with similar neonatal neurobehavioral complications as SSRIs and SNRIs (ACOG, 2008).

OTHER ANTIDEPRESSANTS

Bupropion (Wellbutrin) is an atypical antidepressant that acts as an NDRI. It is used to treat depression as monotherapy or as an adjunctive treatment to other antidepressants. It is thought to have fewer sexual side effects, to be activating (which may worsen anxiety), and may result in weight loss. It is also a therapy for nicotine use disorder and may be helpful in women with comorbid depression and tobacco or nicotine use. Bupropion lowers the seizure threshold and is therefore contraindicated in patients with eating or seizure disorders (ACOG, 2008). Trazodone and mirtazapine (Remeron) are sedating and may be useful in women with comorbid insomnia. Mirtazapine may be useful in women with difficulty gaining weight because it also assists with appetite stimulation and has been studied to be efficacious for women with depression and hyperemesis gravidarum (Abramowitz et al., 2017). There are fewer safety data for bupropion, mirtazapine, and trazodone in pregnancy than there are for other classes of antidepressants, yet there is no evidence to suggest congenital defects or adverse birth outcomes (ACOG, 2008).

ANXIOLYTICS

In addition to antidepressants, sedative–hypnotic medications, or short-acting anxiolytics, are frequently used in the perinatal period to manage anxiety and insomnia for interval or periodic treatment of anxiety as needed. Their rapid onset of action (15–50 minutes) is designed to immediately relieve symptoms. Benzodiazepines and antihistamines act as central nervous system depressants that reduce daytime anxiety and excessive excitement; they also produce drowsiness and promote onset and maintenance of sleep.

The benzodiazepine class of medications has reassuring, yet limited, evidence of safety (e.g., spontaneous abortion and congenital malformations) when used in pregnancy and lactation (Thorsness et al., 2018). When used, lorazepam (Ativan) is generally preferred to alprazolam (Xanax), which can lead to rebound anxiety and/or misuse, and alternatives with longer half-lives (e.g., clonazepam [Klonopin] and diazepam [Valium]; Thorsness et al., 2018). Benzodiazepine use is complicated by the risk of excessive sedation, as well as physiologic tolerance and dependence. Thus, they are avoided in patients with active or historical substance use disorders. When used prior to delivery, intoxication and/or withdrawal syndromes in the neonate may result (ACOG, 2008). In lactation, given the slower metabolism of benzodiazepines by neonates, long-acting benzodiazepines may result in sedation, nausea, and poor feeding, and they are therefore avoided in premature or medically fragile children (Thorsness et al., 2018).

Antihistamines (e.g., hydroxyzine, diphenhydramine, and doxylamine) are not thought to be associated with adverse neonatal outcomes and are frequently used more effectively for insomnia than anxiety. Antihistamines have been associated with lower milk production and are typically used once milk supply has been established.

Due to limited data and unclear benefit, the following medications for anxiety are typically not prescribed during the perinatal period: buspirone, propranolol, zolpidem, eszopiclone, zaleplon, and melatonin (Thorsness et al., 2018).

Alternatives and Adjuncts

For those who do not respond to first-line antidepressants and anxiolytics, there are several alternatives that are utilized in the perinatal period. A select few are mentioned here; detailing the numerous options available is outside of the scope of this chapter.

ANTIPSYCHOTICS

When depression and anxiety do not respond to treatment with psycho-therapy or first-line medications (e.g., antidepressants or anxiolytics), anti-psychotic medications are often used as an adjunctive treatment. In addition, these medications are often used for the treatment of postpartum psychosis and bipolar mania. Medications in this class include second-generation antipsychotics: quetiapine (Seroquel), aripiprazole (Abilify), olanzapine (Zyprexa), and risperidone (Risperdal). Used in lower doses for insomnia and anxiety and at higher doses for mood disturbances, quetiapine is not expected to increase the risk of congenital anomalies; it has also been shown to have limited placental transfer to the fetus. Quetiapine is the preferred second-generation anti-psychotic in lactation based on evidence demonstrating low levels in breast milk, even at higher (e.g., 400 mg) doses (Thorsness et al., 2018). Because of its meta-bolic side effects (e.g., weight gain and insulin insensitivity), quetiapine may cause increased maternal and infant weight, and additional monitoring is considered in late pregnancy.

BREXANOLONE

In March 2019, the U.S. Food and Drug Administration approved a new phar-macological agent specifically for the treatment of postpartum depression, allopregnanolone, a progesterone derivative, under the name brexanolone (Zulresso). Allopregnanolone modulates $GABA_A$ receptors, the primary inhib-itory neurotransmitter in the brain and target of benzodiazepine medications, often implicated in quelling anxiety. Similar to other neurotransmitters, immedi-ately following the birth of the infant and placenta, the level of allopregnanolone drops precipitously and is associated with mood changes. In three randomized, double-blind, placebo-controlled studies, the medication demonstrated rapid re-sponse in symptoms in women experiencing postpartum depression with a lim-ited side effect profile and minimal drug–drug interactions. The medication is administered as an intravenous infusion therapy and requires observation in a hospital setting for 60 hours (Meltzer-Brody et al., 2018). The benefit of this med-ication intervention is that response occurs as soon as the first 24 hours of initia-tion, far faster than the traditional antidepressant therapy. However, accessibility of this treatment is limited due to high cost and requirement of overnight inpa-tient monitoring.

Initiating and Managing Treatment

COUNSELING WOMEN ON IN UTERO EXPOSURE LACTATION RISK

After a careful diagnostic interview is done and the clinician believes the patient may benefit from medication administration, ideally the patient and the clinician would engage in both informed consent and shared decision-making, which are addressed in detail in Chapter 15 of this volume. Shared decision-making goes beyond obtaining informed consent and involves developing an empathic partnership, exchanging information about the available options, allowing time to discuss the potential consequences of each choice, and making a decision by consensus. This model is particularly important in the perinatal population due to the increased complexity of prescribing medication to a woman who may be pregnant or breastfeeding.

As with all medications considered in pregnancy, decisions are made carefully with attention paid to the risks and benefits of use given the potential exposure to the fetus. In order to obtain informed consent, the astute clinician would discuss both the risks of medication use and the risk of untreated psychiatric illness on the fetus or infant. They would also discuss the maternal risks and benefits of medication use. They should suggest alternatives to medication. They should obtain verbal and written consent from the patient if possible, and they should involve the patient's family member(s) in the discussion, if available. It is best to give written information directly to the patient so they can review the risks on their own. The clinician does not need to discuss every possible potential risk from medication use but should summarize major categories of risk, provide written information, and then answer any questions the patient may have.

Gestational age, lactation status, and infant age and health are three important factors in making decisions regarding medication choice. During pregnancy, gestational age is an important clinical consideration because teratogenic effects of medication (e.g., cardiac malformations, cleft lip/palate, and neural tube defects) only occur in the first trimester. In the second and third trimesters, adverse effects could include neurobehavioral development; obstetrics factors such as gestational age, growth restriction, preterm delivery, and risk of preeclampsia; and neonatal complications such as neonatal abstinence syndrome. Infants who are premature or ill may be more likely to have adverse effects of medication from the mother's breast milk due to these infants being more medically fragile. Mothers who breastfeed partially with formula supplementation would have a lower total exposure to their infant.

CASE EXAMPLE

Jenny is 3 weeks postpartum and is having panic attacks at night since her baby was born with a cardiac defect and admitted to the NICU. She is also pumping breast milk, which the infant receives through a gastronomy tube. The panic attacks are very distressing to her, and she fears going to bed at night. This has led to tearfulness and depression throughout the day. The psychiatrist that sees her for an evaluation suggests that she try lorazepam at night to help with panic attacks and sleep. The psychiatrist has already spoken with the pediatrician, who is supportive of this medication in lactation given the infant's medical status. Jenny reports she will not take any medication that is going to make her drowsy, as she fears that she will get called by the NICU in the middle of the night and will be unable to answer the call or respond. The psychiatrist knows that lorazepam could work right away, would provide immediate relief for Jenny, and will likely not cause sedation such that she cannot answer the phone should the NICU call.

In the model of shared decision-making, the psychiatrist should validate Jenny's feelings, even though she may not agree with the risk that Jenny describes. She decided to offer her an alternate medication (sertraline taken in the morning) that may also help with panic attacks but is not likely to cause sedation, even though it will take longer to take effect. A savvy and compassionate clinician should understand the patient's priorities, their comfort with the level of risk, and offer suggestions to reach the goals of both the patient and the clinician.

SIDE EFFECTS, EFFICACY, AND MANAGEMENT

Most medications used to treat anxiety and depression have the most significant side effects at the beginning of treatment, prior to when individuals may observe a positive effect. Further dose adjustments are required for maximum effect. Response to medication is frequently assessed by using validated instruments such as the Edinburgh Postnatal Depression Scale (EPDS) and the Generalized Anxiety Disorder 7 scale after each dose change and in regular intervals (Osborne & Payne, 2017). Sometimes one or more medications may be prescribed to treat different symptoms or treat side effects. For instance, in the previous case example, Jenny may be treated with both a short-acting medication such as lorazepam, which would help with sleep and panic right away, and a long-acting medication such as sertraline, which can be taken daily but will not take effect for a few weeks. Decisions on the choice to treat Jenny would be based on the severity of her symptoms, the presence of risk factors such as suicidal ideation or substance use, past efficacy of medication, and Jenny's comfort with the side effects and treatment plan.

DOSING ADJUSTMENTS

Providers who prescribe medication may take into account several factors when deciding on the dose needed for the individual patient. For instance, physiologic changes in pregnancy often lead to lower drug serum levels as pregnancy progresses. This can lead to a relapse of symptoms of depression, anxiety, panic attacks, or insomnia in the late second or third trimester. Regular monitoring of clinical symptoms and occasional blood levels of medication can help guide when the dose needs to be adjusted. Decreasing the dose of medication prior to delivery is generally not recommended because it is known as a time of increased risk for symptoms onset due to hormonal fluctuation after birth. Medication for insomnia required in late pregnancy may have to be adjusted postpartum if a mother's insomnia resolves or in order for her to wake at night for feedings.

CASE EXAMPLE

Hetal's baby was diagnosed with a fetal anomaly at her 20-week ultrasound. Hetal had significant depressive symptoms set in after this diagnosis that rendered her unable to concentrate at work or parent her 3-year-old. Her obstetrician/gynecologist (OB/GYN) started her on sertraline 25 mg and increased it to 50 mg after 5 days. She felt "much better" after 4 weeks. Her EPDS score decreased from 22 to 10 (above 12 is considered a positive score). At 33 weeks, Hetal returned for a routine prenatal visit and her EPDS score was 18. She reported the medication has "stopped working." Hetal's OB/GYN explained that due to physiologic changes in pregnancy (i.e., increase in total body water and increase renal clearance), her brain was likely not getting the effective dose needed to treat Hetal's depression fully. She recommended increasing sertraline to 100 mg. Two weeks later, the EPDS score drops to 8, and Hetal feels well again. Her OB/GYN plans to continue this dose in the postpartum period as well.

IDEAS WORTH SHARING

- Untreated mental health conditions in mothers of high-risk infants can lead to long-term negative consequences in both the parent and the child.
- Cognitive–behavioral and interpersonal psychotherapies, in an individual or a group setting, are effective in treating anxiety and depression in parents of high-risk infants.
- Major medical organizations throughout the world support the use of medications in pregnant and lactating women because the benefit of treated illness outweighs the risk of untreated illness for the mother and the infant.
- Antidepressants are generally well-tolerated during lactation and passed at low levels to the breast milk.

CONCLUSION

Many treatment options have been studied and are effective for mothers of high-risk infants. The use of psychotherapy and/or medication in pregnancy and postpartum has been proven to be effective. CBT and IPT are effective in reducing depression, anxiety, and PTSD among mothers of preterm and very low birth weight infants. Adjunctive modalities, such as peer support groups, can also be effective in reducing perinatal depression. When anxiety and depression do not respond to psychotherapy alone, antidepressants are widely utilized, evidence-based treatments. Antidepressant use in pregnant women likely does not increase the risk of negative birth outcomes (e.g., stillbirth, spontaneous abortion, and congenital defects), but it may have transient, reversible infant effects after birth. Common symptoms that a mother may experience and possible medication options for her are summarized in Table 11.2.

Table 11.2 SYMPTOMATIC TREATMENT OF PSYCHIATRIC CONDITIONS IN THE
PERINATAL PERIOD

Symptoms	Medication Options	Considerations
Panic attacks	Lorazepam, hydroxyzine SSRIs[a]	Lorazepam and hydroxyzine can be used "as needed" to decrease symptoms within 30 minutes. Lorazepam is the preferred benzodiazepine in the perinatal period. SSRIs are taken daily, may take weeks to take effect, but can prevent recurrence of panic attacks long term.
Insomnia	Doxylamine, trazodone, mirtazapine, lorazepam	Doxylamine, frequently used to treat nausea in pregnancy, assists with onset of sleep and is available without a prescription. Mirtazapine and trazodone are atypical antidepressants that at low doses assist with sleep and are typically taken daily. Lorazepam may be used between nighttime feedings with close monitoring. Bed sharing is discouraged with all sedating medication.
Depression	SSRIs,[a] SNRIs[b]	Initial maternal side effects of SSRIs and SNRIs may include gastrointestinal upset, dizziness, and headaches and typically subside with 3–7 days
Trauma symptoms (flashbacks, nightmares, increased startle)	SSRIs,[a] SNRIs[b]	Antidepressants are compatible with lactation in most cases. Clinicians can use validated instruments to measure the effect of medication on target symptoms (e.g., EPDS, PHQ-9)
Obsessive thoughts or behaviors	SSRIs,[a] SNRIs[b]	Commonly, antidepressants are continued 4–9 months after symptom remission; then a supervised taper may be appropriate.
Generalized anxiety	SSRIs,[a] SNRIs[b] lorazepam short term	

[a]SSRIs include citalopram, escitalopram, sertraline, fluoxetine, fluvoxamine, and paroxetine.

[b]SNRIs include duloxetine, desvenlafaxine, and venlafaxine.

EPDS, Edinburgh Postnatal Depression Scale; PHQ-2, Public Health Questionnaire-2; SNRIs, serotonin norepinephrine reuptake inhibitors; SSRIs, selective serotonin reuptake inhibitors.

REFERENCES

Abramowitz, A., Miller, E. S., & Wisner, K. L. (2017). Treatment options for hyperemesis gravidarum. *Archives of Women's Mental Health, 20*(3), 363–372.

Alvidrez, J., & Azocar, F. (1999). Distressed women's clinic patients: Preferences for mental health treatments and perceived obstacles. *General Hospital Psychiatry, 21*(5), 340–347.

American College of Obstetricians and Gynecologists Committee on Practice Bulletins—Obstetrics. (2008). ACOG practice bulletin: Clinical management guidelines for obstetrician–gynecologists number 92, April 2008 (replaces practice bulletin number 87, November 2007). Use of psychiatric medications during pregnancy and lactation. *Obstetrics and Gynecology, 111*(4), 1001–1020.

Field, T., Diego, M., Delgado, J., & Medina, L. (2013). Peer support and interpersonal psychotherapy groups experienced decreased prenatal depression, anxiety and cortisol. *Early Human Development, 89*(9), 621–624.

Frayne, J., Nguyen, T., Bennett, K., Allen, S., Hauck, Y., & Liira, H. (2017). The effects of gestational use of antidepressants and antipsychotics on neonatal outcomes for women with severe mental illness. *Australian & New Zealand Journal of Obstetrics & Gynaecology, 57*(5), 526–532.

Goodman, J. H. (2009). Women's attitudes, preferences, and perceived barriers to treatment for perinatal depression. *Birth, 36*(1), 60–69.

Hynan, M. T., Steinberg, Z., Baker, L., Cicco, R., Geller, P. A., Lassen, S., Milford, C., Mounts, K. O., Patterson, C., Saxton, S., Segre, L., & Stuebe, A. (2015). Recommendations for mental health professionals in the NICU. *Journal of Perinatology, 35*(1), S14–S18.

Kraljevic, M., & Warnock, F. F. (2013). Early educational and behavioral RCT interventions to reduce maternal symptoms of psychological trauma following preterm birth: A systematic review. *Journal of Perinatal & Neonatal Nursing, 27*(4), 311–327.

Lieberman, K., Le, H. N., & Perry, D. F. (2014). A systematic review of perinatal depression interventions for adolescent mothers. *Journal of Adolescence, 37*(8), 1227–1235.

Marchesi, C., Ossola, P., Amerio, A., Daniel, B. D., Tonna, M., & De Panfilis, C. (2016). Clinical management of perinatal anxiety disorders: A systematic review. *Journal of Affective Disorders, 190*, 543–550.

Meltzer-Brody, S., Colquhoun, H., Riesenberg, R., Epperson, C. N., Deligiannidis, K. M., Rubinow, D. R., Li, H., Sankoh, A. J., Clemson, C., Schacterle, A., Jonas, J., & Kanes, S. (2018). Brexanolone injection in post-partum depression: Two multicentre, double-blind, randomised, placebo-controlled, phase 3 trials. *Lancet, 392*(10152), 1058–1070.

Molenaar, N. M., Kamperman, A. M., Boyce, P., & Berginik, V. (2018). Guidelines on treatment of perinatal depression with antidepressants: An international review. *Australian & New Zealand Journal of Psychiatry, 52*(4), 320–327.

Nillni, Y. I., Mehralizade, A., Mayer, L., & Milanovic, S. (2018). Treatment of depression, anxiety, and trauma-related disorders during the perinatal period: A systematic review. *Clinical Psychology Review, 66*, 136–148.

Osborne, L. M., & Payne, J. L. (2017). Clinical updates in women's health care summary: Mood and anxiety disorders: Primary and preventive care review. *Obstetrics and Gynecology, 130*(3), 674.

Sachs, H. C., & Committee on Drugs. (2013). The transfer of drugs and therapeutics into human breast milk: An update on selected topics. *Pediatrics*, *132*(3), e796–e809.

Shaw, R. J., St. John, N., Lilo, E., Jo, B., Benitz, W., Stevenson, D. K., & Horwitz, S. M. (2014). Prevention of traumatic stress in mothers of preterms: 6-month outcomes. *Pediatrics*, *134*(2), e481–e488.

Sockol, L. E. (2015). A systematic review of the efficacy of cognitive behavioral therapy for treating and preventing perinatal depression. *Journal of Affective Disorders*, *177*, 7–21.

Sockol, L. E. (2018). A systematic review and meta-analysis of interpersonal psychotherapy for perinatal women. *Journal of Affective Disorders*, *232*, 316–328.

Thorsness, K. R., Watson, C., & LaRusso, E. M. (2018). Perinatal anxiety: Approach to diagnosis and management in the obstetric setting. *American Journal of Obstetrics and Gynecology*, *219*(4), 326–345.

Yonkers, K. A., Vigod, S., & Ross, L. E. (2011). Diagnosis, pathophysiology, and management of mood disorders in pregnant and postpartum women. *Obstetrics and Gynecology*, *117*(4), 961–977.

12

TRAUMA AND TRAUMA-INFORMED CARE

MARY COUGHLIN ■

Trauma, by definition, is unbearable and intolerable. (p. 1) . . . We all want
to live in a world that is safe, manageable, and predictable . . . victims remind us that this is not always the case. (p. 194)

—Van Der Kolk (2015)

The American Psychiatric Nurses Association issued a position statement in
March 2017 titled "Whole Health Begins with Mental Health." The organization
posits "mental health promotion, through prevention, recognition and adequate
care and treatment must be the starting point . . . our definition of health must be
transformed to recognize mental health as a foundation for all health." Health is a
state of physical, mental, and social well-being and not merely the absence of disease. Research demonstrates a strong link between early life adversity and mental
and physical health outcomes. Health care experts acknowledge the urgent need
to transform the existing health care paradigm. Health care systems must shift the
focus from "What is wrong with you?" to "What has happened to you?" in order
to reduce the short- and long-term consequences associated with early life adversity. Proactively responding to the unmet needs of the infant and family in crisis
can mitigate the mental health sequelae associated with trauma, improve survival
outcomes, and reduce health care costs.

ADVERSE CHILDHOOD EXPERIENCES

The Adverse Childhood Experiences Study was the largest investigation into the relationship between childhood abuse, neglect, and household dysfunction with adult morbidity and mortality. Replicated across a multitude of demographic populations, the results stand firm. Adversity in childhood negatively impacts health and wellness across the life span. Sixty-one percent of Americans report at least one adverse childhood experience (ACE) during the first 18 years of life, with 25% reporting three or more ACEs. Globally, Carlson et al. (2020) report that two-thirds of youth experience adversity in childhood regardless of where they reside throughout the world.

Adversity in childhood is most often mediated by the child's relationship with adult caregivers and is also referred to as interpersonal trauma. Early life stress and interpersonal trauma are associated with attachment adversity and have been linked to post-traumatic stress disorder and developmental trauma disorder in survivors. Adversity in childhood is associated with significantly poorer health outcomes, risky health behaviors, and socioeconomic challenges (Figure 12.1).

Zarse et al. (2019) published a comprehensive literature review of two decades of research using the Adverse Childhood Experience–Questionnaire (ACE-Q).

ACEs Can Increase Risk for Disease, Early Death, and Poor Social Outcomes

Research shows that **experiencing a higher number of ACEs is** associated with **many of the leading causes of death** like heart disease and cancer.

   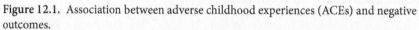

CHRONIC HEALTH CONDITIONS	MENTAL HEALTH CONDITIONS	HEALTH RISK BEHAVIORS	SOCIAL OUTCOMES
• Coronary heart disease • Stroke • Asthma • Chronic obstructive pulmonary disease (COPD) • Cancer • Kidney disease • Diabetes • Obesity	• Depression • Suicide or attempted suicide	• Smoking • Heavy drinking or alcoholism • Substance misuse • Physical inactivity • Risky sexual behavior	• Lack of health insurance • Unemployment • Less than high school diploma or equivalent education

Figure 12.1. Association between adverse childhood experiences (ACEs) and negative outcomes.
Source: Centers for Disease Control and Prevention (https://www.cdc.gov/violencepre vention/aces/resources.html?CDC_AA_refVal=https%3A%2F%2Fwww.cdc.gov%2Fvio lenceprevention%2Facestudy%2Fresources.html#anchor_1626996630 Materials developed by CDC).

The results highlight the dose-dependent, causal relationship between ACEs and mental illness, addictions, adult noncommunicable diseases, disrupted parenting, and insecure childrearing. The perturbations in family integrity leave a transgenerational footprint of the burden of disease associated with early life adversity (Figure 12.2).

THE TRANSGENERATIONAL NATURE OF TRAUMA

The pervasiveness of interpersonal trauma leaves very few unscathed. During sensitive and critical periods of development, life experiences take on new meaning as they direct and disrupt biological processes in the wake of early life adversity. These biological processes, mediated by epigenetic mechanisms, have lifelong implications for an individual's physiologic and psychologic health and well-being. Individuals with a history of interpersonal trauma in childhood are highly susceptible to substance use disorders and mental and physical health challenges. A preoccupation with substance use is one mechanism through which trauma and disrupted attachment is transmitted across generations (Figure 12.3; Meulewaeter et al., 2019).

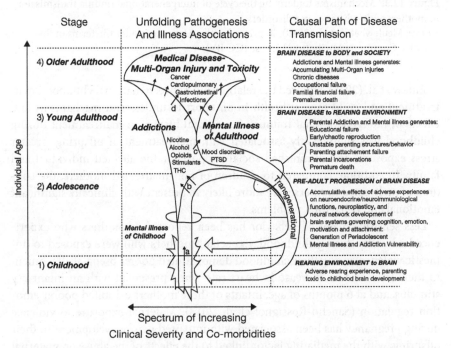

Figure 12.2. Neuroscience-informed causal pathway to adverse childhood experiences comorbidities. PTSD, post-traumatic stress disorder; THC, tetrahydrocannabinol.
Source: Zarse et al. (2019). Reprinted with permission under the Creative Commons Attribution (CC-BY) 4.0 license.

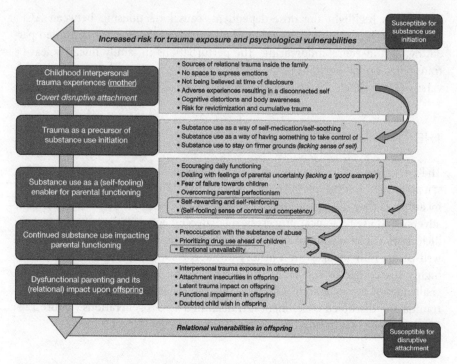

Figure 12.3. Mechanisms underlying the cycle of intergenerational trauma transmission in mothers with substance use disorders.
Source: Meulewaeter et al. (2019). Reprinted with permission under the terms of the Creative Commons Attribution License (CC BY).

Enlow et al. (2018) explored the relationship between maternal childhood maltreatment and child mental health in an effort to understand mechanisms and effects of intergenerational trauma. A maternal history of maltreatment during childhood was significantly associated with maltreatment of offspring, greater stress exposure, and diminished social support for the affected individual and family. In addition, compared to children of non-maltreated mothers, the children of maltreated mothers were more likely to present with clinically significant emotional and behavioral problems.

Less sensitive maternal behavior has been reported in mothers who experienced adversity during childhood. Expectant mothers who were exposed to domestic violence during their childhood demonstrated poorer prenatal attachment to their fetus and an increase in heart rate when presented with an infant-cry stimulus, and at 6 months of age, infants of these mothers exhibited poorer emotion regulation (Sancho-Rossignol et al., 2018). Maternal exposure to violence during pregnancy has been associated with impaired neurodevelopment in their offspring, with the mediating factor linked to the effects of the abuse on maternal mental health.

Adult survivors of childhood abuse exhibit dysregulation of the hypothalamic–pituitary–adrenal (HPA) axis, the hypothalamic–pituitary–thyroid axis, and immune function. These disturbances to maternal biology have been linked to aberrant neurodevelopmental outcomes in their offspring. The experience of chronic stress as a result of early life adversity and the body's biological response with the release of cortisol and a myriad of inflammatory mediators amplifies communication between peripheral inflammation and neural circuitry, leading to chronic low-grade inflammation. This chronic low-grade inflammation predisposes the affected individual to adiposity and insulin resistance while also acting on cortico-amygdala and cortico-basal ganglia threat and reward circuits that lead to self-medicating behaviors such as smoking, drug use, and the consumption of high-fat diets. The combination of inflammation/neuroinflammation and these self-medicating behaviors results in significant physical and emotional pathology, morbidity, and mortality.

TRAUMA AND THE NEONATAL INTENSIVE CARE UNIT

Infants make meaning out of the world based on how the world makes them feel. Does the infant feel safe, secure, and/or connected, or does the infant feel unsafe, insecure, and/or isolated? These feelings create cellular memories mediated primarily by maternal caregiving experiences that influence HPA axis reactivity and affect the developmental trajectory of the infant's lifelong health and well-being (Lucero, 2018). Mitigating the iatrogenic psychological effects of medical care in the neonatal intensive care unit (NICU) and beyond is a moral and ethical imperative for quality health care delivery. Understanding the concepts of infant medical traumatic stress and its association with alterations in brain growth and development highlights the biologic relevance of a trauma-informed developmental approach (Coughlin, 2021).

THE FIVE GUIDING PRINCIPLES OF A TRAUMA-INFORMED APPROACH

Physical and emotional health, economic and social resources, culture, medical establishments, social policy, and structural injustice impact the behaviors of high-risk mothers and families (Figure 12.4) (Krieger, 2020). The hierarchical structure of health care often silences the voice of the patient and family, and this is compounded by social discrimination (Griscti et al., 2017). Social discrimination differentiates the treatment of an individual based on their actual or perceived characteristics; is an added burden for socially disadvantaged groups; and threatens the health and well-being of individuals, the family, and society at large (D'Anna et al., 2018). Adopting a trauma-informed care paradigm shifts the focus from "What's wrong with you?" to "What happened to you?" and is guided by five principles that strive to mitigate systemic and structural barriers to compassionate quality health care: safety, choice, collaboration, empowerment, and trustworthiness.

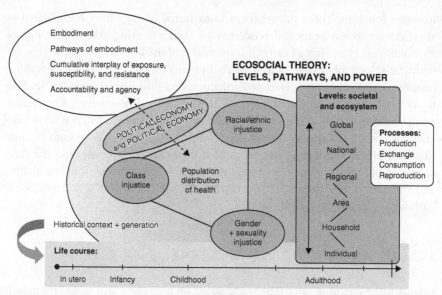

Figure 12.4. Ecosocial theory of disease distribution conceptualizing health inequities in relation to power, levels, life course, historical generation, biology, and ecosystems. *Source:* Krieger (2020). Reprinted with permission under the Creative Commons Attribution 4.0 International License.

Safety within a trauma-informed paradigm refers to the extent to which the service ensures the physical and emotional safety of the vulnerable individuals it serves. This includes not only protecting the individual(s) from harm but also protection from re-traumatization. *Choice* for the patient and family is crucial within the context of trauma-informed care. Choice begins by informing patients and their families about treatment options and their associated advantages and disadvantages compassionately, authentically, and without bias. *Collaboration* is to work jointly—to cooperate with and willingly assist a group to achieve together. Collaboration without compassion produces technically correct results but misses the mark in meeting the individual's emotional, spiritual, and psychosocial needs (Lown et al., 2016). Collaborative care prioritizes respectful caring relationships, emotional support, authentic communication, and shared empowerment. *Empowerment* includes sharing power with the patient and family while encouraging and facilitating patient and family partnership in decision-making throughout their health care journey. *Trustworthiness* focuses on transparency and creating clear expectations. Cultivating trust demands the health care professional be truly aligned with their purpose and their mission of service to others.

TRAUMA-INFORMED CARE AND THE PROFESSIONAL

Partnering with families in crisis hinges on the emotional intelligence, well-being, and healing intention of the health care professional. It requires the professional to cultivate personal wholeness by practicing self-compassion and self-kindness. One cannot give what one does not have: "We have to treat ourselves with gentleness, loving kindness, equanimity and dignity before we can respect and care for others with gentleness, kindness, equanimity and dignity" (Watson & Nelson, 2012). Personal wholeness enables the individual to find comfort with the discomfort in life, acknowledging and embracing the shared human experience.

In caring for critically ill infants and their families, the goal is to help these vulnerable individuals live wholly—live through their disease, through the crisis, and through the trauma—not just to survive the experience but to thrive and to flourish. This aspect of caring demands a connection with the concept of unitary caring science, an evolved worldview of one humanity, one heart, and one world (Watson, 2018). The admonishment of "First, do no harm" reminds the interprofessional team to align with purpose, passion, and mission to ensure care delivery is both competent and compassionate in order to meet the whole person needs of the infant and family in crisis from birth through discharge to home and beyond. Availability of responsive social support networks, mental health resources, transportation options, adequate nutrition, and shelter is life sustaining for the family in crisis, and it is the responsibility of each health care professional to ensure access.

TRAUMA-INFORMED CARE PRACTICES

Mitigating the trauma experience for high-risk infants and families goes beyond the day-to-day medical care. Survivors of complex trauma endure a legacy that impacts attachment, biology, affect, psychology, behavior control, cognition, and sense of self. Van der Kolk (2015) notes that "social support is a biological necessity, not an option, and this reality should be the backbone of all prevention and treatment" (p. 169). Showing up with patience, compassion, presence, and a healing intention is the antidote to complex trauma and toxic stress for the infant, parent, family, and professional.

Trauma-informed care practices must reflect an organizational culture that is aligned with the five guiding principles of a trauma-informed paradigm. Coughlin (2021) has updated the original core measures for developmental care to reflect a trauma-informed approach to the care of the high-risk infant, family, and health care professional. The five core measures for trauma-informed care encompass the healing environment; protected sleep; pain and stress prevention and management; activities of daily living; and compassionate family collaborative care.

The Healing Environment Core Measure

The attributes of the healing environment include a physical environment that is soothing, spacious, and aesthetically pleasing; a human environment emanating compassion, authenticity, and healing intention; and an organizational component that reflects a commitment to healing spaces and experiences that align with a trauma-informed approach while fostering ecological sustainability in support for a healthy planet.

HEALING ENVIRONMENT FOR THE INFANT

A healing environment for the infant accommodates the 24-hour presence of the infant's family, recognizes and acknowledges the infant's repertoire of pre-verbal communication as a guide for all caregiving encounters, and adopts the core measures for trauma-informed developmental care as the standard by which all care is provided.

HEALING ENVIRONMENT FOR THE FAMILY

The healing environment for family ensures personal space, privacy, and community access; verifies that parental presence and partnerships are a system-wide priority; and guarantees that parents enjoy unrestricted access to their infant throughout the hospital stay. Care is coordinated during the hospital stay and through the post-discharge experience while families have access to physical, emotional, financial, and spiritual resources supporting them through their hospital experience.

HEALING ENVIRONMENT FOR THE HEALTH CARE PROFESSIONAL

A healing environment for the health care professional supports efficiency in workflow and provides protected space for staff rest and recovery while promoting collaboration and community. There is zero tolerance for behaviors that under-mine safety, compromise respectful relationships, and/or threaten the environ-ment (internally, interpersonally, and externally). In addition, the organization must ensure health care professionals have appropriate resources to support their holistic health and well-being while on duty to include, but not limited to, clean and restful locations to take respite, access to healthy nourishment around the clock, and dedicated nap areas for shift workers.

The Protected Sleep Core Measure

The attributes of the protected sleep core measure focus on (a) protecting sleep in-tegrity and circadian rhythmicity for infants, families, and health care professionals; (b) supporting sleep strategies that are integral for health; and (c) ensuring that safe sleep practices for infants, families, and health care professionals are adopted, modeled, and incorporated into daily routine.

PROTECTED SLEEP FOR THE INFANT

This component includes providing routine, non-emergent care during wakeful states; ensuring that skin-to-skin care and/or skin-to-skin contact with the parent is an integral component in the infant's daily care; and warrants that infants are transitioned to safe sleep practices in the hospital setting with consistency and reliability.

Protected Sleep for Families

Single-family rooms should be equipped with sleep protection resources such as cycled lighting, recommended sound levels should be adhered to, and comfortable sleeping surfaces should be available. Education on the importance of sleep hygiene routines for infants and families should be provided, and parents should demonstrate competency in safe sleep practices for their infant and themselves prior to discharge. Supportive sleep routines are endorsed and encouraged by staff and their organization. Infant sleep routines are developed in partnership with family and documented to ensure consistency.

Protected Sleep for the Health Care Professional

Shift workers are provided with sleep education for self-health and safety. Strategies to ensure staff safety regarding the sleep displacement/disruption associated with shift work are supported by staff, peers, and the organization at large.

The Pain and Stress Prevention and Management Core Measures

Attributes of this core measure begin with an expressed goal to prevent pain and stress for infants, families, and health care professionals. The presence of pain and/or stress is assessed, managed, and reassessed continuously for infants, families, and health care professionals. Family and/or social networks are utilized as nonpharmacologic strategies and interventions to manage and mitigate pain and/or stress.

Pain and Stress Prevention and Management for the Infant

This begins with a shared expressed goal by the health care team to prevent pain and stress with each care encounter and utilize a validated, age-appropriate, and contextually accurate tool to assess the presence of pain and/or stress. This assessment of pain and/or stress guides interventions and strategies aimed at managing and mitigating the infant's experience of pain and/or stress and ensuring the consistent presence of a dedicated comfort person, ideally the parents, to support the infant during times of distress and disease.

Pain and Stress Prevention and Management for the Family

Families receive education and resources to effectively reduce their pain and distress during their hospital experience. Families receive competency-based education on infant pain and stress cues along with effective comfort measures for their infant. In addition, families are able to recognize and respond to their own pain and stress, adopting effective strategies to optimize their own health and wellness. Finally, families, in partnership with the health care team, identify social and/or medical supports and resources that will assist them in managing and mitigating pain, stress, and distress throughout their hospital stay and beyond discharge.

Pain and Stress Prevention and Management for the Health Care Professional

Staff adopt effective proactive strategies aimed at managing and mitigating the pain and stress they experience as part of their daily life and their work. Staff and team members support each other in managing and mitigating the pain and/or stress experienced on duty (i.e., "code lavender"). Strategies to ensure a healthy work environment are supported and cultivated by staff and the organizational leadership.

The Activities of Daily Living Core Measure

This core measure refers to posture and play, eating and nourishment, and skin care and hygiene. Appropriate postural alignment, mobility, and play ensure comfort, safety, and physiologic and emotional stability to support optimal neuromotor integrity and health. Eating experiences are positive, pleasant, nurturing, and nourishing. Appropriate hygiene and skin care routines preserve barrier function and tissue integrity while also ensuring a calming and nurturing experience.

Activities of Daily Living for the Infant

Examples include skin-to-skin care in the side-lying diagonal position to promote optimal postural alignment and facilitate play with the parent through face-to-face experiences. All infant eating experiences (i.e., breast, bottle, or tube) are guided and directed by the infant's level of readiness and engagement and supported within an age-appropriate environmental milieu. Infants experience tender touch from all caregivers with gentle direct skin contact and skin-to-skin encounters that support a healthy microbiome; nonsterile glove use is reserved for encounters with blood and body fluids.

Activities of Daily Living for the Family

Accessible supportive seating for parents ensures postural alignment and comfort during attachment and play encounters with their hospitalized infant. Parents receive education on healthy nutrition for infants and families and have open access to healthy, nutritious meals in a quiet, clean, and relaxed setting during the hospital stay. Food security is assessed, and appropriate resources and counseling services are activated to restore food security prior to discharge. Swaddled infant bathing is provided by parents on a weekly basis, when safely possible.

Activities of Daily Living for the Health Care Professional

Ergonomic guidelines are established to protect the musculoskeletal health of the health care professionals. Organizations provide resources and benefits that promote physical activity and well-being for staff. Cost-conscious, nutritious food options are available 24/7, and vending machines provide access to healthy snack and beverage options. Staff comply with hand-hygiene protocol and the appropriate use of infection control procedures. In addition, staff have easy access to alcohol-based hand sanitizers and appropriate emollients to preserve their skin integrity.

The Compassionate Collaborative Care Core Measure

The attributes of this core measure include assessing and supporting the emotional well-being of the infant, family, and health care professional; developing strategies to cultivate and maintain self-efficacy; and ensuring that all communication is consistent, compassionate, and reciprocated with respectful active listening.

COMPASSIONATE COLLABORATIVE CARE FOR THE INFANT

Parents are the infant's primary caregivers; supporting parental presence through their physical and emotional proximity is a priority. Infant behavioral cues and developmental capabilities are nurtured in partnership with parents and clinicians over the hospital experience. All infant caring encounters are guided by the infant's behavioral and physiological cues for readiness and engagement.

COMPASSIONATE COLLABORATIVE CARE FOR THE FAMILY

The emotional and psychological well-being of the family in crisis is assessed routinely; there is a process for appropriate referral, care, and support. Formal and informal parent education processes with opportunities for return demonstration to confirm competence and confidence in skill acquisition are well established within the organization. Parents are valued and respected partners in care. They receive compassionate, consistent information, and they collaborate in shared decision-making with the health care team.

COMPASSIONATE COLLABORATIVE CARE FOR THE HEALTH
CARE PROFESSIONAL

Behaviors that reflect burnout and/or staff responses indicative of trauma exposure are responded to compassionately and in a timely manner. Staff are mentored, coached, and supported to adopt new knowledge and skills, while fostering an attitude that ensures the highest quality of care delivery. All staff receive compassionate communication training and exemplify the tenets of compassionate communication with their patients, the families, and each other.

ATTRIBUTES OF A TRAUMA-INFORMED PROFESSIONAL

In addition to the previously discussed core measures and the principles of a trauma-informed approach, attributes of a trauma informed professional have also been identified to support the adoption and integration of a trauma informed paradigm. The attributes of a trauma informed professional are: knowledgeable, healing intention, personal wholeness, courage, advocacy, role modeling and mentorship, scholarship, and leadership for change. These attributes form the core curriculum for the Trauma Informed Professional Assessment-Based Certificate Program.

The Trauma Informed Professional Assessment-based Certificate Program developed by Caring Essentials Collaborative, LLC (https://www.caringessentials. net/) combines self-assessment and reflection with didactics, self-paced online learning, and masterminding sessions to facilitate the learner's personal journey to self-discovery and growth. The premise of the program is that becoming trauma informed begins with self; unbundling one's own story allows for true connection with the shared human experience of others. Connection opens the door to a deeper understanding and knowing to support and alleviate suffering.

The program is divided into eight modules, each module focuses on a specific attribute and learning objective. For example, the module examining the attribute of knowledgeable introduces the learner to all ways of knowing to include intuitive, empirical, ethical, personal, experimental, technical, aesthetic, and metaphysical/spiritual knowing. The program has been designed in accordance with the standards established by the Institute for Credentialing Excellence. This program is open to health care professionals, parents, and others interested in developing their therapeutic value and uncovering higher expressions of self.

SCREENING, ASSESSMENT, AND INTERVENTION

A universal approach to trauma screening is a recommended best practice. Screening not only for a trauma history but also prospectively for trauma potential, which can set the stage to minimize morbidity and break the transgenerational cycle of trauma. Assessing for trauma potential in the NICU setting requires the health care team to fully understand the infant's family dynamics, resources, and the vulnerability of the NICU graduate to non-accidental trauma in the first 6-months post hospital discharge. When adopting a screening strategy, there must be a very clear and consistent response to the screening results. All team members, including parents must be informed of the process.

Recognizing signs and symptoms of trauma in infants, families, and clinicians is a first step to arrest and address the consequences of toxic stress exposure. Toxic stress is the biological response to trauma. All stress is not bad. In fact, positive stress is a normal and essential part of health development supporting adaptation and learning. Toxic stress is the prolonged activation of the stress response system in the absence of the buffering effect of protective relationships.

Signs and Symptoms of Toxic Stress Exposure in the Infant

Infants express their exposure to toxic stress through a variety of behavioral and physiologic responses, including an exaggerated response to acute stress through intense fight-or-flight responses; hyporeactivity and/or immobilization to escalating stress; and fright and freeze responses. Feeding intolerance, poor weight gain, arousal of the sympathetic nervous system, and dysregulation of the autonomic nervous system have also been described in the literature as expressions of toxic stress exposure.

Recognizing stress behaviors early enables the parent or clinician to respond, pause, make adjustments, and/or offer additional support to prevent further stress and dysregulation. Early stress behaviors include raising one or both eyebrows, gaze aversion, blinking or fluttering of the eyes, finger splay, clenched toes and/or fists, furrowed brow, a worried look, and hiccups or yawning. An infant who is not adequately supported or is unable to competently use the support that is provided may experience more serious and lasting consequences.

Signs and Symptoms of Toxic Stress Exposure in the Family

Parents verbalize feelings of guilt, inadequacy, protracted sadness, and worry in the setting of trauma and toxic stress. The following have also been reported: diminished affection and responsiveness to their infant; withdrawn, flat parental affect; and hostility or intrusiveness with their infant. Cynicism, withdrawal, emotional lability, anxiety, fatigue, sleep disturbances, and symptoms consistent with post-traumatic stress disorder have been described in parents who have experienced a NICU hospitalization. Trauma-aware and trauma-informed health care professionals are able to recognize these signs and symptoms and respond authentically, compassionately, and effectively to buffer the trauma experience.

Signs and Symptoms of Toxic Stress Exposure in the Health Care Professional

In addition to screening and assessing infants and families, clinicians must be monitored for signs and symptoms of their trauma exposure as a consequence of bearing witness to the suffering of those they serve. Van Dernoot Lipsky (2009) delineates 16 trauma exposure responses. Onset of these trauma exposure responses is insidious and may be overlooked, misunderstood, or even ignored in settings that lack trauma awareness. Trauma exposure responses include feelings of helplessness and hopelessness, a sense that one can never do enough, hypervigilance, diminished creativity, an inability to embrace complexity, minimizing, chronic exhaustion and physical ailments, an inability to listen, dissociative moments, a sense of persecution, guilt, fear, anger and cynicism, an inability to empathize, addictions, and grandiosity or an inflated sense of importance related to one's work. Adopting a trauma-informed culture begins with trauma awareness.

IDEAS WORTH SHARING

The National Perinatal Association has developed trauma-informed care scripts for the neonatal intensive care experience that can be accessed through https:// www.myperinatalnetwork.org/my-nicu-network.html. These resources provide examples of what not to say and include trauma-informed alternatives. Scripts introduce trauma-informed language across a variety of scenarios. In addition, the NICU Parent Network (https://nicuparentnetwork.org) has developed resources for multidisciplinary clinicians to guide and support the adoption of trauma-informed language across the perinatal continuum.

Awareness of the experience of trauma for medically fragile infants, their families, and clinicians is a first step to transform and humanize the health care experience. Trauma-informed care is an effective, compassionate, and evidence-based strategy. Through this paradigm, health care professionals are invited to actively buffer the trauma experienced by the infants and families they serve in the NICU and beyond.

> I swore never to be silent whenever and wherever human beings endure suffering and humiliation. We must take sides. Neutrality helps the oppressor, never the victim. Silence encourages the tormentor, never the tormented. (p. 134)
>
> —ELIE WIESEL (2017)

REFERENCES

American Psychiatric Nurses Association. (2017). *Whole health begins with mental health* [Position statement]. https://www.apna.org/files/public/Whole-Health-Beg ins-With-Mental-Health-Position-Paper.pdf

Carlson, J. S., Yohannan, J., Darr, C. L., Turley, M. R., Larez, N. A., & Perfect, M. M. (2020). Prevalence of adverse childhood experiences in school-aged youth: A systematic review (1990–2015). *International Journal of School & Educational Psychology, 8,* 2–23. https://doi.org/10.1080/21683603.2018.1548397

Coughlin, M. (2021). *Transformative nursing in the NICU: Trauma-informed age-appropriate care.* Springer.

D'Anna, L. H., Hansen, M., Mull, B., Canjura, C., Lee, E., & Sumstine, S. (2018). Social discrimination and health care: A multidimensional framework of experiences among a low-income multiethnic sample. *Social Work in Public Health, 33*(3), 187–201. doi:10.1080/19371918.2018.1434584

Enlow, M. B., Englund, M. M., & Egeland, B. (2018). Maternal childhood maltreatment history and child mental health: Mechanisms in intergenerational effects. *Journal of Clinical Child and Adolescent Psychology, 47*(Suppl.), S47–S62. doi:10.1080/ 15374416.2016.1144189

Griscti, O., Aston, M., Warner, G., Martin-Misener, R., & McLeod, D. (2017). Power and resistance within the hospital's hierarchical system: The experiences of chronically ill patients. *Journal of Clinical Nursing, 26*(1–2), 238–247. doi:10.1111/jocn.13382

Krieger, N. (2020). Measures of racism, sexism, heterosexism, and gender binarism: From structural injustice to embodied harm—an ecosocial analysis. *Annual Review of Public Health, 41,* 37–62. doi:10.1146/annurev-publhealth-040119-094017

Lown, B. A., McIntosh, S., Gaines, M. E., McGuinn, K., & Hatem, D. S. (2016). Integrating compassionate, collaborative care ("triple C") into health professional education to advance the triple aim of health care. *Academic Medicine, 91*(3), 310–316. doi:10.1097/ACM.0000000000001077

Lucero, I. (2018). Written in the body? Healing the epigenetic molecular wounds of complex trauma through empathy and kindness. *Journal of Child & Adolescent Trauma, 11*(4), 443–455. doi:10.1007/s40653-018-0205-0

Meulewaeter, F., De Pauw, S. S. W., & Vanderplasschen, W. (2019). Mothering, substance use disorders and intergenerational trauma transmission: An attachment-based perspective. *Frontiers in Psychiatry, 10,* 728. doi:10.3389/fpsyt.2019.00728

Sancho-Rossignol, A., Schilliger, Z., Cordero, M. I., Rusconi Serpa, S., Epiney, M., Huppi, P., Ansermet, F., & Schechter, D. S. (2018). The association of maternal exposure to domestic violence during childhood with prenatal attachment, maternal–fetal heart rate and infant behavioral regulation. *Frontiers in Psychiatry, 9,* 358. doi:10.3389/fpsyt.2018.00358

Van der Kolk, B. (2015). *The body keeps the score: Brain, mind, and body in the healing of trauma.* Penguin.

Van Dernoot Lipsky, L. (2009). *Trauma stewardship.* Berrett-Koehler.

Watson, J. (2018). *Unitary caring science: The philosophy and praxis of nursing.* University Press of Colorado.

Watson, J., & Nelson, J. (2012). *Measuring Caring: International Research on Caritas as Healing.* United States: Springer Publishing Company.

Wiesel, E. (2017). *Night: Memorial Edition.* United States: Farrar, Straus and Giroux.

Zarse, E. M., Neff, M. R., Yoder, R., Hulvershorn, L., Chambers, J. E., & Chambers, R. A. (2019). The Adverse Childhood Experiences Questionnaire: Two decades of research on childhood trauma as a primary cause of adult mental illness, addiction, and medical diseases. *Cogent Medicine, 6*(1), 1581447. https://doi.org/10.1080/2331205X.2019.1581447

13

ADDRESSING PERINATAL SUBSTANCE USE ACROSS THE CONTINUUM OF CARE

JENNIFER J. PAUL, JESSALYN KELLEHER,
SUSANNE KLAWETTER, AND SARAH NAGLE-YANG ■

Substance use during pregnancy and the postpartum period is a critical public health concern with high potential for negative effects on maternal and infant/early childhood health and well-being. Although research shows long-standing problematic use of substances such as alcohol and tobacco during the perinatal period, the current "opioid epidemic" reflects escalating medical and nonmedical use of substances during and after pregnancy. Perinatal substance use increases risks for maternal mortality, morbidity, and delivery complications. It is associated with infant mortality, low birth weight, preterm birth, congenital anomalies, and impaired child development (Kotelchuck et al., 2017). Perinatal substance use may also impede maternal–infant attachment, which serves as a powerful developmental catalyst (Lowell et al., 2020). Optimal maternal–infant attachment is especially critical for those impacted by prenatal substance use due to increased rates of infant prematurity and medical complexities. In overview of this chapter, it is important to offer a statement about the chosen terminology related to substance use. Many degrees exist under the broad umbrella of substance use, ranging from social use of substances that may not impact functioning or have problematic sequelae through substance misuse that leads to significant health, psychosocial functioning, legal, or other consequences. In this chapter, when specifically referring to substance misuse that reaches a degree meeting criteria for clinical diagnosis, the terms substance use disorder (SUD) or substance use disorders (SUDs) are utilized.

SUBSTANCE USE AND TRAUMA

Research shows a clear correlation between substance use and trauma. Among the general population, approximately half of people with post-traumatic stress disorder (PTSD) also have a SUD (McCauley et al., 2012; Substance Abuse and Mental Health Services Administration [SAMHSA], 2014b). Co-occurrence of PTSD and SUDs may be higher among those seeking substance use treatment, with up to 60% of those engaged in treatment also having PTSD. In addition, those with co-occurring SUDs and PTSD tend to have more severe substance use and PTSD symptoms, less SUD treatment engagement and adherence, and poorer SUD treatment outcomes (McCauley et al., 2012).

Substance use treatment outcomes are gendered, meaning that women are less likely to receive substance use treatment than men (Meyer et al., 2019). Trauma prevalence is also gendered. Men are more likely to experience trauma than women, but women are more likely to develop PTSD. Women are more likely to experience physical and sexual assault, know their perpetrator, and their traumatic events are more likely to occur in private (SAMHSA, 2014b). Evidence suggests increased risk of PTSD during the perinatal period, particularly among pregnant women who have experienced child maltreatment and/or prior medical trauma (Shenai et al., 2019).

Trauma-Informed Care Approaches to Addressing Substance Use in the Perinatal Period

Although perinatal substance use negatively affects maternal and infant health, research also shows that the perinatal period provides unique opportunities to address problematic substance use or substance misuse. Pregnant women demonstrate a decrease in substance use, especially in the third trimester. Pregnancy may promote substance misuse recovery because women may experience increased motivation to make positive changes on behalf of their infant's well-being. Thus, pregnancy is a critical time for substance use intervention (Shenai et al., 2019). Given the relationship between substance use and trauma, as well as the effects of gender on trauma exposure and substance use, trauma-informed care serves as a useful framework for addressing perinatal substance use (Meyer et al., 2019).

Trauma-informed care (TIC) recognizes the potential presence of trauma—past or current—and adapts service delivery to avoid retraumatization, prevent emotional activation, reduce severity of trauma symptoms, and ultimately improve quality of care (SAMHSA, 2014b). Developed in response to mounting evidence of the prevalence of trauma and the co-occurrence of trauma exposure, substance misuse, and mental health disorders, TIC rests on a foundation of four key assumptions: (a) Realize the prevalence of trauma and its effects on individuals, families, communities, and organizations; (b) recognize trauma presentation/symptomatology; (c) respond using principles of TIC; and (d) resist retraumatization of all persons present in the system, including consumers/ clients/patients and staff (SAMHSA, 2014a).

These assumptions are applied through the following six key principles: safety; trustworthiness and transparency; peer support; collaboration and mutuality; empowerment, voice, and choice; and cultural, historical, and gender issues (SAMHSA, 2014a). *Safety* requires health care systems to provide physically and emotionally safe services and environments for both patients and staff. Health care systems must strive for *trustworthiness* and *transparency* between all levels of the system, including administrators, staff, and patients. TIC values *peer support* among patients and trauma survivors so that opportunities for peer support are utilized when appropriate and available. *Collaboration* and *mutuality* refer to acknowledging and reducing power differentials between administrators, staff, and patients so that all people within the health care system are viewed as potential healers and team members. Wherever possible, health care should promote *empowerment, voice,* and *choice.* Trauma-informed approaches require health care systems to ensure people understand treatment options, actively seek to understand patients' goals and ideas about healing, and incorporate those ideas into treatment planning. Finally, health care systems must attend to *cultural, historical,* and *gender issues,* including examining bias and structural determinants of disparities, increasing access to care among marginalized groups, recognizing historical trauma in systematically targeted communities, and integrating culturally responsive practices (SAMHSA, 2014a).

TIC's key principles are broad enough to serve as a useful guide for tailoring service delivery across diverse practice settings. In the context of perinatal health care for people with SUDs, TIC may be thought of as a corrective lens—a tool through which perinatal care providers can adapt techniques and utilize different strategies to optimize maternal and child health outcomes. This framework may be particularly useful when applied in the neonatal intensive care unit (NICU) given its potential for high levels of distress and traumatic experiences for infants, parents and families, and providers and other staff. It may also inform policy and practice for pregnancy and postpartum care, as well as health care during infancy and early childhood, given the stressors and opportunities these critical developmental transitions offer.

PREGNANCY AND SUBSTANCE USE

Rates/Incidence

Approximately 40% of individuals with a SUD in the United States are women, with the highest lifetime period of risk overlapping with peak reproductive years (ages 18–29 years; Forray, 2016). Although most substance using individuals achieve abstinence during pregnancy, a significant minority continue use. The National Survey on Drug Use and Health found that 5.9% of pregnant people were using illicit substances during the years 2011 and 2012, in contrast to 10.7%

of women of reproductive age who were not pregnant (Brandt et al., 2014). Risk factors for continued use during pregnancy include younger age, unemployment, being unmarried, or having a comorbid psychiatric disorder (Havens et al., 2009). Polysubstance use is common; the majority of pregnant persons who use cannabis or opioids also smoke tobacco (Brandt et al., 2014; Forray, 2016).

Tobacco is commonly reported as the most used substance during pregnancy. Between 12% and 25% of pregnant individuals use tobacco, and less than one-third of those who smoke prior to pregnancy achieve abstinence during pregnancy. Conversely, although alcohol use is common among reproductive-aged women, the large majority of women who use alcohol heavily prior to pregnancy are able to achieve abstinence once pregnant (96%), and rates of binge drinking (defined as five or more drinks on one occasion) and heavy drinking (defined as binge drinking on at least 5 out of 30 days) during pregnancy are relatively low (2.7% and 0.3%, respectively) (Brandt et al., 2014; Forray, 2016). Because many states have legalized cannabis for both medical and recreational use, the prevalence of cannabis use in the United States has increased in both the general population and among pregnant individuals, with increases of 200% and 65%, respectively, between 2002 and 2014 (Brown et al., 2017). Recent data suggest that the prevalence of cannabis use has approached or exceeded that of tobacco use and that approximately 70% of pregnant women believe that cannabis use in pregnancy is "safe" (Rodriguez & Smith, 2019). Opioid and methamphetamine use in pregnancy has similarly risen sharply during the past decade along with comparable trends in the general population (Havens et al., 2009). Table 13.1 provides estimated prevalence rates for use of specific substances during pregnancy.

Clinical Outcomes

Substance use during pregnancy is often accompanied by psychosocial factors and/or medical comorbidities that further increase risk for adverse obstetrical outcomes (Brandt et al., 2014; Forray, 2016). When considering assessment and treatment, obstetrical clinicians should assess for poor nutrition, barriers to engagement in prenatal care, intimate partner violence, and chronic medical conditions such as hepatitis C or HIV. Notably, women with SUDs have very high levels of psychiatric comorbidity (estimates range from 50% to 75%), with both depression and unintentional overdose increasingly understood as leading contributors to maternal mortality (Brandt et al., 2014; Colorado Department of Public Health and Environment, 2020).

Although substance use during pregnancy generally carries elevated direct and/or indirect risks for maternal and fetal health, the degree and type of associated risk vary considerably between individual substances. Heavy alcohol use during pregnancy has well-established pervasive neurodevelopmental risks, and fetal alcohol syndrome is the most common and preventable cause of intellectual disability in the United States (McLafferty et al., 2016). Research has established links between perinatal tobacco use and adverse obstetric outcomes, as well as

Table 13.1 SPECIFIC SUBSTANCE PREGNANCY PREVALENCE RATES, ASSOCIATED OBSTETRICAL RISKS, AND FETAL/INFANT OUTCOMES

Substance	US Rates of Use in Pregnancy (%)	Associated Increase in Obstetrical Risk	Fetal/Infant Outcomes
Tobacco	12–25	PTD, LBW, SGA, IUGR, PPROM, placental abruption, placenta previa, miscarriage, IUFD	Increased infant mortality, major congenital malformations, SIDS, asthma, ear infections, respiratory illness
Cannabis	10–49	Stillbirth, PTD, IUGR, LBW	Neurobehavioral problems, poor executive functioning
Alcohol	Any drink the past 30 days: 7.6 Binge drinking: 2.7 Heavy drinking 0.3	PTD, LBW, SGA, miscarriage, IUFD	Increased infant mortality; fetal alcohol syndrome: abnormal facial features, short statues, microcephaly, cognitive deficits, seizure, and behavioral dysregulation
Opioids	Any filled prescription for an opioid: 14–28 Opioid use disorder at delivery: 0.2	PCL, IUGR, placental insufficiency and abruption, PROM, PPH, PTD, IUFD, oligohydramnios, cesarean delivery	Low Apgar scores, NAS, SIDS, microcephaly, growth deficiency and neurobehavioral problems
Cocaine	1% at any time during pregnancy	PROM, placental abruption; PTD, LBW, SGA, IUGR	Inconsistent finding of delays in cognitive, motor, and language development
Methamphetamine	5.2% in specific regions of the United States	PTD, LBW, PCL, gHTN, IUFD	Inconsistent finding of delays in cognitive, motor, and language development

gHTN, gestational hypertension; IUFD, intrauterine fetal demise; IUGR, intrauterine growth restriction; LBW, low birth weight; NAS, neonatal abstinence syndrome; PPH, postpartum hemorrhage; PPROM, preterm premature rupture of membranes; PROM, premature rupture of membranes; PTD, preterm delivery; SGA, small for gestational age; SIDS, sudden infant death syndrome.

Sources: Brandt et al. (2014), Havens et al. (2009), and McLafferty et al.(2016).

increased risk for sudden infant death syndrome. In addition, perinatal cocaine use is associated with increased obstetric risks (e.g., placental abnormalities, preterm birth, and low birth weight), although recent evidence suggests that early adverse findings regarding long-term neurodevelopmental effects in the setting of antenatal cocaine use were likely confounded by postnatal environmental factors such as caregiving environment. Despite perceptions that cannabis use is harmless or even "safe" in pregnancy, current evidence points to associations between antenatal cannabis exposure and impaired executive functioning and academic achievement in childhood (McLafferty et al., 2016). Finally, neonatal abstinence syndrome (NAS), a well-known potential consequence of prenatal opioid exposure, is associated with high levels of neonatal morbidity and increased health care utilization rates (Forray, 2016). See Table 13.1 for a summary of associated adverse effects reported with specific substances of misuse.

Screening

Identification of substance use during pregnancy can allow obstetrical care providers to proactively monitor for associated obstetrical risk, evaluate a patient's motivation for change, and refer to specialty levels of care. The American College of Obstetrics, the American Academy of Pediatrics (AAP), and the American Medical Association all recommend universal substance use screening as a part of routine obstetric care. Screening should occur at the first prenatal visit and be repeated at least once per trimester for those who report past use. However, pregnant individuals may face multiple barriers to reporting substance use to health care providers, including stigma, guilt, fear of child custody loss, or legal consequences (McLafferty et al., 2016).

To align with TIC, providers should screen for substance use in a nonjudgmental, compassionate, and collaborative manner. The screening process must establish a sense of trust, engage the patient in recommended preventative care, and assess patient motivation and treatment preferences. Commonly used screening tools that can be incorporated into existing practice workflows are the Substance Use Profile–Pregnancy, 4Ps, and NIDA Quick Screen (not validated in pregnancy but widely used in practice). Although it is common practice for obstetric clinicians to utilize urine drug screening (UDS), this practice has significant limitations and potential for harm. A "positive" on a UDS shows evidence of use but cannot provide information about chronicity, frequency, or extent of use when considered in isolation. Similarly, it does not rule out more occasional use or the use of substances not usually captured by standard UDS panels, such as synthetic cannabinoids or opioids. Therefore, current recommendations urge clinicians not to use UDS as a primary method for screening in obstetric practice and only include UDS with the patient's knowledge and consent. Finally, although all U.S. health care providers are required to notify child protective services when caring for an infant who has been affected by substance misuse, specifics of reporting requirements in the perinatal period vary by state. All obstetric and pediatric clinicians should be familiar with the reporting requirements in their state and, to the extent possible by the law, approach the screening and treatment of perinatal substance misuse as a health care issue. Furthermore, clinicians should carefully consider the reality of racial disparities in reporting and carefully examine policies and practices to avoid exacerbating inequities.

Treatment

The SUD treatment needs of pregnant individuals are undeniably complex; however, pregnancy also represents an important window of opportunity for prevention and treatment engagement. Pregnant people with SUDs are often highly motivated by the desire for a healthy pregnancy; more likely to have health insurance than during other times of life; and, in some geographic locations, more likely to have access to SUD treatment compared to nonpregnant individuals. Behavioral interventions are a mainstay of treatment of SUDs both in pregnancy and in the general population. Existing evidence-based treatments with data supporting their use in pregnancy include motivational interviewing, contingency management, and cognitive–behavioral therapy (Forray, 2016).

Limited pharmacologic treatment options are available for SUDs. Nicotine replacement therapy is commonly used to support smoking cessation in pregnant women, especially in the case of heavy tobacco use, although its reproductive safety is uncertain. Evidence supports the efficacy of bupropion for smoking cessation during pregnancy. Bupropion has less established safety data during pregnancy relative to other antidepressants; however, existing evidence suggests it is unlikely to be a major teratogen or have considerable obstetrical risk. The existing level of data regarding varenicline in pregnancy does not allow for a meaningful conclusion about reproductive risk or efficacy during pregnancy (Turner et al., 2019).

Opioid agonist therapy is widely regarded as the preferred treatment for opioid use disorder in pregnancy. Agonist treatment is an effective and powerful tool shown to decrease relapse risk, prevent intoxication and withdrawal states, decrease high-risk behaviors associated with addiction, and improve obstetric and neonatal outcomes in women with opioid use disorder (Forray, 2016; McLafferty et al., 2016). Although both buprenorphine and methadone are widely considered to be safe and effective treatment options during pregnancy, recent data suggest infants exposed to buprenorphine need lower doses of morphine to treat NAS and have shorter hospital stays compared to infants exposed to methadone. Treatment with buprenorphine has additional potential advantages, including increased privacy and the convenience of office-based care. However, at least one randomized controlled trial reported high attrition rates for women prescribed buprenorphine compared to methadone, although this may have been more related to underdosing of women prescribed in the buprenorphine arm of the study than a true limitation of buprenorphine (McLafferty et al., 2016).

Women with opioid use disorder often face pain management challenges during and after childbirth due to increased pain sensitivity as well as tolerance to opioid pain medication. Particularly after cesarean or complicated vaginal delivery, obstetric providers must proactively develop postpartum pain management pathways in partnership with patients that account for these needs. Common approaches include continuation of opioid analgesics in combination with a fixed regimen of acetaminophen and nonsteroidal anti-inflammatory agents, neuraxial or regional blocks, and other non-opioid agents. When continuation of opioid pain medications is required in the postpartum period, obstetric clinicians should provide prescriptions with a limited quantity of pills, identify a clear plan for taper, and arrange early and close follow-up of postpartum pain control (Krans et al., 2019). Finally, clinicians need to ensure coordination of care with pediatric and substance use treatment providers. Given the complex nature of caring for individuals with SUDs during and after pregnancy, a patient-centered approach can allow for greater alignment and coordination between specialist providers and a cohesive plan of care for both the patient and her infant.

NEONATAL PERIOD

Rates/Incidence

Neonatal abstinence syndrome broadly describes the clinical presentation of neonatal withdrawal from in utero substance exposure. Due to the dramatic increase in the number of infants exposed to opioids, neonatal opioid withdrawal syndrome is also commonly used to describe neonatal substance withdrawal symptoms, and the two terms are often used interchangeably. According to the Healthcare Cost and Utilization Project, the national incidence of NAS in 2017 (the most recent year for which data are available) was 7.3 per 1,000 live births, up from 2.2 per 1,000 live births in 2008 (Agency for Healthcare Research and Quality [AHRQ], 2020). Rates of NAS have grown for all income quartiles, ethnicities, and communities. In addition, infants with NAS require more health care than typical newborns, with length of stay (LOS) averaging 11 days in 2017 for infants experiencing NAS compared to 2 days for typical infants (AHRQ, 2020). Longer LOS involves increased costs for hospitals and payers. In 2017, the average hospital stay for a newborn with NAS was $9,200, whereas the average cost for a typical newborn was $1,200 (AHRQ, 2020).

Clinical Presentation

Infants experiencing withdrawal from in utero substance exposure may exhibit a variety of symptoms. For example, infants exposed to opioids typically exhibit symptoms related to the nervous system and/or digestive system because these areas contain large numbers of opioid receptors (Patrick et al., 2020). Common withdrawal symptoms observed in substance-exposed newborns include irritability, continuous crying, tremors, hypertonicity, seizures, tachypnea, difficulty feeding, loose stools, and respiratory problems. Infants experiencing these withdrawal responses may be perceived by caregivers as "difficult" because they can be hard to soothe, and many caregivers endorse confusion regarding reading and responding to their infants' cues.

Implications for Breastfeeding

The AAP (2012) considers breastfeeding and human milk as the standard for infant feeding and nutrition. Maternal substance use is one of the few identified potential contraindications for breastfeeding; however, recommendations vary depending on the type and amount of substance as well as timing between use and feeding (Reece-Stretman & Marinelli, 2015). Typically, mothers who have been treated via methadone maintenance or buprenorphine during pregnancy for opioid dependence are encouraged to breastfeed because human milk and breastfeeding have been shown to decrease LOS and symptom severity for infants experiencing NAS (Reece-Stremtan & Marinelli, 2015). Information and guidelines are less clear for other opioid use and substances such as cannabis and alcohol. Without clear protocols, there is higher risk for subjectivity and judgment in assessment, intervention, and recommendations, including race-based bias, when working with mothers who use substances while breastfeeding. Mothers who use substances and who wish to breastfeed must be supported and counseled as early as possible, ideally prior to conception or early in pregnancy, around risk reduction, benefits of breastfeeding, and available substance-specific and mental health resources.

Assessment and Treatment

In the United States, infants with withdrawal symptoms have traditionally been assessed using the Finnegan Neonatal Abstinence Scoring System (FNASS), a scale based on severity for 21 of the most commonly experienced symptoms. Infants scoring 8 points or higher are treated with pharmacological intervention. Clinically, the FNASS can be difficult to use, requires extensive training, has shown weak support for validity and reliability in studies, and has led to unnecessary opioid treatment for some infants (Grisham et al., 2019).

Grossman and colleagues (2018) developed a model for the management of NAS called Eat, Sleep, Console (ESC) that focuses on determining if withdrawal symptoms interfere with the vital processes of feeding, sleeping, and soothing. An infant who is able to eat an appropriate amount for their gestational age, demonstrates undisturbed sleep for a minimum of 1 hour, and can be consoled within 10 minutes would not receive pharmacologic intervention (Grisham et al., 2019). This approach aligns with family-centered care initiatives that have gained prominence in NICU settings during the past decade. Emphasis is placed on structural, environmental, and social changes designed to support both the infant and the family unit. Many NICUs now encourage family participation in daily rounds, prioritize consistent communication, and encourage practices such as kangaroo care and breastfeeding. The ESC model extends this approach by encouraging families to spend as much time with their infant as possible either at the bedside or through rooming-in to learn their infant's cues and developmental needs as well as provide comfort and enhance bonding. A study by McRae et al. (2021) showed favorable parental perception of the ESC model, with parents highlighting their appreciation of fewer interventions, the ability to take charge of infant care, and encouragement from staff.

Despite emphasis on nonpharmacologic intervention, some infants will need medication to manage withdrawal symptoms. Typically, this occurs when infants have severe symptoms, including seizures and intense dehydration as a result of vomiting and/or diarrhea, or when supportive care has not led to decrease in symptom intensity and frequency (Kocherlakota, 2014). These infants are often treated with morphine, which has the desired effect on neurological and gastrointestinal symptoms at the cost of increased LOS. Phenobarbital, methadone, and buprenorphine are common alternatives to morphine and may be used in specific situations (e.g., if mothers receive buprenorphine during pregnancy, providers will often choose it to manage infant withdrawal symptoms for consistency).

NICU Support for Neonates and Families

Families may face many barriers to engaging with their infant while in the NICU. Transportation, finances, child care for siblings, lack of paid and unpaid parental leave, and maternal medical recovery can impede a family's ability to be present at the bedside. In addition, caregivers with current or prior substance misuse may fear judgment from providers and staff, feel intense guilt or shame, or experience co-occurring mental health concerns. All personnel in NICU settings can support families by utilizing TIC concepts to provide psychological safety and avoid retraumatization. Engaging with caregivers in a nonjudgmental and gentle way can help them self-regulate enough to then co-regulate with their infant, which leads to more successful outcomes for both caregivers and infants. Staff and providers can facilitate active caregiver engagement by scaffolding skill development, validation of experiences, and providing grounding and containment when needed.

INFANCY AND EARLY CHILDHOOD

NICU Post-Discharge Follow-Up

The needs of infants and families impacted by perinatal caregiver substance misuse or SUDs do not end upon discharge from the NICU. Infants exposed to substances in utero and whose parents continue to struggle with substance misuse into the postpartum period are at increased risk for negative outcomes across emotional, behavioral, physical, cognitive, academic, and social domains (Straussner & Fewell, 2018). Mothers with SUDs often require continued medical and mental health care. Infants may have a wide range of post-discharge needs, including more frequent pediatrician visits, general developmental follow-up, early intervention services, and later specialized educational support. The heightened rate of maternal mortality for this population also means that these infants are at greater risk for losing their maternal caregiver early in life (Patrick et al., 2020).

In addition, the impact of exposure for infants with NAS must account for potential effects of maternal prenatal medication-assisted treatment (MAT) utilizing methadone or buprenorphine as well as direct infant pharmacologic intervention to manage withdrawal symptoms. However, small sample sizes, varying research methodologies, and numerous confounding variables make it difficult to precisely determine what, if any, long-term effects can be expected following prenatal MAT (Behnke et al., 2013). Findings are also discordant for pharmacologic intervention sequelae for infants experiencing withdrawal. Despite the absence of clear outcome data, an opportunity exists to enhance protective factors. Straussner and Fewell (2018) highlight that parent–child bonding, self-regulation competence, and social support may buffer potential negative outcomes for these infants.

Assessment and Treatment in Early Childhood

Perinatal substance use has short- and long-term consequences for infants (see Table 13.1), although the research findings regarding long-term outcomes of in utero exposure are inconsistent and, at times, contradictory. Children are often exposed to more than one substance in utero, so it can be difficult to tease apart potential teratogenic effects of a single substance. Furthermore, it can be challenging to detangle the impact of substance exposure from that of the postnatal rearing environment (Jaekel et al., 2021). Behnke and colleagues (2013) completed a synthesis of the existing literature at the time, including hundreds of peer-reviewed articles published between 1968 and 2006, to provide better understanding of the impact of individual substances on physical and developmental outcomes. They provide a useful summary of both short-term and longer term effects by substance across a variety of domains based on their review: clear evidence for negative impacts of nicotine and alcohol on cognition, behavior, language, and achievement; some effects for marijuana exposure on behavior, cognition, and achievement, but not language or growth; effects for cocaine on behavior, cognition, and language, but not other domains; and limited data or lack of consensus on impacts of opioids and methamphetamines (Behnke et al., 2013). The research in this area is evolving and much remains to be learned. Given the likelihood of exposure to multiple substances, taking a polysubstance exposure approach that accounts for biopsychosocial factors in understanding broad developmental effects may be most useful to inform assessment and treatment.

Boris and colleagues (2019) suggest that families be screened across a variety of domains and that the impact of parental substance misuse or SUDs is multifaceted and can be assessed along three dimensions: (a) direct effects of in utero exposure on development, (b) genetic effects influencing parenting behavior, and (c) associated risk conditions impacting the infant's social environment. From a longitudinal perspective, data suggest that opioid-exposed children's emotional and behavioral difficulties significantly worsen over time and that these difficulties are greatest for those with higher prenatal risk, those raised in families characterized by unstable caregiving, and those whose mothers had high levels of social adversity and psychosocial risk (Jaekel et al., 2021). Consequently, a "no wrong door" approach is critical when screening and assessing for the presence and impact of substance misuse. In other words, every point of contact across multiple systems, including adult and pediatric primary care, mental health care, educational, developmental, and home visiting, is an opportunity for screening. Providers should assess children if a mother is symptomatic, and they should assess caregivers/parents if children are symptomatic.

Assessment and treatment of families impacted by substance misuse are not a sprint but, rather, more akin to an intergenerational marathon. Based on an analysis of policies and procedures spanning multiple states and years, SAMHSA developed the Five Points of Family Intervention guidance for serving families impacted by parental substance misuse. The Five Points identifies critical time points from pregnancy through childhood/adolescence to prevent prenatal substance exposure, address the needs of pregnant and parenting individuals with SUDs, and creatively respond to the needs of affected children through cross-system collaboration (Young et al., 2009). Table 13.2 presents highlights of strategies recommended at each key time point.

Planning ongoing support from the first point of contact with a pregnant individual or substance-exposed newborn is critical to ensure treatment services meet complex medical needs through access to uniquely suited health care services, support optimal development, and mitigate the impact of trauma over time (Patrick et al., 2020). Similar to screening and assessment, successful treatment across the early childhood period must include partnering with parents to address inconsistent, disengaged, or harsh parenting practices (Straussner & Fewell, 2018). Untreated parental mental health disorders, including trauma, must also be directly addressed in conjunction with child-focused treatment because they are risk factors for recurring substance misuse and maternal mortality (Brandt et al., 2014) and influence parent–child interactions (Lowell et al., 2020). Evidence-based interventions such as MAT, behavioral therapies, and recovery support services have been shown to reduce perinatal substance use and improve outcomes. Very young children require access to nurturing and safe caregivers with the capacity to respond to their attachment needs. The most effective treatment will support parents in recognizing the impact that substance misuse has on their ability to appropriately read and respond to their children's cues, expand parental capacity to bond with their children, empower parents to become active participants in their children's medical and social–emotional

Table 13.2 FOCUS AND STRATEGIES AT KEY INTERVENTION POINTS IN SUPPORT
OF FAMILIES IMPACTED BY SUBSTANCE USE

Intervention Point	Focus	Strategies
Pre-pregnancy	Prevent and treat SUDs prior to pregnancy	Promote public awareness and education on the risks and effects of substance use Screen women of child-bearing age for SUDs during annual exams using evidence-based tools; use prescription monitoring services and standardized prescribing practices Facilitate referrals to trauma-informed substance use treatment
Prenatal	Screen/assess pregnant women to identify SUDs and provide effective treatment to support recovery	Educate pregnant women about NAS and other potential effects of prenatal substance use on infants and prepare women for delivery and pain management Universally screen all pregnant women for SUDs at each trimester as part of routine prenatal care Facilitate supported referrals to evidence-based treatment that is trauma-informed, gender-responsive, and accessible, and maintain ongoing coordination of care across providers Utilize a Plan of Safe Care developed collaboratively with the pregnant woman and care providers when needed
Birth	Identify and address the multifaceted needs of substance-exposed newborns	Universally screen all women for SUDs verbally at delivery and develop nonbiased guidelines around mother and infant toxicology testing Educate providers about child protective services notification requirements and develop clear guidelines around child welfare responses to substance-exposed newborns Assess and treat infants with suspected prenatal exposure with evidence-based nonpharmacological and pharmacological interventions as needed, and train providers/ staff on these approaches as well as the impact of stigma and bias on outcomes

Table 13.2 CONTINUED

Intervention Point	Focus	Strategies
		Ensure hospital discharge plans address maternal substance use, MAT, home safety, parenting skills, home visitation, pediatric and childcare enrollment, and coordination of care with community providers prior to discharge Offer families information on what to expect following delivery and support for mother/infant Utilize a Plan of Safe Care developed collaboratively with the mother and all care providers
Neonatal/postpartum	Ensure the infant's safety and utilize a comprehensive, family-centered approach to respond to infant, parent, and family needs	Educate providers across systems on evidence-based and best-practice approaches to working with parents with SUDs and infants with prenatal substance exposure, including training about the effects of stigma and bias on outcomes for women and infants Encourage increased well-woman visits in the first year postpartum and screen for postpartum mood/anxiety disorders, SUDs, trauma, and intimate partner violence at both maternal and pediatric visits Ensure mothers with infants receive accessible referrals and have priority access to evidence-based SUD treatment services and community-based supports, including those focused on bonding, attachment, and early parenting Ensure mothers are connected to supports for their infants, including regular developmental screenings, early intervention services, and enrollment in high-quality child care Continue implementation of the Plan of Safe Care through collaboration between all providers and services, including targeted prevention services Share relevant information with child protective services to protect infants from abuse and neglect and ensure child welfare safety plans include consideration of both mother and infant needs across domains

(continued)

Table 13.2 CONTINUED

Intervention Point	Focus	Strategies
Childhood and adolescence	Utilize comprehensive family-centered approach to identify and respond to the unique developmental and service needs of the prenatally substance-exposed toddler, preschooler, child, and adolescent	Monitor progress and provide referrals to appropriate services for all family members Utilize pediatric health care, adult health care, and SUD treatment settings to provide integrated parenting education and support services Screen for unmet psychosocial needs at pediatric, well-woman, and SUD treatment visits Implement routine developmental screenings and facilitate referrals for specialized care Provide SUD, trauma, and mental health screenings and treatment referrals for children and adolescents as needed Collaborate across child welfare, early intervention, educational, home visiting, health care, and mental health care settings and services to address cognitive, behavioral, and social–emotional needs and ensure appropriate support and intervention are provided to children and adolescents

MAT, medication-assisted treatment; NAS, neonatal abstinence syndrome; SUDs, substance use disorders.

Sources: Young et al. (2009) and the National Center on Substance Abuse and Child Welfare (https://ncsacw.samhsa.gov/files/five-points-family-intervention-infants-with-prenatal-substance-exposure-and-their-families.pdf).

care, and assist parents in re-establishing trust and promoting secure attachment in their children.

Child Welfare System Involvement

Due to the multiple impacts of problematic substance use on the family system and caregiving practices, many children whose parents struggle with substance misuse become involved with the child welfare system (CWS). In fact, parental substance misuse is one of the most common reasons children enter child welfare; children younger than age 5 years make up half of the child welfare population, and children younger than age 1 year represent the largest single age group entering CWS (U.S. Department of Health & Human Services [DHHS], 2021). It is critical to note that in comparison with White families, Black, Indigenous, and people of color (BIPOC) families are disproportionately represented in the CWS and are more likely to experience negative outcomes, including child removal. BIPOC children are less likely to be reunified with their birth families or establish permanent placement. They are more likely to have multiple placements, group care and poorer behavioral, educational, and social outcomes. Therefore, medical, behavioral health, and other community providers working with BIPOC families must carefully consider CWS involvement with BIPOC populations and critically evaluate disparities in reporting and referral practices.

Contemporary practice places more focus on providing the support families need to maintain care of their children, including implementing family-centered approaches such as a Plan of Safe Care (POSC). A POSC recognizes that although a child may be the identified client within the CWS, it is critical to support the safety and well-being of the entire family through collaboration with community partners addressing the health and SUD treatment needs of both infant and the affected caregiver/family (DHHS, 2021). In 2009, SAMHSA and the National Center on Substance Abuse and Child Welfare introduced three guiding principles aimed at improving outcomes for children exposed to substances prenatally by supporting the family systems in which they live: (a) Recognize multiple intervention opportunities, (b) engage in cross-system collaboration, and (c) utilize family-centered approaches (Young et al., 2009). We must address the needs of parents in order to facilitate enduring and secure attachment for infants and young children.

Not only has parental substance misuse been a leading reason for CWS involvement but also it is a top contributing factor for removal of children from parental care. This trend has been on the rise due to the opioid epidemic. Data from the most recent DHHS annual report indicate that for children entering foster care, parental substance use as a contributing factor increased from 26% in 2009 to 34% in 2016—claiming the largest percentage increase among reasons for removal (DHHS, 2021). This may be due to direct risk to the child from the presence of substances in the home or to the influence of substance use on parenting behaviors. Mothers with SUDs have reduced capacity to meet their children's needs in a supportive and responsive way, contributing to the intergenerational transmission of SUDs (Boris et al., 2019). Data suggest that childrearing environment may have an even greater impact on outcome for children than exposure to substances in utero (Straussner & Fewell, 2018).

Although removal from parental care may be necessary to maintain safety, this event causes a disruption in caregiving and can interrupt the attachment process. Providers must consider how to best support children navigating transitions between biological parental care and foster care, especially for very young children who may be preverbal and have limited ability to communicate their needs and experience. In a suite of resources developed for various adults who engage with children in foster care, the Committee on Child Welfare within the Harris Professional Development Network (2020) stresses that it is critical to implement meaningful family time with parents and their very young children and that the time families spend together must be guided by consideration of early childhood development, neuroscience, attachment, trauma, implicit bias and oppression, and resilience to increase opportunities for meaningful interactions and development of healthy connections.

IDEAS WORTH SHARING

- Trauma exposure often accompanies the presence of perinatal substance use. TIC can guide services across the perinatal continuum of care in order to improve substance use treatment as well as maternal and infant/ early childhood outcomes.
- All perinatal individuals should be screened for SUDs during routine prenatal and postpartum care. Clinicians should implement screening in a nonjudgmental manner by utilizing screening tools such as the Substance Use Profile–Pregnancy, 4Ps, or NIDA Quick Screen and avoiding use of urine drug testing as a primary screening method.
- Family-centered care in NICU settings must include comprehensive supports for families impacted by substance use. This includes, but is not limited to, opportunities for caregiver–infant dyads to interact and bond, psychosocial resources, consistent parent–provider communication, and TIC.
- Approaches for recurrent assessment and treatment must be tailored to the perinatal period to uniquely address needs of families combating substance misuse, including SUDs. Key intervention time points traverse the life span, including pre-pregnancy, prenatal, birth, postpartum, neonatal/infancy, and childhood/adolescence.

CONCLUSION

Substance use during the perinatal period is a critical public health concern with high potential for negative effects on maternal and infant/early childhood health and well-being. A TIC approach must inform policy and practice across the life span, and especially for perinatal care and during infancy and early childhood given the unique stressors and opportunities these critical developmental transitions offer. For families impacted by substance misuse, it is imperative to utilize collaborative, family-centered, and trauma-informed care that incorporates intentional efforts to reduce stigma and bias in screening, assessment, and treatment across systems to optimize positive outcomes.

REFERENCES

Agency for Healthcare Research and Quality. (2020). *Neonatal abstinence syndrome (NAS) among newborn hospitalizations.* https://www.hcup-us.ahrq.gov/faststats/ NASMap?setting=IP

American Academy of Pediatrics, Section on Breastfeeding. (2012). Breastfeeding and the use of human milk. *Pediatrics, 129*(3), e827–3841. https://doi.org/10.1542/peds.2011-3552

Behnke, M., Smith, V. C.; Committee on Substance Abuse & Committee on Fetus and Newborn (2013). Prenatal substance abuse: Short- and long-term effects on the exposed fetus. *Pediatrics, 131*(3), e1009–e1024. https://doi.org/10.1542/peds.2012-3931

Boris, N. W., Renk, K., Lowell, A., & Kolomeyer, E. (2019). Parental substance abuse. In C. H. Zeanah (Ed.), *Handbook of infant mental health* (4th ed., pp. 187–202). Guilford.

Brandt, L., Leifheit, A. K., Finnegan, L. P., & Fischer, G. (2014). Management of substance abuse in pregnancy: Maternal and neonatal aspects. In M. Galbally, M. Snellen, & A. Lewis (Eds.), *Psychopharmacology and pregnancy* (pp. 169–195). Springer.

Brown, Q. L., Sarvet, A. L., Shmulewitz, D., Martins, S. S., Wall, M. M., & Hasin, D. S. (2017). Trends in marijuana use among pregnant and nonpregnant reproductive-aged women, 2002–2014. *JAMA, 317*(2), 207–209. https://doi.org/10.1001/jama.2016.17383

Colorado Department of Public Health and Environment. (2020). *Colorado maternal mortality prevention program legislative report 2014–2016.*

Forray, A. (2016). Substance use during pregnancy. *F1000Research, 5,* 887. https://doi.org/10.12688/f1000research.7645.1

Grisham, L. M., Stephen, M. M., Coykendall, M. R., Kane, M. F., Maurer, J. A., & Bader, M. Y. (2019). Eat, sleep, console approach. *Advances in Neonatal Care, 19*(2), 138–144. https://doi.org/10.1097/anc.0000000000000581

Grossman, M. R., Lipshaw, M. J., Osborn, R. R., & Berkwitt, A. K. (2018). A novel approach to assessing infants with neonatal abstinence syndrome. *Hospital Pediatrics, 8*(1), 1–6. https://doi.org/10.1542/hpeds.2017-0128

Harris Professional Development Network, Committee on Child Welfare. (2020). *Meaningful family time suite of resources.* https://www.irvingharrisfdn.org/meaningful-family-time

Havens, J. R., Simmons, L. A., Shannon, L. M., & Hansen, W. F. (2009). Factors associated with substance use during pregnancy: Results from a national sample. *Drug and Alcohol Dependence, 99*(1–3), 89–95. https://doi.org/10.1016/j.drugalcdep.2008.07.010

Jaekel, J., Kim, H. M., Lee, S. J., Schwartz, A., Henderson, J., & Woodward, L. J. (2021). Emotional and behavioral trajectories of 2 to 9 years old children born to opioid-dependent mothers. *Research on Child and Adolescent Psychopathology, 49*(4), 443–457. https://doi.org/10.1007/s10802-020-00766-w

Kocherlakota, P. (2014). Neonatal abstinence syndrome. *Pediatrics, 134*(2), e547–e561. https://doi.org/10.1542/peds.2013-3524

Kotelchuck, M., Cheng, E. R., Belanoff, C., Cabral, H. J., Babakhanlou-Chase, H., Derrington, T. M., Diop, H., Evans, S. R., & Bernstein, J. (2017). The prevalence and impact of substance use disorder and treatment on maternal obstetric experiences and birth outcomes among singleton deliveries in Massachusetts. *Maternal Child Health Journal, 21*(4), 893–902. https://doi.org/10.1007/s10995-016-2190-y

Krans, E. E., Campopiano, M., Cleveland, L. M., Goodman, D., Kilday, D., Kendig, S., Leffert, L. R., Main, E. K., Mitchell, K. T., O'Gurek, D. T., D'Oria, R., McDaniel, D., & Terplan, M. (2019). National partnership for maternal safety: Consensus bundle on obstetric care for women with opioid use disorder. *Obstetrics & Gynecology, 134*(2), 365–375. https://doi.org/10.1097/AOG.0000000000003381

Lowell, A. F., Maupin, A. N., Landi, N., Potenza, M. N., Mayes, L. C., & Rutherford, H. J. V. (2020). Substance use and mothers' neural responses to infant cues. *Infant Mental Health Journal*, *41*(2), 264–277. https://doi.org/10.1002/imhj.21835

McCauley, J. L., Killeen, T., Gros, D. F., Brady, K. T., & Back, S. E. (2012). Posttraumatic stress disorder and co-occurring substance use disorders: Advances in assessment and treatment. *Clinical Psychology: Science and Practice*, *19*(3), 283–304. https://doi.org/10.1111/cpsp.12006

McLafferty, L. P., Becker, M., Dresner, N., Meltzer-Brody, S., Gopalan, P., Glance, J., St. Victor, G., Mittal, L., Marshalek, P., Lander, L., & Worley, L. L. M. (2016). Guidelines for the management of pregnant women with substance use disorders. *Psychosomatics*, *57*(2), 115–130. https://doi.org/10.1016/j.psym.2015.12.001

McRae, K., Sebastian, T., Grossman, M., & Loyal, J. (2021). Parent perspectives on the eat, sleep, console approach for the care of opioid-exposed infants. *Hospital Pediatrics*, *11*(4), 358–365. https://doi.org/10.1542/hpeds.2020-002139

Meyer, J. P., Isaacs, K., El-Shahawy, O., Burlew, A. K., & Wechsberg, W. (2019). Research on women with substance use disorders: Reviewing progress and developing a research and implementation roadmap. *Drug and Alcohol Dependence*, *197*, 158–163. https://doi.org/10.1016/j.drugalcdep.2019.01.017

Patrick, S. W., Barfield, W. D., Poindexter, B. B.; Committee on Fetus and Newborn & Committee on Substance Abuse and Prevention. (2020). Neonatal opioid withdrawal syndrome. *Pediatrics*, *146*(5), e2020029074. https://doi.org/10.1542/peds.2020-029074

Reece-Stremtan, S., & Marinelli, K. A. (2015). ABM clinical protocol #21: Guidelines for breastfeeding and substance use or substance use disorder, revised 2015. *Breastfeeding Medicine*, *10*(3), 135–141. https://doi.org/10.1089/bfm.2015.9992

Rodriguez, J. J., & Smith, V. C. (2019). Epidemiology of perinatal substance use: Exploring trends in maternal substance use. *Seminars in Fetal and Neonatal Medicine*, *24*(2), 86–89. https://doi.org/10.1016/j.siny.2019.01.006

Shenai, N., Gopalan, P., & Glance, J. (2019). Integrated brief intervention for PTSD and substance use in an antepartum unit. *Maternal Child Health Journal*, *23*(5), 592–596. https://doi.org/10.1007/s10995-018-2686-8

Straussner, S. L. A., & Fewell, C. H. (2018). A review of recent literature on the impact of parental substance use disorders on children and the provision of effective services. *Current Opinion in Psychiatry*, *31*(4), 363–367 doi:10.1097/YCO.0000000000000421

Substance Abuse and Mental Health Services Administration. (2014a). *SAMHSA's concept of trauma and guidance for a trauma-informed approach* [HHS Publication No. (SMA) 14-4884].

Substance Abuse and Mental Health Services Administration. (2014b). *Trauma-informed care in behavioral health services* [Treatment Improvement Protocol Series 57, HHS Publication No. (SMA) 13-4801].

Turner, E., Jones, M., Vaz, L. R., & Coleman, T. (2019). Systematic review and meta-analysis to assess the safety of bupropion and varenicline in pregnancy. *Nicotine & Tobacco Research*, *21*(8), 1001–1010. https://doi.org/10.1093/ntr/nty055

U.S. Department of Health & Human Services, Administration for Children and Families, Children's Bureau. (2021). *Child maltreatment 2019*. https://www.acf.hhs.gov/cb/research-data-technology/statistics-research/child-maltreatment

Young, N. K., Gardner, S., Otero, C., Dennis, K., Chang, R., Earle, K., & Amatetti, S. (2009). *Substance-exposed infants: State responses to the problem* [HHS Publication No. (SMA) 09-4369]. Substance Abuse and Mental Health Services Administration.

14

HUMAN MILK
AND BREASTFEEDING

DIANE L. SPATZ AND ELIZABETH D. MORRIS ■

WHY DOES HUMAN MILK AND BREASTFEEDING MATTER?

The use of human milk and breastfeeding is a life-saving medical intervention for infants who require time in the neonatal intensive care unit (NICU). The research is clear that human milk decreases morbidity and mortality and improves long-term health and developmental outcomes. Health care providers have an ethical obligation to ensure that families are aware of the need for human milk (Froh & Spatz, 2014). However, despite modest increases in breastfeeding initiation rates in the United States, exclusive human milk rates at 6 months continue to be only approximately 25%. In particular, health care providers must be aware of the tremendous disparities in breastfeeding rates, with many low-income groups and persons of color not having the opportunity to make informed feeding decisions. The Spatz 10-step model for human milk and breastfeeding in vulnerable infants has been implemented in NICUs throughout the United States and the world (American Academy of Nursing, n.d.; Fugate et al, 2015; Spatz, 2004, 2018; Takato et al., 2020). Although not all infants will be able to feed directly at the breast, it is important to assess for parent goals for infant feeding and help facilitate a process so that parents can meet their breastfeeding goals (Table 14.1).

SPATZ 10-STEP MODEL FOR HUMAN MILK AND BREASTFEEDING

Step 1: Informed Decision

At the first meeting with a family, health care professionals should assess the family's exposure and experience with breastfeeding. A good leading question is

Table 14.1 Ten Steps to Promote and Protect Human Milk and Breastfeeding in Vulnerable Infants

1. Informed decision	6. Non-nutritive sucking at the breast
2. Establishment and maintenance of milk supply	7. Transition to breast
3. Human milk management	8. Measuring milk transfer
4. Oral care and feeding of human milk	9. Preparation for discharge
5. Skin-to-skin care	10. Appropriate follow-up

"What have you heard about human milk? or "What are your experiences with breastfeeding?" It is important to note that if a family comes from a background in which no one has ever breastfed, the idea of even considering the topic may be foreign and unknown. This is why presenting families with the science of human milk is of paramount importance (Table 14.2).

In addition, health care providers must give parents appropriate anticipatory prenatal education to initiate lactation. It will take time, work, and effort to establish lactation. Health care providers should assess for maternal risk factors that may impact the ability of the mother to effectively come to volume or develop a full milk supply (Spatz & Miller, 2021). For example, if the mother has abnormal breast tissue development (i.e., glandular hypoplasia/insufficient glandular tissue) or has had breast reduction surgery, in which the entire areola is removed and reattached, it is unrealistic to expect that a full milk volume will be achieved (Spatz & Miller, 2021). These mothers should be educated about this prior to birth and be counseled that every drop of milk that they produce for their infant is an important medical intervention. In addition, there should be a plan in place prenatally to ensure that the infant could be supplemented with pasteurized donor human milk (PDHM) during the NICU stay. It is also important to note that in the United States there are a few contraindications to breastfeeding/provision of own parent's milk (i.e., active illegal substance abuse and HIV-positive status). In these cases, the infant should be afforded the opportunity to receive PDHM.

It is crucial to teach families the specific ways in which human milk protects their infant from morbidity during their NICU stay and beyond. Parents also should be taught about the unique components of human milk that are not present in infant formula. Our role as health care providers is to ensure that families are well educated about the critical role that human milk plays in both short- and long-term health outcomes. When families learn about the science of human milk as well as the physiology of lactation, they may not only make the decision to provide milk but also will likely have high human milk rates for their infants at discharge. In a qualitative project, families who participated in group prenatal care (the centering model) and received education from a PhD-prepared nurse scientist in lactation had a 100% pumping/breastfeeding initiation rate and 87% of their infants were discharged from intensive care units on human milk (Froh et al., 2020).

Table 14.2 BENEFITS OF HUMAN MILK AND BREASTFEEDING FOR CHILDREN

Benefits Specific to Hospitalized Infants	Additional Benefits for All Children
Decrease in mortality	Decrease in mortality Reduction in sudden infant death
Reduction in incidence and severity of necrotizing enterocolitis	Long-term protection of gastrointestinal track (decreased risk of Crohn's disease, irritable bowel syndrome, and celiac disease)
Decrease incidence of sepsis	Decreased incidence and severity of infections (ear, respiratory, gastrointestinal, and urinary tract)
Improved feeding tolerance, enhanced advancement of feeds, and less days of total parental nutrition	Decreased diarrhea, reflux, and constipation
Reduction in bronchopulmonary dysplasia	Decreased asthma Decreased respiratory syncytial virus
Reduction in retinopathy of prematurity	Improved visual acuity
Improved brain development and developmental outcomes	Improved brain development and developmental outcomes
Decrease in hospital costs	Decrease in medical costs and in sick kid visits and rehospitalizations
	Decrease in obesity and diabetes in adulthood
	Decrease in hypertension and heart disease in adulthood
	Reduction in childhood cancers

Adapted from Spatz (2017) and Spatz and Edwards (2015).

Step 2: Establishment and Maintenance of Milk Supply

In order to effectively establish milk supply, mothers should pump within 1 hour of their infant being born and pump every 2 or 3 hours for a goal of eight pumping sessions per 24-hour period (AAN, 2015; Fugate et al., 2015; Spatz, 2014, 2018; Takato et al., 2020). Nurses must assist with milk expression as soon as possible after birth. The nurse could also empower the family members for assistance, including giving the partner or family a job list to support the mother in pumping. The individual can assist with pump assembly, operation of the pump, labeling the milk, and washing and sanitizing the pump kit. Families enjoy being involved in this process and are empowered to help with all other care of the mother (Spatz et al., 2015). When other families are involved in supporting the lactation process, the lactating parent has more time to focus on milk expression, visiting her infant, and her physical recovery.

Target milk volume should be at least 500–1,000 ml per 24-hour period by days 7–10 post birth (AAN, 2015; Fugate et al., 2015; Spatz, 2014, 2018; Takato et al., 2020). All mothers (including those with preterm infants) should be able to come to volume unless they have identified risks. It is important to note that the pregnant person begins secreting milk at 16 weeks of pregnancy. Hospital staff should track time until the first pumping session as well as the total number of pumping sessions per 24 hours. During the first 4 days of milk expression, the volume of milk is not as important as establishing a schedule. By days 5–7, a normal milk production should be in the range of 500–1,000 ml per 24-hour period. There is a critical window of opportunity (i.e., the first hours and days) to ensure coming to volume and a copious milk supply through discharge of her infant from the NICU and beyond.

Step 3: Human Milk Management

Research indicates that mother's own human milk (fresh or refrigerated) is optimal (AAN, 2015; Fugate et al., 2015; Spatz, 2014, 2018; Takato et al., 2020). If fresh milk is not available, then frozen thawed milk should be used. Once milk is frozen, the immunologic components of milk are not as potent, and frozen thawed milk is at higher risk for bacterial proliferation because the majority of white blood cells are killed with freezing (Akinbi et al., 2010). Every day as part of the nurse-to-nurse report, the nurse should be aware of the number of times per day the mother is pumping, her 24-hour daily milk production, how often she plans to come to the NICU, and the volume of fresh milk on hand at the hospital. Daily conversation between the bedside nurse and parent is essential to prioritize a 100% fresh milk diet. If there is an inadequate maternal milk supply, PDHM should be prioritized over infant formula. Research on a cohort of 281 infants in a NICU demonstrated that the cost of PDHM is quite low in comparison to the cost of total parental nutrition (Spatz et al., 2018). Therefore, hospitals should prioritize having PDHM available as a bridge to mother's own milk. Unfortunately, there remain persistent health disparities, with hospitals that serve primarily African American/Black families being less likely to have PDHM available.

Step 4: Oral Care and Feeding of Human Milk

As soon as possible after birth, human milk oral care should be initiated with the infants. Human milk oral care should be done during the entire time that an infant is nil per oz, as well as until the infant is able to receive oral feeds by mouth. Human milk oral care should be done with freshly expressed colostrum, transitional milk, or mature milk. A small oral syringe with 0.2 ml of milk or less or a petite swab can be used for oral care. The inside of the infant's mouth and buccal mucosa is coated with mother's own milk (AAN, 2015; Fugate et al., 2015; Spatz, 2014, 2018). The infant receives bioactive components of the milk through oral care, and human milk oral care can significantly reduce the risk of sepsis for the infant. In addition, human milk oral care is a positive oral experience for the infant and may help facilitate direct breastfeeding at the breast once the infant is ready. Research also shows that when families perform the human milk oral care, they experience feelings of positive progress, they feel involved in their infant's care, and they feel attached to their infant. Mothers also report that by seeing their infant respond to human milk oral care, it motivates them to want to pump and build their milk supply (Froh et al., 2015). Once an infant is ready to receive enteral feedings, colostrum should be fed first in the order that it was pumped (even if it was frozen and thawed). The infant should receive colostrum for 48–96 hours to mimic what would happen for a healthy term infant.

Step 5: Skin-to-Skin Contact

There are multiple systematic reviews and meta-analyses regarding skin-to-skin contact (SSC). All available evidence demonstrates that SSC is both safe and critical for health outcomes of both healthy and sick infants (Conde-Agudelo & Díaz-Rossello, 2016; Moore et al., 2012). The major barrier in NICUs is that often SSC is not prioritized due to staffing, a lack of education, or fear of having an accidental extubation. Health care professionals must prioritize the routine implementation of SSC even for stable intubated infants. At the authors' institution, a parent and staff educational DVD was developed that covers the science behind skin to skin, how to safely transfer an infant for SSC, as well as candid interviews from parents about how meaningful it is to participate in SSC. There are exclusions to SSC, including the infant who is on extracorporeal membrane oxygenation, some infants prior to surgery (abdominal wall defects), or any infant who is physiologically unstable.

Step 6: Non-Nutritive Sucking at the Breast

Often, infants who require NICU hospitalization are not afforded adequate opportunity to engage in non-nutritive sucking (NNS) at the breast. If the infant never requires ventilator support, NNS can be initiated from the day of birth provided the infant is stable from an oxygenation and heart rate standpoint. If the infant is intubated for any period, NNS should begin as soon as feasible (ideally the same day) after extubation. In order to ensure no milk transfer, instruct mothers to pump with a hospital-grade electric breast pump until they see no further jetting of milk from the breast and then continue to express for an extra 2 minutes. This ensures complete breast emptying. Now the infant should be positioned at the breast. The ideal time to do this is during a tube feeding session. While participating in NNS, the infant is able to smell the milk, taste the milk, and begin to learn about the oral feeding experience.

Step 7: Transition to Breast

There is no research to support that infants need to be a certain weight or gestational age to feed directly at the breast. As soon as the infant shows physiological stability (heart rate and oxygenation), direct feeding at the breast should commence. Infants can demonstrate suckling as early as 29 weeks of gestation (Nyqvist, 2008). The mother should be encouraged to breastfeed at least once per day, but ideally as many times of the day as the infant is showing feeding readiness cues. Infant-driven feeding (cue-based feeding) is associated with improved breastfeeding outcomes, as well as shorter length of stay (Chrupcala et al., 2015). In order to best support direct breastfeeding at the breast, NICUs should consider making infant-driven feeding the standard of care (Chrupcala et al., 2015). When using a "transition to breast pathway," even the most complex infants with surgical anomalies can effectively transition to direct breastfeeding prior to discharge (Edwards & Spatz, 2010).

Step 8: Measuring Milk Transfer

Many health care professionals rely on clinical cues to evaluate a breastfeeding session, and a variety of tools exist that are used for healthy term infants. However, with vulnerable infants, pre- and post-weights with a precise electronic scale (accurate to at least ± 2 g) are essential to ensure that the infants are not under- or overfed. Infants may appear to be "breastfeeding" without transferring milk. Pre- and post-weights increase maternal confidence in their ability to care for their infant. In addition, it allows the mother to effectively feed their infant on cue and supplement appropriately if the infant is unable to take the full volume directly from the breast.

Step 9: Preparation for Discharge

As NICU discharge approaches, it is important to empower the family to care for the infant. Empowering the parents to be involved in all aspects of their infant's care is essential. If the mother's goal is to breastfeed, providers should encourage the mother to spend as many hours of the day (or night) at the child's bedside as possible so that she can breastfeed on cue. Parents should be provided a comfortable chair at each bedside for breastfeeding, a hospital-grade pump (so that the mother can pump before feed to elicit release of oxytocin and milk flow), a Baby Weigh scale for pre- and post-weights, and a warmer to warm any additional milk that may be needed after a breastfeeding session. It is important that the family develop confidence in caring for their infant and/or for the mother to have plenty of opportunities to breastfeed prior to discharge.

Step 10: Appropriate Follow-Up

At time of infant discharge, an infant may not be transferring all of their feeds at the breast dependent on maternal milk volume, the amount of opportunity the infant has to participate in SSC and NNS, and/or the number of direct breastfeeding sessions afforded to the dyad. Special circumstances are addressed later in relation to other potential challenges that can occur with long-term NICU stays. However, almost all challenges that families may experience with the provision of human milk and breastfeeding would be avoided with appropriate evidence-based lactation education, assessment, care, and support. The entire health professional team should be partners in helping families cope with breastfeeding difficulties.

NICU INFANT FEEDING DIFFICULTIES

Many NICU infants require feeding tubes for initial enteral feeds. Thus, direct breast feeds are not feasible. Despite this, health care professionals should prioritize the use of human milk for all enteral feeds. It is important to note that infants could receive feeds via nasogastric tube, gastrostomy tube, and/or jejunostomy tube. Feeding tubes can be a significant source of infection. Therefore, if the infant requires a feeding tube, human milk plays a significant role in preventing bacterial overgrowth on the feeding tube (Mehall et al., 2002). Feeding tubes can serve as a significant source of nosocomial infections (Mehall et al., 2002). Therefore, human milk should be viewed as an essential and protective factor when infants require feeding tubes. In addition, if the infant has been receiving human milk oral care, this will help prepare the infant for eventual direct breast feeds.

The most common cause of infant feeding difficulties in the NICU relates to long=term intubation. Infants may develop feeding aversion and/or may fatigue quickly. In some instances, a swallow test may be ordered to determine if the infant is having silent aspiration. Speech–language therapists, occupational therapists, and lactation specialists should be consulted to assist with oral feeding. Optimal activities to promote oral feeding skills include human milk oral care, SSC, and NNS. Some infants will tire easily with oral feeds; therefore, Lau (2020) recommends an individualized approach. If the infant is able transfer 80% of feedings orally, it is best to allow for self-maturation. If the infant is transferring less than 80% of feeds, one can consider the following interventions to improve oral feeding skills: positioning, non-nutritive oral motor training, tactile–kinesthetic/massage, and changing feeding positions (Lau, 2020). It is recommended to offer interventions in 2-day blocks to allow for self-maturation of the infant.

POST-DISCHARGE CARE

Discharge planning begins at NICU admission. The Spatz 10-step model for human milk and breastfeeding has proven research outcomes that demonstrated human milk feeds at discharge can be significantly increased if this model is utilized (Fugate, 2015; Spatz, 2004; Takako et al., 2020). However, in many NICUs, direct at-breast feeds are not prioritized for vulnerable infants, so many infants end up being fed expressed milk or formula by bottle. Therefore, health care providers must prioritize support for parents who have the goal to directly feed at the breast. Even if an infant cannot feed at the breast or the mother only wishes to feed expressed milk, the need for SSC and holding and touching of their infant should be emphasized and prioritized. If the infant will be discharged home with some or all feeds via a bottle, it is important that infants gain competence in this skill. Pados and colleagues (2019) demonstrate that there is tremendous variability among bottle nipples. Slow-flow nipples allow the infant to have better heart rate and oxygen stability. Parents should be instructed on infant feeding cues and how to perform "paced bottle feeding."

Another concern post-discharge is infant growth. There are highly accurate scales that can be rented for use post-discharge. The BabyWeigh scales are accurate to ± 2 g and can hold infants up to 10,000 g (22 pounds). Some hospitals provide these scales to parents at discharge free of charge on a loaner basis. Parents can also rent these scales in the community and may be able to receive insurance reimbursement with a prescription. The scale is extremely beneficial to parents who wish to directly feed at the breast. It allows the parents to know exactly how much milk the infant is taking at every feeding session, thus preventing overfeeding or underfeeding of the child. The family can also weigh their infant weekly to track infant weight gain.

RELATIONSHIP TO PARENTAL COPING

Whereas the physical benefits to infants and mothers have been widely known and even referred to as "mutual caregiving," less has been captured in the literature about the effects of the provision of human milk and/or breastfeeding on parental coping in the NICU. Breastfeeding has been reported to impact mood and stress reactivity in mothers. Specifically, breastfeeding mothers report reductions in anxiety, negative mood, and stress compared to formula-feeding mothers (Krol & Grossmann, 2018). The NICU environment as the point of entry to parenthood often creates an immediate tension at a most sensitive time in the postnatal period; breastfeeding/pumping can be the antidote to that most poisonous of periods.

The NICU setting is one that understandably leaves parents feeling frightened and powerless while their infant is obscured by equipment undergoing testing and procedures. In the Children's Hospital of Philadelphia NICU, that they have felt they became passive, useless observers to their infant while a team of medical providers satellite around the infant. Breastfeeding can help facilitate maternal sensitivity and secure attachment between mother and infant. In fact, research has shown that breastfeeding mothers have a tendency to touch their infants more often and spend more time in mutual gaze with their infants compared to bottle-feeding mother–infant dyads (Krol & Grossmann, 2018). The very act of breastfeeding/pumping installs parents, and mothers specifically, as an integral and necessary part of the caregiving team. As previously mentioned, almost all mothers can provide milk for their infants, and there are few contraindications to breastfeeding (i.e., HIV-positive and active illegal drug use). Mothers for whom breastfeeding is contraindicated should be encouraged to participate in SSC and touching and holding of their child. There are also mothers who may wish to express milk for their child but do not wish to directly feed at the breast. Hamdam and Tamim (2012) demonstrated in a prospective study that breastfeeding mothers have lower scores on the Edinburgh Postnatal Depression Scale. It follows that principally in a NICU setting, rates of postpartum mood and anxiety disorders would be higher due to the uncertainty of the infant's condition, prognosis, and required interventions.

The entire multidisciplinary team should be involved in helping parents meet their personal goals for the provision of human milk and breastfeeding. This includes, but is not limited to, lactation specialists, nurses, social workers, physicians, occupational therapists, speech–language pathologists, registered dietitians, and psychologists. The social worker can play a key role in the perinatal period by conducting a thorough and detailed psychosocial assessment. The family's biopsychosocial situation is of paramount importance, specifically who compromises their support system, mental health history, the family construct (e.g., other children), employment, and insurance/entitlement benefits. This information contributes to developing a stable post birth plan that accounts for the entire patient and family situation. Specific attention should be paid to the family's knowledge about human milk and breastfeeding and factors that they believe will contribute positively or negatively to the experience. The information should be housed in the maternal electronic medical record so that it can be accessible to all providers.

IDEAS WORTH SHARING

Traditionally, perinatal social workers are associated with connecting patients with needed resources. Often, this is limited/restricted to structural supports such as providing referrals to the Women, Infants, and Children program and provision of food stamps and car seats. Perinatal social workers are committed to breastfeeding with the same level of passion found in the medical staff but for unique reasons. The National Association of Social Workers (2017) Code of Ethics articulated on the first page that the profession's primary mission is to "enhance human well-being and help meet the basic human needs of all people with particular attention to the needs and empowerment of people who are vulnerable, oppressed and living in poverty." The association identified six core values that guide this practice: service, social justice, importance of human relationships, dignity and worth of the person, integrity, and competence. The following case example highlights an intervention that incorporates the core values utilized to support a mother's choice to breastfeed.

CASE EXAMPLE

Denise is a 21-year-old pregnant, incarcerated female with a 2-year-old son in the foster care system. Denise is disenfranchised both from her family of origin and from the baby's father. She has not seen her son in the past 12 months. Her current pregnancy is complicated by the presence of an extremely large left lower lobe extralobar bronchial pulmonary sequestration.

Denise experienced a high-risk pregnancy and cesarean-section delivery to immediate postnatal resection. Through multiple meetings with Denise, it was clear that she has sustained trauma in her life, abandonment by those who should have protected her, and is now in the prison system believing that her ability to be independent and parent her children is improbable. She is not able to stay in the hospital with her infant son and will need to place him in foster care. His medical condition and need for surgery were not well known by the staff, and she could be present in the NICU only when accompanied by a prison guard. Her pre-existing mental health disorders in combination with her psychosocial situation were clear risk factors for a perinatal mood and anxiety disorder and limited opportunity to bond with her infant.

The role of the social worker was to capitalize on Denise's strengths and abilities. In performing the assessment, it became clear how poorly Denise thought of herself and how little she felt she had to offer. After rapport had been established and the subject of breastfeeding had been broached, it became clear that this was the single area that Denise found she could contribute to her son's health and well-being. She had been reluctant to consider lactation while incarcerated because there were no breast pumps in the prison. Working closely with the lactation team and mother's milk bank at the birth hospital allowed her to leave with a free hospital-grade pump. Social work coordinated with the prison and the NICU staff for maternal visits from the prison, with the guards transporting the pumped milk with the mother.

This case example makes evident the role that breastfeeding played in social work–guided practice with this patient. The six core values were each considered when designing the intervention. Social workers provided supportive *service* to the patient in the interview process of gathering important psychosocial information. Aspects of *social justice* were accounted for as this patient remained eligible for the opportunities of other mothers in society (despite incarceration, she was able to pump). An acknowledgment of her desire to create a meaningful *human relationship* with her infant was the cornerstone from which the intervention was designed. When Denise came in for her prenatal care appointments, though under guard, *the dignity and worth of her as a person* were upheld in eliciting what she needed as an expectant mother. The multidisciplinary team maintained *integrity* always in the unified vision to uphold the maternal–infant bond despite the challenges presented by the justice and foster care systems. The lactation program and social work teamed up during and after birth to empower the patient to capitalize on her inherent *competency* as a lactating mother providing sustenance for her infant. This involved prioritizing time with her infant and ensuring early frequent milk expression.

CONCLUSION

There is a dearth of information in the literature about the role of social workers in supporting breastfeeding, which is both surprising and disappointing. There are abundant opportunities for collaboration across the health care and political spectrum to become involved beyond the very important task of making structural/concrete referrals. Lactation nurses and social workers create a powerful dyad to engage parents in the provision of human milk and breastfeeding. Social workers are ideally suited and trained to view the parent within the context of their family and society at large. This makes for an unrivaled partnership in the pursuit of helping families reach their personal breastfeeding goals.

REFERENCES

Akinbi, H., Meinzen-Derr, J., Auer, C., Ma, Y., Pullum, D., Kusano, R., Reszka, K. J., & Zimmerly, K. (2010). Alterations in the host defense properties of human milk following prolonged storage or pasteurization. *Journal of Pediatric Gastroenterology and Nutrition*, 51(3), 347–352. doi:10.1097/MPG.0b013e3181e07f0a

American Academy of Nursing. (n.d.). *10 Steps to promote and protect human milk and breastfeeding in vulnerable infants*. http://www.aannet.org/initiatives/edge-runners/profiles/edge-runners--10-steps-to-promote-and-protect-human-milk

Chrupcala, K. A., Edwards, T. M., & Spatz, D. L. (2015). A continuous quality improvement project to implement infant-driven feeding as a standard of practice in the newborn/infant intensive care unit. *Journal of Obstetric, Gynecologic, and Neonatal Nursing*, 44(5), 654–664. doi:10.1111/1552-6909.12727

Conde-Agudelo, A., & Díaz-Rossello, J. L. (2016). Kangaroo mother care to reduce morbidity and mortality in low birthweight infants. *Cochrane Database of Systematic Reviews*, 2016(8), CD002771. https://doi.org/10.1002/14651858.CD002771.pub4c

Edwards, T. E., & Spatz, D. L. (2010). An innovative model for achieving breastfeeding success in infants with complex surgical anomalies. *Journal of Perinatal and Neonatal Nursing*, 24(3), 246–253. doi:10.1097/JPN.0b013e3181e8d517

Froh, E. B., Deatrick, J. A., Curley, M. A., & Spatz, D. L. (2015). Making meaning of pumping for mothers of infants with congenital diaphragmatic hernia. *Journal of Obstetric, Gynecologic, and Neonatal Nursing*, 44(3), 439–449. https://doi.org/10.1111/1552-6909.12564

Froh, E. B., Schwarz, J., & Spatz, D. L. (2020). Lactation outcomes among dyads following participation in a model of group prenatal care for patients with prenatally diagnosed fetal anomalies. *Breastfeeding Medicine*, 15(11), 698–702. https://doi.org/10.1089/bfm.2020.0061

Froh, E. B., & Spatz, D. L. (2014). An ethical case for the provision of human milk in the NICU. *Advances in Neonatal Care*, 14(4), 269–273. https://doi.org/10.1097/ANC.0000000000000109

Fugate, K., Hernandez, I., Ashmeade, T., Miladinovic, B., & Spatz, D. L. (2015). Improving human milk and breastfeeding practices in the NICU. *Journal of Obstetric, Gynecologic, and Neonatal Nursing, 44*(3), 426–438. doi:10.1111/1552-6909.12563

Hamdam, A., & Tamim, H. (2012). The relationship between postpartum depression and breastfeeding. *International Journal of Psychiatry in Medicine, 43*(3), 243–259. doi:10.2190/PM.43.3.d

Krol, K. M., & Grossmann, T. (2018). Psychologische Effekte des Stillens auf Kinder und Mütter [Psychological effects of breastfeeding on children and mothers]. *Bundesgesundheitsblatt, Gesundheitsforschung, Gesundheitsschutz, 61*(8), 977–985. https://doi.org/10.1007/s00103-018-2769-0

Lau, C. (2020). To individualize the management care of high-risk infants with oral feeding challenges: What do we know? What can we do? *Frontiers in Pediatrics, 8,* 296. https://doi.org/10.3389/fped.2020.00296

Mehall, J. R., Kite, C. A., Gilliam, C. H., Jackson, R. J., & Smith, S. D. (2002). Enteral feeding tubes are a reservoir for nosocomial antibiotic-resistant pathogens. *Journal of Pediatric Surgery, 37*(7), 1011–1012. https://doi.org/10.1053/jpsu.2002.33831

Moore, E. R., Anderson, G. C., Bergman, N., & Dowswell, T. (2012). Early skin-to-skin contact for mothers and their healthy newborn infants. *Cochrane Database of Systematic Reviews, 5*(5), CD003519. https://doi.org/10.1002/14651858.CD003 519.pub3

National Association of Social Workers. (2017). *Code of ethics.* https://www.socialwork ers.org/about/ethics/code-of-ethics

Nyqvist, K. H. (2008). Early attainment of breastfeeding competence in very preterm infants. *Acta Paediatric, 97*(6), 776–781. https://doi.org/10.1111/j.1651-2227.2008. 00810.x

Pados, B. F., Park, J., & Dodrill, P. (2019). Milk flow rates from bottle nipples used in the hospital and after discharge. *Advances in Neonatal Care, 19*(1), 32–41. https://doi. org/10.1097/ANC.0000000000000538

Spatz, D. L. (2004). Ten steps for promoting and protecting breastfeeding in vulnerable populations. *Journal of Perinatal & Neonatal Nursing, 18*(4), 385–396. https://doi. org/10.1097/00005237-200410000-00009

Spatz, D. L. (2017). SPN position statement: The role of pediatric nurses in the promotion and protection of human milk and breastfeeding. *Journal of Pediatric Nursing, 37,* 136–139.

Spatz, D. L. (2018). Beyond BFHI: The Spatz 10-step and breastfeeding resource nurse model to improve human milk and breastfeeding outcomes. *Journal of Perinatal and Neonatal Nursing, 32*(2), 164–174. doi:10.1097/JPN.0000000000000339

Spatz, D. L., & Edwards, T. M. (2015). *The use of human milk and breastfeeding in the neonatal intensive care unit* [Position statement]. National Association of Neonatal Nurses.

Spatz, D. L., Froh, E. B., Schwarz, J., Houng, K., Brewster, I., Myers, C., Prince, J., & Olkkola, M. (2015). Pump early, pump often: A continuous quality improvement project. *Journal of Perinatal Education, 24*(3), 160–170. https://doi.org/10.1891/ 1058-1243.24.3.160

Spatz, D. L., & Miller, J. (2021). When your breasts might not work: How health care professionals can provide anticipatory guidance. *Journal of Perinatal Education, 30*(1), 13–18.

Spatz, D. L., Robinson, A. C., & Froh, E. B. (2018). Cost and use of pasteurized donor human milk at a children's hospital. *Journal of Obstetric, Gynecologic, and Neonatal Nursing, 47*(4), 583–588. https://doi.org/10.1016/j.jogn.2017.11.004

Takako, H., Mizue, M., Izumi, H., Chie, O., Harue, T., Uchida, M., & Spatz, D. L. (2020). Improving human milk and breastfeeding rates in a perinatal hospital in Japan: A quality improvement project. *Breastfeeding Medicine, 15*(8), 538–545. https://doi.org/10.1089/bfm.2019.0298

15

SHARED DECISION-MAKING
ACROSS SETTINGS

JEANNIE ZUK, KRISTIN CARTER, BETH M. MCMANUS,
AND BROOKE DORSEY HOLLIMAN ■

Fetal care centers and neonatal intensive care units (NICUs) necessitate on-going complex decisions by parents and health care providers about birth plans, prenatal assessments for suspected anomalies, an antenatal diagnostic workup for an infant's condition, treatment options for both the mother and the infant, and infant care following discharge from the hospital. Many of those decisions must be made amid uncertainty with no obvious correct answer. Although parents ultimately have the right to make decisions for their infant with the best interest standard in mind, the decision-making process should not occur in isolation without the support of the health care team. One of the most effective ways to support parents in such situations is to engage them in shared decision-making.

MODEL OF SHARED DECISION-MAKING

In fetal care centers or the neonatal intensive care unit (NICU), many different models of decision-making exist, and each of them relies on the values of the parents or family, the health care provider, or both. In addition to the model of shared decision-making, the paternalistic model, the informed model, and the professional-as-agent model are prominently discussed in the literature (C. Charles et al., 1997). In the paternalistic model, the provider takes a dominating role and does what they consider best with little input from the parents or family. Although the paternalistic model may still have a role in emergent situations, the medical field has largely moved away from this model. The informed model attempts to give the decision-making power to the parents or family while the provider's role is to share technical health information without sharing personal treatment preferences. The professional-as-agent model requires the provider to make decisions based on what the parents or family would have chosen without any influence from the provider's treatment preferences.

However, in the model of shared decision-making, providers and parents engage in two-way communication of information, values, and preferences (C. Charles et al., 1997). According to the National Quality Forum (2017), shared decision-making is "a process of communication in which clinicians and patients work together to make optimal health care decisions that align with what matters most to patients" (p. 1). There are three required components:

- Clear, accurate, and unbiased medical evidence about reasonable alternatives—including no intervention—and the risks and benefits of each;
- clinician expertise in communicating and tailoring that evidence to individual patients; and
- patient values, goals, informed preferences, and concerns, which may include treatment burdens. (p. 1)

The model of shared decision-making is often highlighted as the ideal model for decision-making in medicine, especially when uncertainty exists (C. Charles et al., 1997). In fetal care centers and NICUs, levels of uncertainty can be high, and deciding what is "right" for an infant amid such uncertainty can be incredibly difficult. Gillam (2016) proposed the zone of parental discretion (ZPD), which refers to the gray zone of decision-making that lies between the best interest standard, or optimal decision, and the harm threshold, or harmful decision. Within the ZPD, parents have the right to make decisions for their infants, and shared decision-making can be an effective way to help them do so.

Shared decision-making in fetal care centers and NICUs can be conceptualized in three phases (Lantos, 2018). In the first phase, the provider prepares for meeting with the parents by reflecting on personal biases and then setting those views aside, being open to the parents, and determining a goal of the conversation. The second phase pertains to creating a safe physical and emotional space where the conversation can occur. Finally, the third phase, which is iterative in nature, involves an exploration of the parents' emotions, fears, hopes, goals, and values. Only after that exploration can providers help frame the options for moving forward.

ENCOURAGING POSITIVE FAMILY–TEAM COMMUNICATIONS

Communication is an integral part of shared decision-making and is also an integral part of work in fetal care centers and NICUs. Communication enables the health care team to understand the parents' and family's fears, hopes, and values and also serves as the means through which the health care team can educate about the infant's condition and can comfort parents and family during trying moments (Orzalesi & Aite, 2011). However, numerous factors can make this communication challenging, including the infant's condition, the emotions of the parents and family, the emotions of the health care team that providers often fear sharing with families, the uncertainty of prognoses in the NICU, and the NICU environment (Orzalesi & Aite, 2011).

The infant's medical condition and need for admission to the intensive care unit can initially cause parents tremendous angst and guilt, regardless of the severity of the illness. Parents may have difficulty expressing themselves and become overwhelmed with the amount of medical information shared with them. Communication will be most effective when parents are comfortable with the relationship with the health care team, maintaining trust and honesty. However, if the infant starts to experience some improvement and then declines, the parents are sometimes again devastated by a sudden downward turn of the infant's condition. The ups and downs of the infant's condition can lead to a loss of the parents' trust in the health care team, which presents barriers to open and effective communication (Orzalesi & Aite, 2011).

Uncertainty has been called the uncomfortable companion to decision-making for infants because most diagnoses have a wide range of unpredictable outcomes (Krick et al., 2020). Providers must simultaneously establish trust and give hope to families while effectively communicating the real uncertainty of the situation and supporting families in the ZPD. Finding the balance of those tasks can be quite difficult and can complicate any communication. Furthermore, the uncertainty and differences in provider and parent or family values can cause providers to hide their emotions. By sharing their emotions and values rather than hiding them, providers can help maintain empathetic communication at a time when it is desperately needed by both parents and the health care team (Orzalesi & Aite, 2011).

Finally, the hectic environments in the fetal care center and the NICU, which necessitate the use of unnatural technologies that can overwhelm families and require an extensive health care team that rotates frequently, can create a barrier to effective communication. Each member of the health care team has their own communication style and approach to working with the family, and parents may hear different opinions from different people, which may create confusion and mistrust (Orzalesi & Aite, 2011).

Despite the numerous barriers, positive communication between the parents or family and the health care team in the fetal care center and the NICU is possible and should be encouraged. Some of the key steps to positive communication are outlined in Box 15.1. The steps should be encouraged among all members of the health care team, and their implementation will help develop positive family–team communication and subsequent improvements in patient care and family satisfaction.

Box 15.1

KEY STEPS TO ENSURING POSITIVE FAMILY–TEAM COMMUNICATION IN THE NICU

- Perform introductions of the infant's health care team, along with an explanation of roles.
- Create a safe, welcoming environment by finding a quiet, private room; avoiding interruptions; limiting the number of health care professionals; and sitting during the conversation.
- Speak to the parents with the infant present, if possible.
- Ask the parents how much they want to know.
- Emphasize the positive aspects of the infant's situation and describe the challenges.

- Use nonverbal communication (e.g., eye contact, head nodding, and leaning in during the conversation) and empathy.
- Meet with both parents as soon as possible, which keeps the father/partner from having to be the messenger to the mother as she recovers from the birth process.
- Attempt to maintain continuity of staff.
- Follow up at short time intervals (e.g., later that day or the next day) to assess whether the information has been understood.

Sources: Lantos (2018) and Orzalesi and Aite (2011).

HEALTH LITERACY CONSIDERATIONS

A key part of positive communication and of shared decision-making is an understanding and assessment of health literacy. According to the National Library of Medicine, health literacy is defined as "the degree to which individuals have the capacity to obtain, process, and understand basic health information and services needed to make appropriate health decisions" (Ratzan & Parker, 2000, p. vi). As this definition highlights, health literacy extends well beyond a person's capacity to read. It is composed of listening and speaking skills (known as oral literacy), reading and writing skills (known as print literacy), numeracy, and cultural and conceptual knowledge. It is therefore influenced by an interplay of education, culture and society, and the characteristics of the health care setting (Institute of Medicine, 2004).

Approximately 87% of adults in the United States have limited health literacy (Agency for Healthcare Research and Quality [AHRQ], 2020). People with limited health literacy might have difficulties following a treatment plan, filling out complex forms, sharing their health history, understanding risk and probability, and participating in shared decision-making (AHRQ, 2020). Those difficulties can lead to poor health outcomes, exacerbate health outcome disparities, and contribute to patient/caregiver dissatisfaction with health care providers.

Knowledge of the health literacy of parents of infants in the NICU is limited, but such knowledge may have a vital role in engaging parents or family members in shared decision-making and improving medical communication in a stressful environment, creating appropriate discharge plans, and ensuring caregiver ability to execute discharge plans successfully. One study of parents of newborns found that a higher percentage of parents of infants in the NICU (43%) had suspected limited health literacy (SLHL) compared to parents of infants in the well-baby nursery (25%) (Mackley et al., 2016). Lower educational status, minority race/ethnicity, and female parental gender were associated with increased odds of SLHL, although a notable portion of parents with a college degree had SLHL. Screening for health literacy and numeracy skills in the NICU may be beneficial to increasing awareness of health literacy issues among parents and family members and improving efforts to support caregiver education.

Utilizing the teach-back method, presenting a small amount of information at a time, using pictures, striving to communicate numbers clearly by using frequencies instead of decimals or percentages, giving absolute risk instead of relative risk, framing outcomes in both positive and negative terms, and using the same measurement system as the caregiver can also be helpful in addressing health literacy issues (AHRQ, 2020).

In the teach-back method, the provider shares health information about an important topic and then asks the infant's parents to use their own words to describe the infant's health and the next steps or decisions in the infant's care. The provider can also ask the parents to demonstrate how to do something that is necessary for the care of the infant (e.g., prepare the infant's formula). This technique can increase the parents' ability to remember and understand information and can make them feel more relaxed.

When communicating numbers as frequencies rather than as decimals or percentages, the provider can say "1 out of 100" rather than "0.01" or "1 percent." Furthermore, risk should be communicated as the absolute risk (3 out of 1,000 infants born term will have this condition, whereas 6 out of 1,000 infants born prematurely will have this condition) rather than as the relative risk (preterm infants have two times the risk of this condition compared to term infants). Finally, medicine often utilizes the metric system, but depending on the country, parents may more readily use the customary system. Discussing the parents' preferences and trying to present information to them in that system, when able, will help with their understanding and compliance. These techniques can be employed by any member of the patient's health care team, including behavioral health providers.

COUNSELING CONSIDERATIONS (TEAM–FAMILY COMMUNICATION)

Communication and counseling considerations between families and the clinical team about decisions that need to be made during the perinatal period and following birth can be challenging and should focus on the essence of shared decision-making, whenever possible. Clear and focused communication between parents and the health care team becomes critical when an infant's diagnosis and prognosis are uncertain, with elicitation of parent values and goals for their infant as important as a discussion of information, procedures, and risks.

The most commonly used description of a shared decision-making model (SDM) assumes clear communication about options, or choices, available to parents about their infant's medical course and often downplays the difficulties parents face in making the "best" decision for their infant. This becomes even more important when conflicting information becomes available and the medical plan evolves as the infant's medical status changes. Feudtner and colleagues (2018) describe SDM as a process often obscured by simplicity with parents reviewing a situation with a series of solutions or options they can choose. Communication and counseling are generally health care provider led with a presentation to parents prioritizing the problem and selecting the treatment options. When this works well, clinicians partner with parents to elicit values and goals and incorporate this information into recommendations about treatment options. Some clinicians utilize a type of checklist decision aid to provide information and clarify parent values (Sullivan & Cummings, 2020). In a best-case scenario, as described by Feudtner and colleagues (2018), parents were provided with all the necessary information about a decision for a tracheostomy for their infant daughter, the advantages and disadvantages of the tracheostomy, the implications of caring for a ventilator-dependent infant, and what would happen if the parents chose not to perform the tracheostomy. The parents took time to reflect on the information provided and carefully considered the different scenarios presented in the family meeting. After making their choice for treatment, the parents responded to the team saying they really did not have a decision to make—that the tracheostomy was the only option available because their goal was their daughter's survival no matter the challenges. In this case, the parents stated they participated in decisions each step of the way with clear and consistent input from the clinicians involved with their daughter's care. Shared decision-making became an ongoing process, revisited multiple times throughout the infant's NICU stay rather than a one-time physician-driven decision.

Sometimes the SDM process becomes more complicated with parents who "want to do everything" for their infant (Fry & Frader, 2018) and disagree with the clinician team who may believe that "everything" is not in the best interest of the infant or that some treatment decisions would harm the infant (Saunders, 2021). The definition of what constitutes harm has come under scrutiny, with little agreement among physicians. Such is the worst-case scenario of Charlie Gard and the court battle over the role of parents' decision-making and what constitutes harm. The drawn-out and very public court case highlighted differences of opinions in the United Kingdom and the United States about treatment for severely medically compromised infants and children, parents' role in decision-making, and physicians' clinical judgment (Saunders, 2021).

Charlie Gard was diagnosed with a rare encephalopathic form of mitochondrial DNA depletion syndrome caused by a mutation in the *RRM2B* gene

(Ross, 2020). For the first few months of life, Charlie behaved as a normal, healthy infant, but his parents noticed muscle weakness and failure to thrive, which, after an extensive workup, quickly progressed to paralysis and he was placed on a ventilator. Due to the lack of known treatments for Charlie's condition, his parents did an extensive search for researchers with experience treating mitochondrial diseases, finding a clinical trial underway at Columbia University Medical Center in New York City with Dr. Michio Hirano. Hirano's trial used nucleoside bypass treatment with preliminary, unpublished, evidence of effectiveness treating syndromes such as Charlie's. The medical team caring for Charlie was hesitant to seek approval to use Hirano's nucleoside bypass treatment because of concerns about the drug's effectiveness and the small number of treated patients. Charlie's parents petitioned the doctors treating him at his UK hospital to grant approval to use the experimental treatment from the U.S. clinical trial despite a lack of results. Charlie's condition continued to deteriorate, and the UK physicians recommended withdrawal of what they considered futile care that would only prolong Charlie's suffering while the parents continued to argue for transferring Charlie to the United States to receive the experimental treatment, arguing it was in his best interest to try the treatment. The court case became sensationalized after Charlie's parents raised £1.3 million (approximately $1.8 million) through public donations to pay for transporting Charlie to the United States to receive the experimental treatment. Ultimately, after multiple arguments in UK courts, multiple petitions by his parents, and an examination by Hirano, who traveled to the United Kingdom to examine Charlie, it was determined Charlie would not benefit from the experimental treatment. The court arguments centered around what was in Charlie's best interests and who has the right to determine those interests—the physicians, the court, or the parents. Charlie's parents ultimately accepted Hirano's evaluation and agreed to withdraw ventilator support. Charlie died on July 28, 2017, at 11 months of age.

This extremely difficult and complex worst-case scenario highlights the consequences of conflicting opinions, the role of parents in defining what is in the best interest for their child, physicians determining what is considered futile care, and the limits of SDM for medically fragile infants and children. This case continues to be argued in medical and legal journals, with a range of opinions on the outcome. Truog (2020) argues that the UK courts sought to protect Charlie from his parents' views on what was best for him, whereas U.S. opinion generally sides with greater parental involvement in decision-making. The ZPD model of shared decision-making is commonly cited as justification for allowing parents to make final decisions, whereas other authors have argued for the application of the "harm principle" unless parents' decisions have been determined to cause harm to their child. Wilkinson (2019) calls the issues raised by cases such as that of Charlie Gard vexing and profound; this case continues the discussion of shared decision-making, communication between families and clinicians, and the form of counseling families.

COMMON CHALLENGING DECISIONS

Pregnancy and Fetal Diagnosis

Advances in prenatal screening, diagnosis, and counseling in the past decade have complicated pregnancy-related decision-making and focused on the importance of an SDM process. This process includes multiple conversations between the pregnant woman and clinicians with detailed information about the fetal diagnosis, potential intrauterine treatment options along with treatments available after birth, and a plan for delivery of the infant or, in some cases, termination of the pregnancy. Ideally, most of these physician-led discussions incorporate parent values, goals, and personal beliefs that will influence decisions. However, Paton et al. (2020) emphasize no standard exists on the "right" way to counsel families using SDM principles, particularly given the uncertainty around morbidity, mortality, and prognosis involved with a diagnosis of a serious or severe congenital fetal anomaly. Paton et al. describe parents who participate in a "rational" decision-making process by considering the information about the diagnosis and weighing the risks and benefits of treatment, coming to what these authors describe as a "good" decision. In this scenario, physicians typically controlled the type and amount of information given, expecting parents to use this information to form their decisions. When parents sought information outside of the fetal care center's environment, searched for other opinions, or made what Lotto et al. (2018) refer to as a "heart-led decision," this potentially affected the physician–parent relationship by introducing an element of mistrust in the provided information from the clinical team.

Most fetal centers are able to detect and/or confirm cardiac anomalies, anencephaly, myelomeningocele, renal agenesis, congenital diaphragmatic hernia, trisomies 13 and 18, and skeletal dysplasias. Several of these diagnoses are potentially lethal without intervention, whereas others carry significant morbidity or indicate potentially life-limiting future conditions. All involve difficult and complex decisions with no consistent recommendations on what constitutes a "good" decision (Lotto et al., 2018). For decisions about infants with severe congenital heart disease, for example, parents face weighing the burdens of treatment, multiple corrective surgeries, and long stays in intensive care units with the potential benefits of caring for an infant with heart disease. Lynema et al. (2016) frame their discussions with parents whose infant has critical or moderately severe congenital heart disease in terms of survival to hospital discharge and identifiable risk factors for mortality. Some parents are more willing to take on these risks than others and make their decisions accordingly.

Fetal Interventions

Specialized, multidisciplinary fetal care centers have increased in number internationally and throughout the United States, providing clinical expertise in evaluating and prenatal interventions for a range of fetal anomalies, including congenital diaphragmatic hernia, twin–twin transfusion syndrome, and myelomeningocele. In 2011, the American College of Obstetricians and Gynecologists (ACOG) published a Committee Opinion on maternal–fetal interventions and fetal care centers outlining recommendations about consent for procedures, emphasizing the need for a multidisciplinary team approach to interventions and oversight of fetal care centers. These ACOG recommendations highlighted the importance of differentiating between cutting-edge, innovative interventions and research to gather data on outcomes and best practice. In addition, prospective parents must be provided with information about alternatives to potentially high-risk interventions in order to make the best decisions for their fetus and their family without coercion to participate.

Evaluations at these centers often require the pregnant woman and a support person to travel to the center to meet with a team of experts, including maternal–fetal medicine specialists, fetal surgeons, neonatologists, social workers, and/or psychologists, for an evaluation that includes detailed fetal ultrasounds and echocardiograms; fetal magnetic resonance imaging; genetic screening tests such as cell-free DNA screening, maternal serum screening, and carrier screening; as well as diagnostic tests for some chromosomal abnormalities. Some fetal interventions are only available at a few institutions and are offered within a window of time during the pregnancy, requiring a time-sensitive decision about the intervention. Some parents described the evaluation as impacting their lives because many needed to relocate to the fetal care center in a different state, far from families and their usual support system. These families especially appreciated the SDM process that valued both the information provided and the emotional support for their decisions (Kett et al., 2017).

When considering risky procedures such as intrauterine fetal surgery, many parents made decisions based on the need to "do everything" in an attempt to go home with a live infant and to say they gave their infant every chance to survive rather than rely solely on information provided by their health care providers (Fry & Frader, 2018). Fry and Frader describe blogs in which parents wrote about their experiences with fetal surgery and how they dealt with decisions when facing fetal surgery options. Many parents wrote about needing both guidance and support when faced with difficult decisions after clinicians presented information, risks of the procedures, and outcomes based on their clinical experience. The blogs illustrated that mothers wanted what was "best" for their fetus "perhaps with less regard for their own well-being" (Fry & Frader, 2018, p. 231). Maternal risks were considered secondary to their fetus' survival and a sacrifice they were willing to make, and mothers spoke about fetal surgery decisions as something any good parent would make.

Intrauterine Myelomeningocele Repair

Myelomeningocele (MMC) is one of the most common prenatally diagnosed congenital abnormalities of the central nervous system. Although not typically fatal, MMC is associated with significant postnatal morbidity due to the abnormal development of the central nervous system, resulting in hydrocephaly, hindbrain herniation, and functional motor deficits depending on the level of the spinal lesion. The MOMS trial was a National Institutes of Health–funded prospective, multicenter randomized trial that examined prenatal and postnatal MMC closures to compare outcomes of fetal/neonatal death or placement of a cerebrospinal fluid shunt and also neurodevelopmental/motor outcomes (Moldenhauer & Adzick, 2017). The MOMS trial was halted early for demonstrated efficacy of the prenatal closure, and this has been offered as standard of care at many of the larger fetal care centers. Although the prenatal MMC closure outcomes have shown decreased need for postnatal shunting and reversal of hindbrain herniation with improved motor function, the intervention is not without both maternal and fetal risk, and it requires careful evaluation by the fetal care center team and a discussion of realistic expectations with parents. Ongoing research examining neonatal outcomes following the prenatal closure compared with postnatal repair has demonstrated an increased risk for birth before 30 weeks of gestation but no difference in other prematurity-related complications such as sepsis, necrotizing enterocolitis, and intraventricular hemorrhage (Rintoul et al., 2020).

Although prenatal closure may be considered standard of care at many institutions, the decision about intrauterine MMC surgery is not an easy one for many parents. Ravindra et al. (2020) discuss an active SDM model in which the fetal care team presents parents with information about risks and benefits of both fetal surgery and a postnatal closure to introduce parents to available options before beginning what they refer to as the discussion about what matters most to parents. The definition of what matters most is different for each family, and ideally the SDM process does not pressure parents to choose one approach over the other. Ravindra et al. (2020) found that of 175 referrals, 80 (46%) qualified for repair and 57 patients opted for fetal surgery. Decisions were based not only on the information provided but also on an appraisal of how fetal surgery fit with family needs and values.

Interventions at Labor and Delivery

Shared decision-making at labor and delivery generally focuses on whether a repeat cesarean section is needed, either after a trial of labor or after a previous cesarean section birth, commonly referred to as a VBAC (vaginal birth after cesarean). Many studies report that women who successfully give birth by VBAC experience fewer complications and have a shorter recovery than after a cesarean birth. However, a VBAC comes with risks, including uterine rupture and the possibility of an emergency repeat cesarean birth (Tucker Edmonds et al., 2020). Healthy People 2020 goals included a reduction in the elective cesarean birth rate with an increase in VBAC rates and a trial of labor (Attanasio et al., 2018). Although data concerning women's preferences for VBAC are mixed, according to Attanasio et al., many women desire a vaginal birth, but decisions about attempting VBAC can be complex and must take into consideration perceptions of safety, the convenience of scheduling a cesarean birth, wanting the experience of a vaginal birth, and perceptions of clinician attitudes. Conversely, women who preferred a repeat cesarean birth reported they did not have a choice because their hospital policy dictated birth mode.

The discussion around a cesarean birth, either after a trial of labor (TOLAC) or VBAC, is a discussion about risk and the level of acceptable risk during childbirth (S. Charles & Wolf, 2018). The discussion also centers around the medicalization of childbirth and physician control over the process. S. Charles and Wolf describe women who adamantly desire either a TOLAC or a VBAC traveling miles to a provider who will allow them to make their own decision about how they give birth. Tucker Edmonds et al. (2019) refer to decisions made about the mode of delivery as preference-sensitive decision-making using a collaborative SDM model of open communication that includes frank discussion about risks but also includes the pregnant woman's values and preferences. Women report greater satisfaction with the birth when they are offered options and the conversation between the pregnant woman and her provider includes a discussion of maternal and fetal risks, benefits, and the woman's preferences (Tucker Edmonds et al., 2020). Unfortunately, this model is not uniformly applied, with Black and Latina women and women of lower socioeconomic levels less likely to report SDM and indicating being given fewer options regarding cesarean sections compared to White women (Attanasio et al., 2018). In addition, Black and Latina women have higher rates of cesarean delivery than White women as well as greater use of obstetric procedures, which may contribute to the differences in delivery decision-making.

Interventions at Birth

Tucker Edmonds et al. (2019) describe a gap in understanding the extent to which parents want to participate in SDM and their level of understanding complex medical information about their critically ill infant. The American Academy of Pediatrics published guidelines in 2015 for counseling "periviable" infants born between 22 and 25 weeks of gestation, with recommendations for detailed discussions with parents about resuscitation and comfort care/palliative care (Feltman et al., 2020). However, as treatment and survival for 24- and 25-week infants has improved, the definition of what constitutes periviable has evolved, leading to a change in the conversations between parents and neonatologists. The lack of consensus about appropriate treatments drives variability in how to counsel parents, with differences among institutions throughout the United States. Uncertain survival and the extent of long-term neurobehavioral outcomes add complexity to counseling and the role parents play in decision-making.

Resuscitation decisions about extreme preterm, or periviable, infants made at the time of birth are often guided by institutional policy and have generally been based on gestational age. However, recent studies have argued for considering factors such as weight, sex, and verification of gestational age when assessing outcomes. Feltman et al. (2020) described intervention options offered to mothers for 22- and 23-week deliveries that included parent preference for resuscitation along with a reassessment period in the NICU with an evaluation of prognostic outcomes and risk of further treatment. However, there was variability in the application of SDM, with maternal age, race/ethnicity, education level, and socioeconomic factors influencing the amount of information discussed and the frequency of the communications. Tucker Edmonds et al. (2019) describe parents interviewed during pregnancy as desiring a role in several antenatal treatment decisions, including infant resuscitation and mode of delivery, but wanting the discussion to go beyond information about morbidity and mortality. Factors influencing parents in their decision-making included giving their infant "a fighting chance," avoiding pain and suffering, and doing what they viewed as best for their infant. Parents differed on the potential for long-term disability as influencing their decisions, with some citing prior experience with preterm birth or disability, whereas others described reliance on their faith and acceptance of a higher power. Mercurio and Carter (2020) support transparency in communicating outcomes and potential disability but deferring to parents' values and judgment of what matters to them.

Interventions in the Neonatal Period for Infants with a Poor Prognosis

Long considered lethal, interventions for infants with a prenatal diagnosis of trisomy 13 or 18 (T13 or T18) were not often recommended, and comfort care was the only available option. In the past decade, even when parents sought life-saving interventions, many neonatologists were concerned that some interventions prolonged the infant's suffering without significantly improving quality of life, presenting a burden to the family. This conflict often set up a difficult relationship between the parents and the health care providers (Janvier & Watkins, 2013).

Thiele et al. (2013) reported on three mothers who described their experience trying to make decisions about interventions for their infants diagnosed with T13 or T18 when health care/medical provider recommendations were for termination or palliative care if the pregnancy was not spontaneously interrupted. The women spoke of feeling abandoned by the medical team, requests for information about treatment options were ignored, and attempts at SDM were co-opted by what they described as "physician authoritarian attitudes." Attitudes have significantly changed since Thiele et al's article was published, and what many consider aggressive interventions for infants with T13 or T18 are now becoming more normalized, including parent perspectives and values in the decision-making process. Janvier et al. (2020) describe the importance of supporting parents in their choices while not offering unrealistic hope. Parents may believe a diagnosis such as T13 or T18 leads to a "devaluation" of their infant with an implied judgment of the parents' decision-making abilities. Janvier and colleagues describe establishing trust between parents and clinicians as foundational to SDM and avoiding adversarial interactions when developing a plan of care for infants. Parents described the importance of ongoing discussions with the clinician team in which input from parents was considered valuable and information was personalized.

Recent survival data show a more nuanced picture of T13 and T18 with a discussion on the possibility of what Kett (2020) describes as a self-fulfilling prophecy. Although almost all infants with T13 or T18 who survive infancy experience neurodevelopmental delays, some of which are profound, many of these children achieve developmental milestones, although delayed, and parents describe them as bringing joy to their family. Nevertheless, this more complicated picture of infants with T13 and T18 is not all positive. Leuthner and Acharya (2020) recommend a careful examination of parents who choose aggressive interventions and those choosing termination or palliative care after birth, along with studies on long-term parent responses to their choices, family dynamics and coping, and the financial implications of caring for a child with medical complexity.

Role of Behavioral Health Clinicians in Supporting Families in Their Decision-Making Process

Both the practice of and research on SDM in behavioral health are still in the early stages. Parents are considered the primary decision-makers for their infants, based on our society's moral and legal traditions that uphold the family as the foundation of our values and beliefs. This underscores the importance of behavioral health care professionals and families to engage in effective communication and mutual respect often during highly stressful and emotional periods. Common ethical and moral dilemmas in decision-making are encountered by families and staff during the perinatal period (e.g., selective reduction, pregnancy interruption due to fetal anomaly, and fetal surgery) and neonatal period (e.g., "heroic" life-saving measures and continuation of care vs. withdrawal). The SDM approach allows behavioral health professionals to consider the best available evidence when making suggestions while supporting parents as they consider their options to achieve informed preferences and decisions.

There are concerns about the need for cultural competence in ensuring that SDM is accessible to all families. For example, in many cultures, family members and spiritual leaders may be expected to participate in important decision-making processes and cautioned against promoting models of SDM that are not inclusive of a variety of perspectives, expectations, and values regarding decision-making. In addition, more work needs to be done on the promotion and financing of SDM in the NICU. The use of SDM should be embedded throughout the behavioral health care system so that everyone is trained in the practice of SDM and SDM becomes the model by which decisions are made in the NICU. SDM should be incorporated into and promoted through funding mechanisms that support behavioral health initiatives such as person-centered care and transformation of the behavioral health care system.

IDEAS WORTH SHARING: SUGGESTED MODEL OF APPROACH

Despite the recent focus on increasing family engagement in neonatal care and the growth of interventions to promote SDM, barriers to effective SDM persist (Boland et al., 2019; Wyatt et al., 2015). In this chapter, models of SDM were presented in particular phases to help providers optimize shared decision-making (Lantos, 2018). We also considered the unique challenges of providing care and optimizing SDM in the context of uncertainty and the high-acuity environment of fetal and neonatal intensive care. Last, we emphasized the importance of utilizing a team approach that leverages the expertise of behavioral health providers while simultaneously promoting effective team and team–parent communication.

Here, strategies to integrate these challenges and opportunities to promote effective SDM are considered. Despite the lack of a unified and "best practice" approach to SDM, several approaches to care have been suggested, and in this section we integrate that information to offer guidance for neonatal and fetal care providers. First, Elwyn and colleagues (2012) describe a three-step approach to shared decision-making: (a) choice talk, (b) option talk, and (c) decision talk. During *choice talk*, the provider ensures that parents know the possible choices. To this end, providers can offer and justify choices while being mindful of the parent's understanding and emotional reaction to each of the choices presented. During *option talk*, clinicians provide a greater level of detail about each option. This typically involves describing each option along with its relative trade-offs, risks, and benefits all within the context of the patient's understanding and preferences for specific options. In the third step, *decision talk*, providers weigh patient preferences and facilitate a decision toward what is best for the patient.

Another approach to care that offers concrete actions for providers to promote shared decision-making has been presented and can be integrated into the three-step process described by Elwyn et al. (2012). Specifically, Lantos (2018) suggests that providers use open-ended questions, let parents share what they know and feel, and work toward achieving a "common ground." These actions require that providers speak less and listen more to allow parents the opportunity and space to share their preferences, thoughts, understanding about choices, and emotions regarding care options.

CONCLUSION

As fetal and neonatal critical care continues to evolve, care choices and options for patients will continue to be complex and require effective team communication and shared decision-making. Thus, it will be increasingly important for providers, care teams, and leadership to foster a culture that promotes the attributes of effective SDM. This includes creating genuine opportunities for parents to understand, process, and discuss their options in a context that facilitates active listening and mutual understanding with the goal of a true shared decision-making process.

REFERENCES

Agency for Healthcare Research and Quality. (2020, September). *SHARE approach curriculum tools.*

American College of Obstetricians and Gynecologists. (2011). Committee opinion no. 501: Maternal–fetal intervention and fetal care centers. *Obstetrics and Gynecology, 118*(2 Pt. 1), 405–410. doi:10.1097/AOG.0b013e31822c99af

Attanasio, L. B., Kozhimannil, K. B., & Kjerulff, K. H. (2018). Factors influencing women's perceptions of shared decision making during labor and delivery: Results from a large-scale cohort study of first childbirth. *Patient Education and Counseling, 101*(6), 1130–1136. doi:10.1016/j.pec.2018.01.002

Boland, L., Graham, I. D., Légaré, F., Lewis, K., Jull, J., Shephard, A., Lawson, M. L., Davis, A., Yameogo, A., & Stacey, D. (2019). Barriers and facilitators of pediatric shared decision-making: A systematic review. *Implementation Science, 14*(1), 7. doi:10.1186/s13012-018-0851-5

Charles, C., Gafni, A., & Whelan, T. (1997). Shared decision-making in the medical encounter: What does it mean? (Or it takes at least two to tango). *Social Science and Medicine, 44*(5), 681–692. doi:10.1016/s0277-9536(96)00221-3

Charles, S., & Wolf, A. B. (2018). Whose values? Whose risk? Exploring decision making about trial of labor after cesarean. *Journal of Medical Humanities, 39*(2), 151–164. doi:10.1007/s10912-016-9410-8

Elwyn, G., Frosch, D., Thomson, R., Joseph-Williams, N., Lloyd, A., Kinnersley, P., Cording, E., Tomson, D., Dodd, C., Rollnick, S., Edwards, A., & Barry, M. (2012). Shared decision making: A model for clinical practice. *Journal of General Internal Medicine, 27*(10), 1361–1367. doi:10.1007/s11606-012-2077-6

Feltman, D. M., Fritz, K. A., Datta, A., Carlos, C., Hayslett, D., Tonismae, T., Lawrence, C., Batton, E., Coleman, T., Jain, M., Andrews, B., Famuyide, M., Tucker Edmonds, B., Laventhal, N., & Leuthner, S. (2020). Antenatal periviability counseling and decision making: A retrospective examination by the Investigating Neonatal Decisions for Extremely Early Deliveries Study Group. *American Journal of Perinatology, 37*(2), 184–195. doi:10.1055/s-0039-1694792

Feudtner, C., Schall, T., & Hill, D. (2018). Parental personal sense of duty as a foundation of pediatric medical decision-making. *Pediatrics, 142*(Suppl. 3), S133–S141. doi:10.1542/peds.2018-0516C

Fry, J. T., & Frader, J. E. (2018). "We want to do everything": How parents represent their experiences with maternal–fetal surgery online. *Journal of Perinatology, 38*(3), 226–232. doi:10.1038/s41372-017-0040-4

Gillam, L. (2016). The zone of parental discretion: An ethical tool for dealing with disagreement between parents and doctors about medical treatment for a child. *Clinical Ethics, 11*(1), 1–8. doi:10.1177/1477750915622033

Institute of Medicine. (2004). Health literacy: A prescription to end confusion. National Academies Press.

Janvier, A., Farlow, B., Barrington, K. J., Bourque, C. J., Brazg, T., & Wilfond, B. (2020). Building trust and improving communication with parents of children with trisomy 13 and 18: A mixed-methods study. *Palliative Medicine, 34*(3), 262–271. doi:10.1177/0269216319860662

Janvier, A., & Watkins, A. (2013). Medical interventions for children with trisomy 13 and trisomy 18: What is the value of a short disabled life? *Acta Paediatrica, 102*(12), 1112–1117. doi:10.1111/apa.12424

Kett, J. C. (2020). Who is the next "baby doe"? From trisomy 21 to trisomy 13 and 18 and beyond. *Pediatrics, 146*(Suppl. 1), S9–S12. doi:10.1542/peds.2020-0818D

Kett, J. C., Wolfe, E., Vernon, M. M., Woodrum, D., & Diekema, D. (2017). The multidisciplinary fetal center: Clinical expertise is only part of the experience. *Acta Paediatrica, 106*(6), 930–934. doi:10.1111/apa.13812

Krick, J. A., Hogue, J. S., Reese, T. R., & Studer, M. A. (2020). Uncertainty: An uncomfortable companion to decision-making for infants. *Pediatrics, 146*(Suppl. 1), S13–S17. doi:10.1542/peds.2020-0818E

Lantos, J. D. (2018). Ethical problems in decision making in the neonatal ICU. *New England Journal of Medicine, 379*(19), 1851–1860. doi:10.1056/NEJMra1801063

Leuthner, S. R., & Acharya, K. (2020). Perinatal counseling following a diagnosis of trisomy 13 or 18: Incorporating the facts, parental values, and maintaining choices. *Advances in Neonatal Care, 20*(3), 204–215. doi:10.1097/anc.0000000000000704

Lotto, R., Smith, L. K., & Armstrong, N. (2018). Diagnosis of a severe congenital anomaly: A qualitative analysis of parental decision making and the implications for healthcare encounters. *Health Expectations, 21*(3), 678–684. doi:10.1111/hex.12664

Lynema, S., Fifer, C. G., & Laventhal, N. T. (2016). Perinatal decision making for preterm infants with congenital heart disease: Determinable risk factors for mortality. *Pediatric Cardiology, 37*(5), 938–945. doi:10.1007/s00246-016-1374-y

Mackley, A., Winter, M., Guillen, U., Paul, D. A., & Locke, R. (2016). Health literacy among parents of newborn infants. *Advances in Neonatal Care, 16*(4), 283–288. doi:10.1097/anc.0000000000000295

Mercurio, M. R., & Carter, B. S. (2020). Resuscitation policies for extremely preterm newborns: Finally moving beyond gestational age. *Journal of Perinatology, 40*(12), 1731–1733. doi:10.1038/s41372-020-00843-4

Moldenhauer, J. S., & Adzick, N. S. (2017). Fetal surgery for myelomeningocele: After the Management of Myelomeningocele Study (MOMS). *Seminars in Fetal & Neonatal Medicine, 22*(6), 360–366. doi:10.1016/j.siny.2017.08.004

National Quality Forum. (2017). *NQP shared decision making action brief.* https://www.qualityforum.org/Publications/2017/10/NQP_Shared_Decision_Making_Action_Brief.aspx

Orzalesi, M., & Aite, L. (2011). Communication with parents in neonatal intensive care. *Journal of Maternal-Fetal & Neonatal Medicine, 24*(Suppl. 1), 135–137. doi:10.3109/14767058.2011.607682

Paton, A., Armstrong, N., Smith, L., & Lotto, R. (2020). Parents' decision-making following diagnosis of a severe congenital anomaly in pregnancy: Practical, theoretical and ethical tensions. *Social Science and Medicine, 266*, 113362. doi:10.1016/j.socscimed.2020.113362

Ratzan, S., & Parker, R. (2000). Introduction. In C. Selden, M. Zorn, S. C. Ratzan, & R. M. Parker (Eds.), *National Library of Medicine current bibliographies in medicine: Health literacy* (pp. v–vii). National Library of Medicine.

Ravindra, V. M., Aldave, G., Weiner, H. L., Lee, T., Belfort, M. A., Sanz-Cortes, M., Espinoza, J., Shamshirsaz, A., Nassr, A., & Whitehead, W. E. (2020, February 28). Prenatal counseling for myelomeningocele in the era of fetal surgery: A shared decision-making approach. *Journal of Neurosurgery: Pediatrics.* Advance online publication. doi:10.3171/2019.12.Peds19449

Rintoul, N. E., Keller, R. L., Walsh, W. F., Burrows, P. K., Thom, E. A., Kallan, M. J., Howell, L., & Adzick, N. S. (2020). The Management of Myelomeningocele

Study: Short-term neonatal outcomes. *Fetal Diagnosis and Therapy*, *47*(12), 865–872. doi:10.1159/000509245

Ross, L. F. (2020). Reflections on Charlie Gard and the best interests standard from both sides of the Atlantic Ocean. *Pediatrics*, *146*(Suppl. 1), S60–S65. doi:10.1542/peds.2020-0818L

Saunders, B. (2021). A sufficiency threshold is not a harm principle: A better alternative to best interests for overriding parental decisions. *Bioethics*, *35*(1), 90–97. doi:10.1111/bioe.12796

Sullivan, A., & Cummings, C. (2020). Historical perspectives: Shared decision making in the NICU. *Neoreviews*, *21*(4), e217–e225. doi:10.1542/neo.21-4-e217

Thiele, P., Berg, S. F., & Farlow, B. (2013). More than a diagnosis. *Acta Paediatrica*, *102*(12), 1127–1129. doi:10.1111/apa.12411

Truog, R. D. (2020). Is "best interests" the right standard in cases like that of Charlie Gard? *Journal of Medical Ethics*, *46*(1), 16–17. doi:10.1136/medethics-2019-105808

Tucker Edmonds, B., Hoffman, S. M., Laitano, T., Bhamidipalli, S. S., Jeffries, E., Fadel, W., & Kavanaugh, K. (2020). Values clarification: Eliciting the values that inform and influence parents' treatment decisions for periviable birth. *Paediatric and Perinatal Epidemiology*, *34*(5), 556–564. doi:10.1111/ppe.12590

Tucker Edmonds, B., Hoffman, S. M., Laitano, T., McKenzie, F., Panoch, J., Litwiller, A., & Corcia, M. J. D. (2020). Evaluating shared decision making in trial of labor after cesarean counseling using objective structured clinical examinations. *MedEdPORTAL*, *16*, 10891. doi:10.15766/mep_2374-8265.10891

Tucker Edmonds, B., Savage, T. A., Kimura, R. E., Kilpatrick, S. J., Kuppermann, M., Grobman, W., & Kavanaugh, K. (2019). Prospective parents' perspectives on antenatal decision making for the anticipated birth of a periviable infant. *Journal of Maternal–Fetal & Neonatal Medicine*, *32*(5), 820–825. doi:10.1080/14767058.2017.1393066

Wilkinson, D. (2019). In defense of a conditional harm threshold test for paediatric decision-making. In I. Goold, J. Herring, & C. Auckland (Eds.), *Parental rights, Best interests and significant harm: Medical decision-making on behalf of children post Great Ormond St. vs Yates* (pp. 85–106). Hart.

Wyatt, K. D., List, B., Brinkman, W. B., Prutsky Lopez, G., Asi, N., Erwin, P., Wang, Z., Domecq Garces, J. P., Montori, V. M., & LeBlanc, A. (2015). Shared decision making in pediatrics: A systematic review and meta-analysis. *Academic Pediatrics*, *15*(6), 573–583. doi:10.1016/j.acap.2015.03.011

16

PERINATAL CRISIS AND TRAUMATIC BEREAVEMENT

MARA TESLER STEIN AND DEBORAH L. DAVIS ■

Rikki's first pregnancy was with identical twin girls. She went into premature labor at 24 weeks of gestation, etiology unknown, and recalls a scary first night in the hospital. "I can remember putting both hands on my pregnant belly, patting and stroking my babies. I told them I was very sorry, that I loved them, and then I prepared to say goodbye. All that night I waited. I was sure, no matter what I tried to do, my body would override it, and reject my babies." After a suspected uterine infection was ruled out by amniocentesis, Rikki was hospitalized until giving birth at 30 weeks of gestation after preterm premature rupture of membranes. After 11 weeks of relatively uneventful courses in the neonatal intensive care unit (NICU) but unable to be weaned off oxygen, the twins were discharged home on oxygen by nasal cannula, weighing just over 5 pounds each.

Perinatal crisis is the parent's experience of threat to their infant's well-being during pregnancy, birth, or early infancy. Whether their infant ultimately lives or dies, perinatal crisis is often a frightening violation of parents' expectations, resulting in the intertwining of grief and trauma (Horesh et al., 2021; Sanders & Hall, 2018). This traumatic bereavement can interfere with parent development, such as inhibiting the parent's growing bond with their infant, disrupting their emerging identity as a parent to the child, and complicating otherwise supportive relationships (Davis & Stein, 2013).

Perinatal crisis and traumatic bereavement can occur in the context of infertility, pregnancy complications, prenatal screening, prenatal diagnosis, miscarriage, pregnancy termination, perinatal palliative care, stillbirth, complicated labor (including unexpected induction), surgical birth, parenting in the NICU, neonatal death, and/or taking home an infant with medical or developmental challenges or a life-limiting condition.

This chapter supports perinatal practitioners in their efforts to skillfully support parents experiencing any crisis from prenatal planning through infancy. It begins by examining parents' core developmental tasks and their vulnerability to disruption during this period, in addition to the effects of traumatic bereavement, in order to understand the challenges parents face. It then examines how to recognize traumatic stress in parents, explores the evidence-based practices of "trauma-informed care," and discusses the importance of making referrals to "trauma-focused treatment." Overall, it explores how to think about providing trauma-informed care to parents in developmentally supportive ways, which can lessen the trauma and developmental disruption often associated with perinatal crisis.

PARENTS' CORE DEVELOPMENTAL TASKS DURING THE PERINATAL PERIOD

For many parents, the months of pregnancy, birth, and early infancy include sweeping change and challenging growth. Parents typically tackle three core developmental tasks: (a) regulating powerful emotions, (b) growing into their parental identity with the infant, and (c) managing shifts in relationships (Davis & Stein, 2013). These emotional, psychological, and social developmental tasks foster the parents' growth into the role of mother, father, or co-parent to their new infant. For example,

- During the perinatal period, parents may experience powerful feelings of love, hopeful anticipation, joyful aspirations, and a laser focus on the infant. These emotions emanate from hormonal and neurobiological changes that prime bonding and caregiving (Rilling, 2013).
- Parental identity develops out of this neurobiologically designed devotion to protecting, nurturing, and getting to know the infant. This psychological growth, which gives rise to competent caregiving, flows from experiencing oneself as a capable parent (Flacking et al., 2012).
- Socially, parents may seek peer support from other parents who are pregnant or parenting small children. They may adjust their already established relationships with friends, relatives, and medical caregivers, shifting their focus to those who they can rely on for special support during this time (Côté-Arsenault & Denney-Koelsch, 2016).

These developmental tasks are challenging under the best of circumstances, so when parents are further challenged by a threat to their infant's well-being, they may be especially vulnerable to the disruptive effects of this crisis. For instance, a crisis can be emotionally derailing, as hope and joy turn into shock, fear, uncertainty, and grief, with some parents withdrawing from their infant, afraid to get "too attached" or seeing themselves as agents of harm (Davis & Helzer, 2010l; Davis & Stein, 2013). Crisis can hinder developing identity as "a capable parent" when parents feel powerless to protect their infant from any or all threats (Sanders & Hall, 2018). Crisis can strain relationships, as parents may feel friction with their partner, friends, family, and medical practitioners who may misunderstand this experience and their reactions or do not share common ground (Davis & Stein, 2013). In short, crisis complicates parents' developmental tasks: They now face navigating the intertwining of grief and trauma, which introduces additional challenges in the domains of parental identity, emotional regulation, and shifting relationships.

BEREAVEMENT AND TRAUMATIC BEREAVEMENT

With perinatal crisis, many parents experience bereavement because the threat to their infant's well-being can entail certain losses (Davis & Stein, 2013). For example, parents may lose the expected "blissful pregnancy" or the uncomplicated birth they anticipated. Some lose a sense of control over their lives, lose their faith in a benevolent god, lose hope for having a healthy infant, or lose confidence in their parenting ability. They may mourn the loss of reproductive health or lose trust in their bodies. If their infant dies, parents may grieve for all of the above as well as for this child, often keenly feeling the loss of a significant part of themselves and their future (Davis & Helzer, 2010). If their infant lives with medical or developmental challenges, parents have lost their envisioned healthy infant and their anticipated parenting journey (Davis & Stein, 2013). As Rikki reflects, "Babies aren't supposed to need intensive care. Parents' arms are supposed to be enough."

Many parents experience not just bereavement but *traumatic* bereavement due to the perceived severity of the threat to their infant or reproductive health. This means that even when a practitioner considers something medically inconsequential, such as unexpected test results or changes in an infant's health status, parents can still experience the event as stressful, particularly when their nervous systems have already been impacted by prior trauma. Rikki remembers one incident in particular:

> After my twin girls were born at 30 weeks gestation, about a month into their NICU stay, when I arrived for the day, instead of two isolettes next to each other, there was only one. My heart dropped into my stomach and all I could think was, "Which baby died?" Turns out, one baby had simply been moved across the aisle. Everything was fine, but I was a wreck.

As Rikki demonstrates, perinatal traumatic bereavement has a tangible impact on the parent's nervous system, leaving multilayered distress that can persist far longer than the traumatic events themselves (Hase et al., 2017).

Pathogenic Memories

The brain routinely processes and integrates experiences into long-term memory, but trauma, and even stressful life events, can impair this neurological capacity.

Sometimes, difficult experiences remain unprocessed and maladaptively stored in the nervous system, where they lack access to the adaptive information that would aid in processing and integration into long-term memory (Hase et al., 2017; Shapiro, 2018). Instead, pathogenic memories are formed, resulting in persistent distress, such as flashbacks, hypervigilance, chaos, and hyperreactivity, as well as derailing adaptive growth and development (Hase et al., 2017). In this way, pathogenic memories of a perinatal crisis can fragment the parent's sense of self, relationships, and the ability to manage the distress, thus disrupting the accomplishment of core developmental tasks (Davis & Stein, 2013).

For birthing persons in particular, pregnancy, childbirth, and the postpartum period are powerful physiological and sensory experiences, which can create stronger interoceptive, intrusive memories, putting them at special risk for post-traumatic stress (Harrison et al., 2021). Indeed, mounting evidence suggests that childbearing trauma should be considered a unique subtype of post-traumatic stress that warrants routine screening and specialized care (Horesh et al., 2021).

Recognizing Traumatic Stress

When assessing traumatic stress, the parent's subjective experience is key because the impact of the experience on the nervous system matters far more than the type of experience or even the infant's outcome (Hase et al., 2017; Maddox et al., 2019). Here is an analogy: Imagine a car traveling along a highway, and a pebble hits the windshield. Focusing on the size of the pebble, one might assume a negligible effect. However, depending on the prior state of the windshield and how and where the pebble hits, its effect could range from negligible to a massive shattering. So, in order to determine the effect, instead of focusing on the pebble, focus on what happened to the windshield. Likewise, with perinatal crisis, what matters most are not the objective details of the crisis but, rather, the subjective impact it has on the parent. Many mothers in particular share this shattering effect: "I felt deeply like I hadn't done enough to protect my baby."

What signs of traumatic stress can a practitioner look for? A traumatized parent's report could be anything from "That was really hard" to "I'm fine." However, the parent's nervous system and resulting reactions hold the objective truth about how difficult and disruptive it was, such as when parents repeatedly re-experience the traumatic event(s) or when parents' reactions to current events seem overly intense. Some parents are hypervigilant with their infant, even when others offer reassurance. In contrast, some parents' reactions seem numb, detached, avoidant, or immobilized, such as when parents seem reluctant to engage with their infant. Parents commonly vacillate between these reactions, and many feel disjointed, noticing that although they may know that the crisis is over, they continue to react as if it is not. The impact of the traumatic experience can also be reflected in the chaos some parents experience in the aftermath. After his infant died, Tim observed, "My garage used to always be spotless and organized. It's a metaphor for our life right now. It's a mess. Everything is just kind of helter-skelter. Things are thrown wherever." With post-traumatic stress, the parent's dominant state is reactivity, detachment, and/or disorganization rather than calm curiosity (Hase et al., 2017).

Rikki was first traumatized by early preterm labor, which threatened to end the lives of her twins. During 6 weeks of hospitalization and staving off preterm birth, her brain grew hypervigilant, disrupting her nervous system's ability to digest overwhelming fear and uncertainty as she endured the terror of not knowing whether her pregnancy would last long enough to give her girls a good chance of not just survival but healthy, normal lives. After birth, their NICU courses were not easy. One neonatologist would say, "Never trust a preemie," emphasizing for Rikki the fact that even when nothing scary was currently happening, that could change at any moment. Even after NICU discharge, Rikki remained anxious and hypervigilant because she viscerally understood, "There are still no guarantees that my babies will be okay."

TRAUMA-INFORMED CARE

Trauma-informed care is a philosophy of care that respects trauma's impact on the nervous system and seeks to prevent traumatizing or re-traumatizing the patient. In perinatal practice, the top priority of trauma-informed care is to ensure that all interactions with staff, environmental settings, and institutional policies are appropriately sensitive and geared toward reducing or eliminating distress, largely by supporting the developing parent–infant relationship (Côté-Arsenault & Denney-Koelsch, 2016; Davis & Stein, 2013; Limbo & Kobler, 2016; Sanders & Hall, 2018; Warland et al., 2011). The practitioner is also mindful that trauma is often a consequence of perinatal crisis and seeks to minimize its impact by providing a therapeutic holding environment. When "holding space," the practitioner is a consistently calm, compassionate presence so that parents can feel safe even as they struggle. With the practitioner's trustworthy support, parents can seek calm and gain confidence in their ability to prevail (Sanders & Hall, 2018). For example, being with a dying infant has potential for being a traumatic experience for parents. But with the therapeutic holding of trauma-informed care, which in this case would incorporate the best practices of perinatal hospice and palliative care, parents will face bereavement but not necessarily traumatic bereavement.

It is important to note that trauma-informed care is not the same as trauma-focused care. Although trauma-informed care provides a necessary therapeutic holding, some parents cannot fully heal without also addressing their neurology and pathogenic memories. For example, a parent can appear to be "stuck," still deeply affected by past events and continuing to experience traumatic stress, even as the practitioner tries to support, guide, and comfort them. Whereas trauma-informed care fosters stabilization and adjustment following crisis, trauma-focused treatment addresses pathogenic memories and mobilizes the aspects of adjustment and healing that have been blocked by trauma's impact on the nervous system, making adjustment easier and healing more complete (Cotter et al., 2017).

Whereas effective trauma-focused treatment requires specialized training, trauma-informed care can be practiced in alignment with many, often overlapping, gold-standard philosophies of care, including the following:

- Relationship-centered/family-centered care: Cultivating therapeutic relationships with parents and prioritizing the parent–infant bond can have calming, healing effects (Flacking et al., 2012; Harrison et al., 2021; Limbo & Kobler, 2016; Sanders & Hall, 2018).
- Developmentally supportive care: Supporting parents around their developmental tasks can reduce trauma's disruptiveness during this vulnerable period (Davis & Stein, 2013; Flacking et al., 2012; Sanders & Hall, 2018). The best practices of perinatal hospice and palliative care are developmentally supportive to parents of dying infants (Baughcum et al., 2020; Côté-Arsenault & Denney-Koelsch, 2016).
- Holistic, individualized, culturally competent care: Considering the whole picture and approaching parents with curiosity, respect, and humility can engender the trust needed to inquire about parents' struggles, beliefs, and preferences and tailor their care accordingly, thereby reducing distress and improving outcomes (Harrison et al., 2021; Limbo & Kobler, 2016).
- Compassion-focused care: As a "nonjudgmental witness," the practitioner is a calm and soothing presence, providing effective support by walking alongside parents as their journeys unfold (Beaumont et al., 2016; Limbo & Kobler, 2016; Zaki, 2020).

These philosophies of care involve many complementary practices that are sensitive to parent trauma and key to the implementation of trauma-informed care.

Trauma-Informed Practices

The following evidence-based practices are recommended by leading experts to avert or counteract the deleterious effects of trauma and are therefore beneficial to parents in crisis (Baughcum et al., 2020; Beaumont et al., 2016; Côté-Arsenault & Denney-Koelsch, 2016; Dales & Jerry, 2008; Davis & Helzer, 2010; Davis & Stein, 2013; Harrison et al., 2021; Limbo & Kobler, 2016; Sanders & Hall, 2018; Warland et al., 2011):

- See parents as whole, competent, worthy, and able to prevail—and be aware of practitioner bias. The parents' inexperience, disorientation, pain, and suffering are a result of what happened to them, not an indication of something wrong with them. And when parents do not look like, speak like, or act like the practitioner, it is imperative for the practitioner to be aware that bias can lead to treating parents as "less than" rather than worthy of respect, trust, and care. By being aware of bias, the practitioner can mindfully practice curiosity, compassion, and collaboration rather than being judgmental, dismissive, or directive. When the practitioner sees parents as whole, competent, worthy survivors, this encourages parents to see themselves that way.

- Accept and connect, instead of directing and protecting. To accept is to be a nonjudgmental witness and supportive companion who accepts each parent's journey and respects their pace while walking alongside. To connect means offering relationship-centered care, including building rapport, inquiring about parents' experiences and desires, providing gentle guidance when asked, and respecting parents' choices by remaining curious about their journey rather than judging or second-guessing it. An accepting, connecting mindset also boosts cultural sensitivity because instead of making assumptions about parents' preferences, the practitioner inquires, listens, and responds accordingly.

- Address feelings first. Listening to parents calms their nervous systems, which then lets them absorb information and pinpoint their desires, weigh options, and make decisions. When there is no space to discuss feelings and experiences, parents may not be able to find space for the information from the team. They may also feel dismissed, disrespected, and abandoned, which only adds to their trauma. By asking how parents are doing and then listening with compassion, practitioners show a fearless willingness to accept and connect even in the face of parent distress and suffering.

- Welcome parents to the NICU or hospice care team and then pave the way for their smooth orientation and transition. For example, hold regular team meetings to discuss each family's situation, each infant's current condition, and how best to engage with each parent, such as how much detailed information parents want and their chief concerns, values, priorities, and decisions. This enables the team to individualize care without asking parents to repeatedly express their preferences, decisions, and goals.

- Introduce parents to the idea that they are learning how to be a different kind of parent to a different kind of infant. When parents struggle, they may worry that their fear and confusion may equal incompetence. When practitioners acknowledge that there is much to learn and demonstrate faith in parents' growing competence, they foster development of parental identity.

- Collaborate and involve parents in caregiving and decision-making for their infant. Collaboration shows respect for the parent's role and contributions to their infant's care. When decisions are made *with* them, not *to* them, parents feel seen and valued for who they are and what they bring to the situation. Parental involvement helps parents regain a sense of agency and positive parental identity.

- Recognize that parents vary in how much information they want and need. To individualize care, the practitioner can inquire, "Do you have any questions about what's happening here?" and then give parents plenty of time and opportunity to formulate their questions. The practitioner can also check in with "I have more information; Is now a good time?" Asking permission can gauge the level of detail parents desire and help them manage the flow of information.

- Be mindful of how information is conveyed. There is a major difference between the directive, "Don't touch," and the inviting, "Can I show you the kind of touch your baby responds to?" Another example, "It's just a preemie thing," could feel dismissive. The following is a more reassuring report: "This is common among preemies. Would you like me to explain what I mean?"

- Teach instead of directing parents on what to do with their infant. When teaching parents how to read the infant's cues, what the infant needs, and explaining *why*, the practitioner helps parents learn *how to think* about the many meaningful ways they can connect with their infant. Learning how to think about "parenting this different kind of infant" puts parents in charge of *what to do*. Being in charge boosts parents' feelings of agency, competence, and confidence, and it supports developing parental identity. Teaching parents the *why* also results in truly informed consent, as parents gain clarity and motivation rather than just doing as they are told.

- Have realistic expectations. Naturally, parents in crisis can be overwhelmed by the scary, unfamiliar terrain of a high-risk pregnancy or birth, the NICU environment, or spending time with a deceased infant. Parents typically need multiple opportunities to find equilibrium, trust the team, absorb information, and learn how to apply it to their infant's care.

- Slow down. When the practitioner takes a seat or otherwise conveys that they are not in a hurry, this enables the practitioner to be fully present and shows a willingness to engage and listen to the parent's feelings, thoughts, concerns, and questions.

- Practice self-compassion. Self-compassion is the foundation of self-care. It includes mindfulness, reflective practice, self-kindness, grounding, healthy boundaries, and recognizing shared humanity—all of which enable the practice of compassionate care.

- Practice compassion. Due to limbic resonance and co-regulation, traumatized parents and infants can draw upon the equanimity of the compassionate practitioner to soothe their ramped-up nervous systems, which reduces trauma-induced distress and developmental disruption. Compassion (or empathic concern) is different from emotional empathy. When practitioners practice compassion, they can remain calm in the face of parent suffering, feeling compassion *for*, not empathy *with* (Singer & Klimecki, 2014). As such, compassion does not fatigue; empathy does. In fact, practicing compassion benefits practitioners by warding off vicarious trauma and burnout (Zaki, 2020).

Precious Little Should Come Between Parents and Their Infants

When thinking about perinatal crisis and parent development, a compassionate and developmentally supportive priority of trauma-informed care is that precious little should come between parents and their infants. Following this tenet can significantly improve outcomes for parents (as well as for the infants who survive) because it can lessen the trauma suffered due to the crisis (Bergman, 2019; Davis & Stein, 2013).

During and after perinatal crisis, parents may struggle to feel like capable parents to their infants. Trauma derails their developing parental identity due to feeling inadequate and disconnected from their infant. Their despair can deepen further when they are denied full and easy access to their little one—for instance, when the infant is taken away for observation or intensive care or, in the case of death, taken away too soon for autopsy or burial. These barriers to parenting are devastating and re-traumatizing to parents who struggle to feel worthy and who long to nurture their infant or take care of their infant's body—even if only for a short time. Barriers can also feel senseless and distressing during this critical time when parents are biologically primed to envelop their infant in a close embrace (Bergman, 2019).

When parents can care for their infant in personally meaningful ways that show their love, they can start to heal trauma's wounds to their developing parental identity. If their infant survives, their emotional healing can help them overcome or avoid blocks to their caregiving as they raise their child. If their infant dies, this healing of their parental identity becomes part of their mourning, adjustment, and meaning making, and it can help them overcome or avoid blocks to caregiving of their other children, including those born subsequently (Davis & Helzer, 2010).

When parental connection with their infant is prioritized, developmental disruption through trauma is lessened in three ways: (a) by supporting parents' efforts to manage powerful feelings of grief, fear, and uncertainty; (b) by encouraging parents' growth into their parenting role and identity; and (c) by strengthening the therapeutic nature of the relationship between practitioners and parents (Bergman, 2019; Davis & Stein, 2013).

In these ways, trauma-informed care by itself, particularly in the form of supportive relationships that facilitate a parent's agency and identity, can send many parents along a healing path of growth and meaning making. But for many parents who are traumatized, growth and meaning making are elusive without trauma-focused treatment.

TRAUMA-FOCUSED TREATMENT

Sometimes, parents can manage the traumatic stress triggered by pathogenic memories by learning skills that recruit the neocortex or "thinking brain" to boost coping. However, trauma can damage the bridge between the processing capacities of the neocortex and the pathogenic memories. As a result, new information, reframing, or supportive words cannot reliably modify the pathogenic memory network (Hase et al., 2017; Maddox et al., 2019). In contrast, neurologically based treatments directly access pathogenic memories at their source. It is thought that these treatments work because they mobilize the nervous system to rebuild the bridge between thoughtful, reflective capacity and limbic disarray (Hase et al., 2017; Maddox et al., 2019; Shapiro, 2018). Rebuilding the bridge recruits the brain's hardwired capacity for integration, healing, and meaning making, allowing traumatic experiences and pathogenic memories to be processed and adaptively integrated into long-term memory (Maddox et al., 2019; Shapiro, 2018).

Rikki reflects on her progress after receiving neurologically based, trauma-focused treatment:

Even after lots of different therapy over the years, I couldn't shake the feeling that my twins' premature birth was my fault. That I'd screwed up the most important job I'd ever been given. No matter how many times others told me it wasn't my fault. I sort of believed them, in that I knew I should know it wasn't my fault, that I'm a good mom, I'm a capable parent, I deserve good things, I can trust my judgment, I'm competent—yeah, yeah. I know, in my head. But when push comes to shove, I'm not feeling it. Like I couldn't believe it viscerally. I can't trust myself. Maybe I'll screw up this too. But after [trauma-focused] treatment, what was so profound was to viscerally experience the knowing, the realization, the understanding of my worth and goodness as a parent. The knowing went from my head, all the way down to my gut. It went from an abstract knowing to a genuine, internal believing. As if the therapy untangled the knots—knots that had kept my chest constricted, my head low, my eyes down—freeing me to having my head up and seeing the light and knowing that it was for me.

As an adjunct to the therapeutic holding of trauma-informed care, trauma-focused treatment is necessary for many parents, especially those who have suffered repeated or prolonged trauma. Some parents may eventually heal without trauma-focused therapy, but early treatment can make grieving and adjustment less agonizing and healing more timely and complete (Cotter et al., 2017).

IDEAS WORTH SHARING

Here are three examples of how a practitioner (nurse, physician, behavioral health specialist, etc.) might think about providing trauma-informed care to parents when an infant is in the NICU, dying, or deceased. These examples demonstrate how to be mindful of the compassionate, developmentally supportive priority of "precious little should come between parents and their babies." The first-person pronouns are intentional to invite the reader into the experience. Note also how the compassion behind this priority might ward off burnout, and why providing this developmental support to parents not only helps them but also can make the practitioner's job easier. These examples are a synthesis of the work by thought leaders in the field of perinatal care:

1. With parents of infants in the NICU, I see their distress and confusion as the result of trauma. I don't critique their efforts at caregiving as I don't want to reinforce their fears that they are incompetent or agents of harm, which would only add to their distress and make my job harder. My job is easier when I encourage and orient parents with, "Your baby needs special handling. And I'm sure you want to know what will help your infant thrive. Is now a good time to share what I've learned?" Then, I can mentor them in reading their infant's cues and the many ways they can connect in developmentally supportive ways, especially kangaroo care. Slowing down is key, making it possible for me to hold space for parents to express feelings, absorb information, ask questions, practice, and gain confidence. The more attuned a parent is to their infant's cues, the more likely they are to become a confident, "good-enough parent," which also fosters secure attachment, and their infant thriving beyond the NICU. I strive to tune into parents' cues, too, suggesting trauma-focused treatment as needed to boost their capacity for parenting their infant, free from the burden of trauma.

2. With parents of dying infants, I don't direct, "Let's do this with your baby," or "Why don't you go get some sleep?" as that would put me in charge of how they spend this fleeting and precious time, which makes my job harder. My job is easier when parents remain in charge of their own experience. To support them, I slow down, and ask, "How are you feeling? What are you noticing about your baby? What are your concerns? Which comfort care measures make sense to you? What would be meaningful and memorable for you to do with your baby?" I normalize their experience by sharing, "Many parents find that holding their baby skin-to-skin is soothing for the baby as well as themselves, and you can think about doing that too." And then I breathe, hold space for parents' thoughts and feelings, listen to what comes up for them, and support them in making comfort care decisions, determining what they value, and creating meaningful experiences during the last weeks, days, or moments of their infant's life. I help traumatized parents access trauma-focused treatment, to boost their ability to be present with their dying infant and/or foster resilience as they grieve.

3. With the parents of deceased infants, I don't direct, "You should spend time with your baby's body and take pictures," as this might impose seemingly morbid tasks, which could elevate their distress, which makes my job harder. Nor do I ask "yes or no" questions, as distressed

parents are prone to reflexively respond "No." My job is easier when I get to know each parent by asking open-ended questions about their pregnancy, infant, and thoughts or feelings about being parents. I can normalize spending time with the infant by sharing *why* other parents have done so—for example, "They get to show their love and to act and feel like parents." Especially for parents who are hesitant to spend time with their infant, "the why" helps them make sense of traditional mourning rituals such as holding their infant against their skin, taking care of their infant's body, taking their infant home, gathering keepsakes, and making commemorative photos. By continuing to engage with parents over time and listening as they recall family traditions or identify their own heartfelt desires, I help them bring their vision into focus. Finally, I accept their ideas and decisions with equanimity, accepting that it's their journey to make. I encourage parents to access trauma-focused treatment, to reduce unnecessary suffering as they grieve and to boost their resilience so that they can parent their present and perhaps future children.

These three snapshots show how trauma-informed care is also compassionate, holistic, developmentally supportive, and relationship-centered. Specifically, practitioners can mitigate the effects of trauma when they slow down; accept and connect with parents; see parents as competent collaborators; hold space for parents' feelings, thoughts, and questions; and respect the parents' pace while walking alongside. See Further Reading and Resources for resources that support this practice.

CONCLUSION

During the perinatal period, parents typically engage in core developmental tasks that lead to emotional, psychological, and social growth as they become parents to their new infant. This time of transition leaves them vulnerable to trauma, so when a crisis occurs, parents can benefit from compassionate, developmentally supportive, trauma-informed care provided by the health care team. Although trauma-informed care can soften the effects of perinatal trauma, many parents require trauma-focused care that directly treats trauma's neurological repercussions and pathogenic memories. Thus, a key part of trauma-informed care is making referrals to behavioral health specialists who are trained to provide neurologically based trauma-focused treatment.

FURTHER READING AND RESOURCES

The following are additional resources for cultivating the perinatal practice of compassion-focused, developmentally supportive, trauma-informed care.

Articles, Full Text Available Online

Coutts, S., Woldring, A., Pederson, A., et al. (2021). What is stopping us? An implementation science study of kangaroo care in British Columbia's neonatal intensive care units. *BMC Pregnancy and Childbirth, 21*, 52. doi:10.1186/s12884-020-03488-5

Dowling, T. (2018). Compassion does not fatigue! *Canadian Veterinary Journal, 59*(7), 749–750.

Feldman, R. (2020). What is resilience: An affiliative neuroscience approach. *World Psychiatry, 19*(2), 132–150. https//doi.org/10.1002/wps.20729

Klimecki, O. M., Leiberg, S., Lamm, C., & Singer, T. (2013). Functional neural plasticity and associated changes in positive affect after compassion training. *Cerebral Cortex, 23*(7), 1552–15561. doi:10.1093/cercor/bhs142

Nijdam, M., Gersons, B., Reitsma, J., De Jongh, A., & Olff, M. (2012). Brief eclectic psychotherapy v. eye movement desensitisation and reprocessing therapy for post-traumatic stress disorder: Randomised controlled trial. *British Journal of Psychiatry, 200*(3), 224–231. doi:10.1192/bjp.bp.111.099234

O'Leary, J., Warland, J., & Parker, L. (2011). Prenatal parenthood. *Journal of Perinatal Education, 20*(4), 218–220. doi:10.1891/1058-1243.20.4.218

Ramezani, T., Hadian Shirazi, Z., Sabet Sarvestani, R., & Moattari, M. (2014). Family-centered care in neonatal intensive care unit: A concept analysis. *International Journal of Community Based Nursing and Midwifery, 2*(4), 268–278.

Solomon, R. M. (2018). EMDR treatment of grief and mourning. *Clinical Neuropsychiatry, 15*, 173–186. https://www.clinicalneuropsychiatry.org/download/emdr-treatment-of-grief-and-mourning

Suttle, M. L., Jenkins, T. L., & Tamburro, R. F. (2017). End-of-life and bereavement care in pediatric intensive care units. *Pediatric Clinics of North America, 64*(5), 1167–1183. doi:10.1016/j.pcl.2017.06.012

Wool, C., & Parravicini, E. (2020). The Neonatal Comfort Care Program: Origin and growth over 10 years. *Frontiers in Pediatrics, 8*, 588432. doi:10.3389/fped.2020.588432

Books

Davis, D. L. (2002). *Loving and letting go: For parents who decided to turn away from aggressive medical intervention for their critically ill newborn* (Rev. ed.). Centering.

Davis, D L. (2016). *Empty cradle, broken heart: Surviving the death of your baby* (3rd ed.). Fulcrum.

Davis, D. L. (2020). *When courage lies in letting go: Turning toward "palliative care only" for your child's life-limiting condition* (3rd ed.). Centering.

Davis, D. L. & Stein, M. T. (2004). *Parenting your premature baby and child: The emotional journey.* Fulcrum.

Dworkin, M. (2006). *EMDR and the relational imperative: The therapeutic relationship in EMDR treatment.* Routledge.

Hughes, D. A., & Baylin, J. (2012). *Brain-based parenting: The neuroscience of caregiving for healthy attachment.* Norton.

Koloroutis, M. (Ed.). (2004). *Relationship-based care: A model for transforming practice.* Creative Health Care Management.

Kuebelbeck, A., & Davis, D. L. (2011). *A gift of time: Continuing your pregnancy when your baby's life is expected to be brief.* Johns Hopkins University Press.

Youngson, R. (2012). *Time to care: How to love your patients and your job*. Rebelheart.

PROGRAMS

Carry You with Me. *Navigating life after loss*. A self-guided program of videos and reflective exercises for parents grieving the perinatal death of a baby. Created by Alanna Knobben. https://carryyouwithme.com/cywm-program

NIDCAP. A comprehensive resource that promotes family-centered, evidence-based, developmentally supportive care for hospitalized infants and their parents. Originated by Heidelise Als, PhD. https://nidcap.org

The Schwartz Center for Compassionate Health Care. Offers innovative programs, education, and advocacy to support caregivers, health care leaders, and others in bringing compassion into every healthcare experience. https://www.theschwartzcenter.org

The Touchstone Institute for Psychotherapy and Training. Offers workshops for professionals who work in the field of perinatal mental health, including introductory and advanced training in trauma-focused treatment. Originated by Mara Tesler Stein, PsyD. https://www.touchstoneinstitute.org

ONLINE VIDEOS

Palliative. An award-winning documentary that explores conversations with parents during end-of-life care, with pediatric palliative care specialist, Dr. Nadia Tremonti. https://www.palliativefilm.com. A free 22-minute version of this film, titled *Dying in Your Mother's Arms*, is available at https://vimeo.com/446832129

The Touchstone Institute maintains a list of curated videos that offer a deeper dive into some of the topics addressed in this chapter. It includes the classic, Colorado Collective for Medical Decisions video, *You Are Not Alone*, including its accompanying instructions and CCMD Neonatal Guidelines. https://www.touchstoneinstitute.org/video

REFERENCES

Baughcum, A. E., Fortney, C. A., Winning, A. M., Dunnells, Z. D., Humphrey, L. M., & Gerhardt, C. A. (2020). Healthcare satisfaction and unmet needs among bereaved parents in the NICU. *Advances in Neonatal Care, 20*(2), 118–126. https://doi.org/10.1097/anc.0000000000000677

Beaumont, D., Irons, C., Rayner, G., & Dagnall, N. (2016). Does compassion-focused therapy training for health care educators and providers increase self-compassion and reduce self-persecution and self-criticism? *Journal of Continuing Education in the Health Professions, 36*(1), 4–10. https://doi.org/10.1097/CEH.0000000000000023

Bergman, N. J. (2019). Birth practices: Maternal–neonate separation as a source of toxic stress. *Birth Defects Research, 111*(15), 1087–1109. https://doi.org/10.1002/bdr2.1530

Côté-Arsenault, D., & Denney-Koelsch, E. (2016). "Have no regrets": Parents' experiences and developmental tasks in pregnancy with a lethal fetal diagnosis.

Social Science and Medicine, *154*, 100–109. https://doi.org/10.1016/j.socsci
med.2016.02.033

Cotter, P., Meysner, L., & Lee, C. W. (2017). Participant experiences of eye movement desensitisation and reprocessing vs. cognitive behavioural therapy for
grief: Similarities and differences. *European Journal of Psychotraumatology*, *8*(1),
1375838. https://doi.org/10.1080/20008198.2017.1375838

Dales, S., & Jerry, P. (2008). Attachment, affect regulation and mutual synchrony in adult
psychotherapy. *American Journal of Psychotherapy*, *62*(3), 283–312. https://doi.org/
10.1176/appi.psychotherapy.2008.62.3.283

Davis, D. L., & Helzer, S. (2010). Perinatal death and bereavement care. In E. S.
Gilbert (Ed.), *Manual of high risk pregnancy & delivery* (5th ed., pp. 149–169).
Elsevier.

Davis, D. L., & Stein, M. T. (2013). *Intensive parenting: Surviving the emotional journey
through the NICU*. Fulcrum.

Flacking, R., Lehtonen, L., Thomson, G., Axelin, A., Ahlqvist, S., Moran, V. H.,
Ewald, U., & Dykes, F. (2012). Closeness and separation in neonatal intensive care. *Acta Paediatrica*, *101*(10), 1032–1037. https://doi.org/10.1111/
j.1651-2227.2012.02787.x

Harrison, S., Ayers, S., Quigley, M., Stein, A., & Alderdice, F. (2021). Prevalence and
factors associated with postpartum posttraumatic stress in a population-based maternity survey in England. *Journal of Affective Disorders*, *279*, 749–756. https://doi.
org/10.1016/j.jad.2020.11.102

Hase, M., Balmaceda, U. M., Ostacoli, L., Liebermann, P., & Hofmann, A. (2017). The
AIP model of EMDR therapy and pathogenic memories. *Frontiers in Psychology*, *8*,
1578. https://doi.org/10.3389/fpsyg.2017.01578

Horesh, D., Garthus-Niegel, S., & Horsch A. (2021). Childbirth-related PTSD: Is it a
unique post-traumatic disorder? *Journal of Reproductive and Infant Psychology*,
39(3), 221–224. https://doi.org/10.1080/02646838.2021.1930739

Limbo, R., & Kobler, K. (2016). Moments matter: Exploring the evidence of caring for
grieving families and self. In B. P. Black, P. M. Wright, & R. Limbo (Eds.), *Perinatal
and pediatric bereavement in nursing and other health professions* (pp. 345–372).
Springer. https://doi.org/10.1891/9780826129277.0018

Maddox, S. A., Hartmann, J., Ross, R. A., & Ressler, K. J. (2019). Deconstructing the
gestalt: Mechanisms of fear, threat, and trauma memory encoding. *Neuron*, *102*(1),
60–74. https://doi.org/10.1016/j.neuron.2019.03.017

Rilling, J. K. (2013). The neural and hormonal bases of human parental care.
Neuropsychologia, *51*(4), 731–747. https://doi.org/10.1016/j.neuropsycholo
gia.2012.12.017

Sanders, M. R., & Hall, S. L. (2018). Trauma-informed care in the newborn intensive
care unit: Promoting safety, security and connectedness. *Journal of Perinatology*,
38(1), 3–10. https://doi.org/10.1038/jp.2017.124

Shapiro, F. (2018). *Eye movement desensitization and reprocessing (EMDR) therapy: Basic
principles, protocols, and procedures*. Guilford.

Singer, T., & Klimecki, O. (2014). Empathy and compassion. *Current Biology*, *24*, R875–
R878. https://doi.org/10.1016/j.cub.2014.06.054

Warland, J., Davis, D. L., et al. (2011). *Caring for families experiencing stillbirth: A unified position statement on contact with the baby. An international collaboration*.

https://www.researchgate.net/publication/275623852_Caring_for_Families_
Experiencing_Stillbirth_A_Unified_Position_Statement_on_Contact_with_the_B
aby#read

Zaki, J. (2020). The caregiver's dilemma: In search of sustainable medical empathy.
Lancet, *396*(10249), 458–459. https://doi.org/10.1016/s0140-6736(20)31685-8

17

THE VALUE OF PEER SUPPORT FOR HIGH-RISK PREGNANT WOMEN AND THEIR NICU INFANTS

SUE L. HALL, JENNY LANDRY, AND ERIN THATCHER ∎

THE RATIONALE FOR PEER SUPPORT

Peer support can be defined as the provision of emotional, informational, practical, and social support and mentoring by one person to another who is currently going through a similar experience (G. Thomson & Balaam, 2019). The shared lived experience enables the person providing support to have knowledge of the stresses the other person is facing and to understand what they are going through in a way that the professional health care staff cannot (Ardal et al., 2011; Preyde & Ardal, 2003). A key goal of peer support is to enhance the well-being and resilience of the person receiving the support.

Twenty-two percent of women have high-risk pregnancies; conditions include preterm labor, preterm premature rupture of the membranes and/or prolonged rupture of the membranes, preeclampsia/eclampsia, infection, and carrying a fetus with an anomaly. These women are known to be at increased risk of stress, anxiety, and depression compared with women whose pregnancies are uncomplicated; antepartum hospitalization, with its confinement and prescriptions for bed rest, can heighten their anxiety (Rodrigues et al., 2016). Some of these maternal conditions may lead to birth of their infant, which can be preterm or ill, necessitating a stay in the neonatal intensive care unit (NICU). NICU mothers have elevated levels of parental stress, depression, and anxiety (Soghier et al., 2018) compared with mothers of healthy, term infants, and they are at risk of short- and long-term sequelae that include an elevated incidence of anxiety disorders, postpartum depression (Rogers et al., 2013), acute stress disorder (Shaw et al., 2006), and post-traumatic stress disorder (PTSD) (Callahan et al., 2006).

Although professional mental health clinicians are increasingly becoming integrated into perinatal health care settings, not every woman's distress will rise to the level needing professional intervention; peer mentors may be particularly helpful in these instances. The use of trained volunteers to supplement or provide alternatives to traditional social and psychological support services has a long history in the United States; several notable examples include Alcoholics Anonymous and the National Alliance on Mental Illness. Although a support intervention provided by nurses to women who were hospitalized in Singapore with preterm labor demonstrated reduced rates of anxiety and depression among the women (Kao et al., 2019), we identified no studies in which peer mentors delivered support to hospitalized women with high-risk conditions of pregnancy. Peer support has been implemented in NICU settings to a much greater degree, with G. Thomson and Balaam (2019) reporting on 48 peer support organizations in 16 countries. Parents who provide peer support to other parents, are variously referred to as "mentor," "veteran," "alumni," "buddy," "facilitator," or "resource" parents (Dahan et al., 2020; Preyde & Ardal, 2003; S. Thomson et al., 2015).

NICU parents may find that their usual support systems of family and friends "just don't understand" or want them to "get over it and move on" (Ardal et al., 2011), or their family and friends may be too far away or too busy with their own lives to provide them with needed support. Grandparents may themselves be grieving their grandchild's plight, and they may not be able to be adequately supportive of their now adult children. NICU parents may not feel comfortable sharing their innermost thoughts and vulnerabilities with NICU staff because the parents want to be perceived in the best light possible. In addition, NICU staff, including the doctors, nurses, social workers, and psychologists, may be too overwhelmed with their many responsibilities to always be able to provide individual families with all the support they need when they need it. Similarly, women who are hospitalized during the antepartum period may find themselves isolated from their support networks amid busy professional staff members who may struggle to fulfill all of their clinical responsibilities, including meeting all of the emotional needs of the women in their care.

A mentor matched with a woman who has a high-risk pregnancy or a premature or sick infant according to similarities in the status of their pregnancies and/or their infant's clinical condition (similar weeks of gestational age and similar clinical issues), their socioeconomic, educational, geographic, and cultural backgrounds, and/or their family composition may be best positioned to offer ongoing support. This supportive relationship can begin in the antepartum period, when it is anticipated that the infant of a high-risk pregnant woman may require NICU admission, and can continue through and even beyond the NICU (Ardal et al., 2011). Having similar health issues rather than similar sociodemographic backgrounds was the most common parameter on which mentor matches were made in an international study of peer support by G. Thomson and Balaam (2019). Continuity of care and continuity of relationships are especially important considerations for parents, given how many transitions in caregivers that parents go through, beginning with their obstetric providers and continuing through their labor and delivery team, postpartum staff, NICU staff, and community agency staff after discharge.

Pregnant women and NICU parents ideally share their experiences with mentors without feeling judged, in a relationship in which they are respected by the mentor (Preyde & Ardal, 2003). Mentors can help new parents feel both safe and more comfortable in the foreign environment of the NICU and to accept their situation. Mentors can also help parents navigate their experience, provide them with practical tips and guidance, and encourage them to become advocates for their infants. Some relatively small studies of primarily mothers have demonstrated that NICU parents who receive peer support learn to cope and deal with stress more effectively (Ardal et al., 2011); are less stressed, less anxious, and less depressed (Preyde & Ardal, 2003); and become more optimistic and hopeful. In addition, they are more likely to visit their infant and become involved in his or her care to a greater degree while in the NICU (Boukydis, 2000). Through these actions, parents develop improved relationships with their infants, become more confident in their roles as parents, and gain increased self-esteem. Peer mentors also help parents become better prepared for discharge by helping them become more knowledgeable about resources they might need (Kerr & McIntosh, 2000); this may facilitate a shorter hospital stay and earlier discharge.

Peer support should be viewed by both antepartum and NICU clinicians as a supplement to what the professional staff offers parents, not as a replacement. Hospital clinicians should continue to screen and monitor pregnant women and new parents for postpartum depression and other perinatal mood and anxiety disorders, and they should make appropriate referrals to behavioral health services as indicated. In addition, an important component of peer mentor training includes the identification of criteria that would lead a mentor to refer their matched parent to a mental health professional, in collaboration with the person supervising the peer support program. A parent receiving peer support can be engaged with formal therapy from a trained mental health professional at the same time.

Recognizing the value that peer support can provide to parents, the American Academy of Pediatrics (2012) recommends that "pediatricians should encourage and facilitate peer-to-peer support and networking, particularly with children and families of similar cultural and linguistic backgrounds or with the same type of medical condition" (p. 399). Although peer support should be firmly anchored as a core principle of family-centered care in NICUs, such programs are not universally a part of NICU care either in the United States or throughout the world.

MODELS OF PEER SUPPORT

Peer support can be offered to women with high-risk pregnancies and to NICU parents in a variety of formats, and it is best if a peer support organization can offer a "menu" of services to meet a range of needs of the families they are serving. Table 17.1 provides a listing of perinatal peer support "umbrella" organizations in the United States and abroad. Some of the member programs of each of the broader organizations provide services primarily for women who have specific high-risk conditions during the antepartum period of pregnancy; however, the majority of programs provide services locally, regionally, or nationally to parents with infants in the NICU and/or to recently bereaved parents of newborns.

The types of support offered by these programs may include in-person meetings between peer mentors and their matches; telephone, text, or email connections; in-person group meetings; or virtual (online) support groups or Facebook pages where parents can interact (Hall et al., 2015). In addition, support programs may offer parents practical types of support, including financial or material support based on need.

One-to-One Support

One-to-one connections can be made in person or via telephone or text messages. For in-person connections, mentors can introduce themselves to expectant or new parents during formal or informal rounds either on the antepartum ward or in the NICU and invite parents to get involved as well as give them brochures detailing the peer support services available to them. Outreach materials should be prepared in several languages depending on the makeup of the community being served. Alternatively, parents can be asked by those on the care team, including physicians, nurses, social workers, and psychologists, if they want to be matched with a mentor. Within an institution, this responsibility may be designated to a particular clinician or group of clinicians to ensure that it is carried out. Ideally, parents whose infants are admitted to the NICU should be offered mentors early in their NICU stay. If a parent is not initially interested in having a mentor, they

Table 17.1 PEER SUPPORT UMBRELLA ORGANIZATIONS

Organization	URL	Services Provided
NICU Parent Network	https://nicuparentnetwork.org/member-directory	Lists more than 40 perinatal peer support organizations in the United States
European Foundation for the Care of Newborn Infants	https://www.efcni.org/parent-and-patient-org-2	Lists perinatal peer support organizations in Europe
Canadian Premature Babies Foundation	https://www.cpbf-fbpc.org/peer-support-for-nicu-families	Lists perinatal peer support organizations in Canada

can be offered one at a later date if their situation changes and it seems appropriate to remind them of the opportunity to become matched with a mentor.

Support Groups

Some parents may not want their "own" mentor but may be interested in and willing to attend an informal activity or a support or education group held either in the hospital or in a community location. Women who are hospitalized during the antepartum period may enjoy having time to gather with others going through similar experiences to share feelings or to engage in a simple activity such as crafting or knitting. Hospital social workers or psychologists can provide these experiences on their own or in partnership with members of a peer support program. In the NICU, parents can come together in group meetings to informally share a meal while discussing their role as parents, the reality of having their infant in the NICU, and their associated emotions. Having more than one moderator at a group meeting, as well as a diversity of moderators including fathers and parents whose infants have diagnoses other than prematurity, is important to participants (Dahan et al., 2020). Mentor parents may team up with NICU professionals to offer sessions on a variety of topics, such as infant development or feeding issues; NICU staff can present information while the peer support leaders moderate the discussion (Boukydis, 2000). Parents who have taken their infants home from the NICU may find benefit in returning to the support groups even after discharge.

Meetings with NICU parents may be better attended if they are in the hospital, eliminating transportation barriers and minimizing the time required for parents to be away from their infant's bedside. Parents are also more likely to participate if the word "support" is not used when describing a meeting (Dahan et al., 2020). Some parents may not join because they might feel uncomfortable sharing in front of a group, and some may not want to hear other parents' stories.

Online Support

Some parents may prefer to access support on one of the many Facebook pages or websites of either local or national peer support organizations. They may choose internet support because they can participate anonymously by reading discussion boards to learn but do not have to contribute to the discussion if they are not ready. Parents can also access the resources at a time and place of their choosing and without requiring child care and/or transportation to do so.

STARTING AND SUSTAINING A PEER-TO-PEER SUPPORT PROGRAM

NICUs may be approached by graduate NICU parents wanting to "give back" to the community of NICU parents by establishing a peer support program, or a NICU may choose to start its own program after recognizing the need or responding to a recommendation from its parent advisory committee. Another option is for NICUs to develop collaborative relationships and to contract for services with programs that offer peer support either nationally or regionally. Mental health staff providing services to antepartum and NICU families should familiarize themselves with the variety of organizations to which they can refer women and their families for specific support needs, and they should maintain an up-to-date referral directory of organizations and contacts. Some families may need assistance to overcome technology hurdles (e.g., obtaining internet access) to be able to participate.

Whether a peer support program is hospital-based or community-based, it is important that a strong collaborative relationship be established between NICU administration, NICU staff, and the peer support volunteers and/or employees. Identifying internal "champions" in the hospital staff, whether they are clinicians or administrators, is critical to the success and longevity of peer support programs. Creating a paid position for a parent support coordinator who will serve as the liaison with the peer support group can also contribute to program success. Hiring a parent-to-parent manager has made it possible for one hospital to develop and manage multiple initiatives to offer both their families and their staff continuing support and education (Voos et al., 2015). Peer support programs are more likely to be sustainable and to offer more support services if they have dual commitment from professional NICU staff and volunteer mentor parents (Boukydis, 2000). The breadth of services offered by peer support programs or funded by a hospital will vary according to the size of each program, the number of families being served, as well as the program's personnel and financial resources.

Time constraints, transportation limitations, childcare issues, technology hurdles, postpartum health challenges, and simple lack of awareness of services may be barriers to parent participation; solutions may need to be sought on an individual basis. NICU staff need to be aware that sometimes NICU parents who do not have premature infants feel like they "don't belong" in parent support groups; all should be welcomed and included. It may be more difficult to sustain a peer support program, and specifically parent support group meetings, in smaller NICUs that tend to have more mature infants with time-limited problems leading to shorter hospital stays.

Selection and Training of Peer Mentors

One key to success of a peer support program depends on having a core group of well-trained, dedicated, and empathetic mentors ready and available to provide support to families in need. Their primary role is to listen and offer support, not to dwell on their own personal story. Their support should empower families to make decisions that are "right" for them. It is never their role to provide medical advice. Most often, mentors will be volunteering their time, and they need to be able to make a significant commitment to the program. They should be screened by personal interview with the program's volunteer director to ensure they have had adequate time to come to terms with their own experience; it is recommended that volunteers have a minimum of 1 or 2 years between their personal lived experience and the time they volunteer. Other topics to cover during interviews include questions to determine their motivation, how they and their family are faring now, as well as how they might cope with challenging situations that they might encounter with mentees. Examples include situations that might trigger their own emotional distress, critical illness or death of a mentee's infant, or a mentee's extreme emotional distress. Applicants' positive personal qualities, such as communication skills and the ability to express empathy, compassion, and confidence, are also considered. Another way to screen volunteers is to give them responsibilities within the peer support program, such as fundraising, until leaders have a chance to get to know them (G. Thomson & Balaam, 2019). After screening volunteers, the next step is to run background checks on them. Then, training must be provided by the program that is selecting the mentors.

All mentors should also go through the hospital's general volunteer training program and be required to meet the hospital's standard volunteer requirements. The support program and/or the hospital's interdisciplinary perinatal or neonatal team can provide training specific to the mentor role through a combination of online and in-person training over a period of time. An intervention manual should be made available to mentors (S. Thomson et al., 2015). In preparation for stepping into their role, mentors should learn about medical situations and procedures about which they may be unfamiliar, and they should hear other mentors' experiential stories. This will help them respond to the stories of their future matches. It may also be a way for them to learn boundaries, including that they should not share inappropriate aspects of their own personal stories that would be stress-inducing or harmful to new parents or aspects that would lead to unfounded hope (G. Thomson & Balaam, 2021).

Mentors should be trained in how to listen and provide support; how to help parents mobilize their own support systems; how to address cultural insensitivities such as racial and ethnic stereotyping and microaggressions; common and expected emotional responses to their situation and to the NICU; premature infant development and parenting strategies; how to address grief and loss; knowledge of the mentoring program, NICU, and hospital policies and procedures; and how to recognize red flags and warning signs among the families with whom they are connected (G. Thomson & Balaam, 2019). This training may be both intellectually and emotionally challenging, another reason for spacing it out over several days or longer (S. Thomson et al., 2015).

Methods of training may include role playing and case discussions (Ardal et al., 2011). Mentors may then spend some time "shadowing" a current mentor before getting their own match. Mentors should also become familiarized with the setting in which they will work (antepartum and/or NICU) and meet staff with whom they may interface. When matched with a pregnant woman or parent to provide support, the mentor will need to negotiate terms of the relationship regarding how much contact to have and in what form. Mentors must also assure their matches that they will maintain confidentiality, with the exception of disclosing a need to contact a supervisor if they believe the person receiving support is potentially a danger to themself or others. In such a case, it would be best if the mentor transparently discussed the referral with their match prior to making it, indicating their belief that a professional should be consulted (G. Thomson & Balaam, 2019).

NICU parent mentors should be supervised regularly for at least the first 6 weeks of a match either by someone in their organization with experience or by someone on the hospital or NICU staff (a social worker or psychologist) to ensure that both parties indicate the match is acceptable to them. Mentors should have access to a clearly identified peer or professional supervisor with whom they can problem-solve, debrief, and process their experience as needed. Most peer support programs gather feedback on their parent mentors from the parents receiving service themselves, other peer mentors, and health care professionals (G. Thomson & Balaam, 2019).

Although peer mentors are matched on as many variables as possible with pregnant women or NICU parents, occasionally matches are not a good fit and may need to change. Reasons may include differences in language, culture, or parents' experiences; in addition, some peer supporters may not be emotionally ready to fulfill their role or may not operate within expected guidelines (G. Thomson & Balaam, 2019). The duration of relationships between mentors and matched parents depends on many factors, including whether mentors' personal, family, or work responsibilities interfere with their ability to maintain their time commitment to the program and its families; relationships may continue after hospital discharge. Some mentors may discontinue their involvement if they experience an untenable emotional burden related to this work; supervisors should be aware of this possibility and be ready to support the mentor as needed. And of course, parents are always free to decline the mentor experience.

Many volunteer mentors experience benefits from their participation, finding their relationships with parents to be mutually supportive as well as healing and affirming of their own journeys. They also feel positively about their ability to help others and may see improved functioning in their own families and in other aspects of their lives through the process of reframing their identity (G. Thomson & Balaam, 2021).

Trust between hospital staff and peer mentors—the peer–professional interface—is yet another key part of the equation. Volunteer mentors should also be viewed by hospital staff as allies sharing the same goal of improving both patient and parent care, patient satisfaction, and family outcomes.

Expanded Roles of Peer Support Programs and Peer Mentors

Members of peer support programs can fulfill many other roles in addition to providing individual or group support to parents. Mentors may host activities for parents, such as crafting and scrapbooking, and holiday events and parties;

distribute gift bags to new parents; host events for siblings, such as supervised weekend visits to the NICU, play groups while parents are visiting their infant, or craft sessions to make special gifts for their NICU sibling; invite grandparents to parent group meetings or host activities for them separately; participate in parent advisory committees and contribute to unit policy development; and offer their input on research projects being undertaken in the unit (Dahan et al., 2020; G. Thomson & Balaam, 2019). They may also find special ways to recognize and honor NICU staff or raise funds to help the NICU afford "extras" it might not otherwise have, such as providing staff education targeted toward helping clinicians provide psychosocial support to parents or purchasing new equipment (G. Thomson & Balaam, 2019). Parent mentors add value to the training of the NICU staff by sharing their stories so that all can gain a more personal appreciation of the challenges that NICU parents face.

Further Considerations When Starting a Peer Support Program

Trickey (2013) provides a comprehensive table listing nine steps for successful operation of peer support programs. In addition to steps already discussed, others include assessing the local culture through meetings with community members, developing an organizational infrastructure, and having a marketing plan that would likely include an informational website to get started. When such a program first forms, it is usually an all-volunteer operation. Membership needs to grow, funds need to be raised, goals need to be identified, and volunteers need to be recruited and trained before service provision can start. Once programs become more mature, a board of directors may be added to bolster community support and fundraising, and a medical advisory board may be added to review any educational information the program puts together to assess its accuracy and reliability. A hospital starting its own program will have to go through most of the same steps, although administration of the group's activities may remain with the hospital and not with mentor parents.

When hospitals collaborate with a community program, a number of issues must be decided; some of these are shown in Box 17.1.

Factors Associated with Sustainability of Peer Support Programs

A critical element in maintaining the stability and sustainability of a peer support program is forging a strong partnership between leaders of the peer organization and the hospital unit (Boukydis, 2000; G. Thomson & Balaam, 2019). If a key person in the hospital/NICU changes jobs, a replacement should be sought immediately to ensure the continuance of the program; its survival should not be dependent on the presence of a single person who has been its champion. Similarly, if the leader of a peer support program decides to opt out of involvement, a best

Box 17.1

QUESTIONS TO CONSIDER WHEN STARTING A PEER SUPPORT PROGRAM

1. Will the hospital start its own program or partner with a community program?

2. Will the program be staffed by any paid personnel, or will it be an all-volunteer program?

3. Who will be the "champion" for the peer support program within the hospital environment?

4. Will the hospital contribute to funding the program, and if so, in what manner (i.e., a general donation or through contracted services)?

5. Will the program be offered space within the hospital as an operational base?

6. How will women or new parents be referred to the support program?

7. Will hospital staff team up with peer support staff to provide training to new mentors?

8. Will mentors be included on medical rounds?

9. What are the guidelines for sharing protected health care information with mentors?

10. Will the hospital's professional clinical team collaborate with mentors to offer educational group discussions?

practice would be for them to identify someone to take over the program and their commitments after they depart.

The final necessary—and often difficult— element in establishing a successful and sustainable peer support program is funding, whether it be provided by a hospital or health care system, private donations, or government or private grants (G. Thomson & Balaam, 2019). Many programs will rely on a combination of funding streams; again, a partnership between the hospital and the support program that ensures shared funding will lead to the best chance of sustainability. Having a peer support program may give a hospital a competitive advantage in the health care marketplace; this point can be proposed to hospital administrators as a reason to help fund such a program, in addition to promoting the idea that such a program should improve patient satisfaction as well as patient/family outcomes.

EXEMPLARS OF CURRENTLY EXISTING PROGRAMS

An example of a program providing peer support to pregnant women with the high-risk condition of preterm premature rupture of the membranes (PPROM) is the nonprofit PPROM Foundation (https://www.aapprom.org), founded in 2013 by a woman who experienced PPROM 12 weeks into her pregnancy with twins. She gave birth at 27 weeks, and her children are now healthy and thriving. The program describes itself as a "partner in expectant management" for pregnant women, whether hospitalized or not, who have experienced rupture of the fetal membranes well before their due date, leaving them and their fetus at risk for infection and/or subsequent preterm delivery and even fetal loss or infant death. Free services that are provided include person-centered advocacy, social and emotional support, educational materials, and other resources to families affected by this condition, which is the leading identifiable cause of preterm birth in the United States. Women can initially access support through a telephone line that is answered 24/7 by a "live" person who will collect intake information on the woman's situation to enable matching with a mentor, which this organization calls an "advocate." Advocates are matched with women primarily on the gestational age of their pregnancy at which the rupture of the membranes occurred and also through any other relevant diagnostic condition. Although this program has volunteers that make bedside visits to hospitalized women in 35 states, most of the advocates provide virtual support by Skype, FaceTime, email, and/or text; 90% of the women they serve are self-referred through internet searches. Peer advocates provide information and support to help families make informed decisions in difficult situations, such as terminating versus continuing an affected pregnancy.

When someone with personal experience wants to become an advocate for the PPROM Foundation, they are screened after completing an interest form. Online training is conducted by the group's leaders. The program maintains a large database of volunteers, which includes their geographic location, specific pregnancy diagnosis, the gestational age at which their membranes ruptured, their availability and flexibility to volunteer, contact information, social media accounts, cultural and demographic information (race, gender, LGBTQIA+ status, etc.), history of fertility treatment, languages spoken, and optional information on income and insurance. Volunteer advocates spend approximately 4 hours per week connecting remotely with their matches; a volunteer supervisor checks in with them monthly, and they have access to a private Facebook group in which they can communicate with one another. Volunteers typically remain active for 2 or 3 years. The PPROM Foundation has a board of directors that meets quarterly and a medical advisor. Members also work with staff in physicians' offices, offering their services as a supplement to what the physicians and their behavioral health staff can provide to women with PPROM.

A NICU peer support program that can serve as an exemplar is the nonprofit Hand to Hold (https://www.handtohold.org), founded in Austin, Texas, in 2010 by a woman who gave birth to her son at 25 weeks and later to her daughter at 34 weeks. Originally providing peer support services to hospitals in the Austin area, Hand to Hold has grown into a national program with more than 200 volunteer peer mentors. Hand to Hold has a successful history of fundraising in its hometown community as well as finding corporate sponsors for its various projects and services, enabling it to have a number of paid employees. Participating hospitals at several locations in Texas contract to have a family support specialist hired by Hand to Hold available to current parents in the NICU at least twice a week, including nights. This specialist informs families about their opportunities to be matched with a peer mentor, conducts formal and informal groups for them, attends the required NICU discharge class, and interfaces with NICU staff in support of families.

Hand to Hold offers services to any NICU family nationwide. Its parent mentor database includes information on both mothers and fathers whose infants have had a wide range of diagnoses, what kind of interventions the infants required, whether they were discharged from the hospital with home equipment, and whether the infants died. Parents contact Hand to Hold through referrals from hospitals and insurance agencies and also through their own internet searches. Some may not connect with the program until after their infant is discharged, which is a time when parents have "lost" the continuous support of the NICU professionals from their hospital experience and are coping with the realities of having what might be a medically fragile infant at home. After discharge, parents may feel socially isolated and may struggle with the emotional sequelae of their NICU experience, including depression and/or PTSD. Hand to Hold offers one-on-one mentor services free of charge; mentors communicate with parents using phone, texts, emails, "live" virtual support groups, and an active Facebook page for parents.

Mentors are recruited by and contact Hand to Hold through its website, weekly newsletter, and personal referrals, or they may have previously been mentored themselves. They undergo typical processes for background screening and training. The program's volunteer coordinator keeps in touch with matched pairs for a 6-week period to ensure the connection is going smoothly; mentors then let the coordinator know when a match has become inactive, at which time the parent who has received mentoring will be surveyed about their satisfaction with the services.

CONCLUSION

Although it may seem that time required to develop a relationship with an antepartum or NICU parent support program is one more demand on an antepartum unit's or a NICU's limited resources, investing in such a program contributes to the well-being of the families being served. Peer supporters can meet the needs for much of the emotional support that families with high-risk pregnancies and/or NICU infants need and deserve, augmenting what the professional clinical staff provides. A well-functioning peer support program can potentially improve outcomes and satisfaction of families in its care, and it can be an important and positive differentiating factor between hospitals in a crowded health care market.

REFERENCES

American Academy of Pediatrics, Committee on Hospital Care, & Institute for Patient- and Family-Centered Care. (2012). Patient- and family-centered care and the pediatrician's role. *Pediatrics*, *129*(2), 394–404. https://doi.org/10.1542/peds.2011-3084

Ardal, F., Sulman, J., & Fuller-Thomson, E. (2011). Support like a walking stick: Parent-buddy matching for language and culture in the NICU. *Neonatal Network*, *30*(2), 89–98. https://doi.org/10.1891/0730-0832.30.2.89

Boukydis, C. (2000). Support services and peer support for parents of at-risk infants: An international perspective. *Children's Health Care*, *29*(2), 129–145.

Callahan, J., Borja, S., & Hynan, M. (2006). Modification of the Perinatal PTSD Questionnaire to enhance clinical utility. *Journal of Perinatology*, *26*(9), 533–539.

Dahan, S., Bourque, C., Reichherzer, M., Prince, J., Mantha, G., Savaria, M., & Janvier, A. (2020). Peer support groups for families in neonatology: Why and how to get started? *Acta Paediatrica*, *109*, 2525–2531. https://doi.org/10.1111/apa.15312

Hall, S., Ryan, D., Beatty, J., & Grubbs, L. (2015). Recommendations for peer-to-peer support for NICU parents. *Journal of Perinatology*, *35*, S9–S13. https://doi.org/10.1038/jp.2015.143

Kao, M.-H., Hsu, P.-F., Tien, S.-F., & Chen, C.-P. (2019). Effects of support interventions in women hospitalized with preterm labor. *Clinical Nursing Research*, *28*(6), 726–743. https://doi.org/10.1177/1054773817744323

Kerr, S., & McIntosh, J. (2000). Coping when a child has a disability: Exploring the impact of parent-to-parent support. *Child Care, Health and Development*, *26*(4), 309–322.

Preyde, M., & Ardal, F. (2003). Effectiveness of a parent "buddy" program for mothers of very preterm infants in a neonatal intensive care unit. *Canadian Medical Association Journal*, *168*(8), 969–973.

Rodrigues, P. B., Zambaldi, C. F., Cantilino, A., & Sougey, E. B. (2016). Special features of high-risk pregnancies as factors in development of mental distress: A review. *Trends in Psychiatry and Psychotherapy*, *38*(3), 136–140. https://doi.org/10.1590/2237-6089-2015-0067

Rogers, C., Kidokoro, H., Wallendorf, M., & Inder, T. (2013). Identifying mothers of very preterm infants at-risk for postpartum depression and anxiety before discharge. *Journal of Perinatology*, *33*(3), 171–176. https://doi.org/10.1038/jp.2012.75

Shaw, R., Deblois, T., Ikuta, L., Ginzburg, K., Fleisher, B., & Koopman, C. (2006). Acute stress disorder among parents of infants in the neonatal intensive care nursery. *Psychosomatics*, *47*, 206–212.

Soghier, L., Kritikos, K., Carty, C., Tuchman, L., Streisand, R., & Fratantoni, K. (2018). Postpartum depressive symptoms in parents at discharge from the neonatal intensive care unit (NICU): Risk factors and association with parental stress. *Pediatrics*, *142*(1), 182.

Thomson, G., & Balaam, M. (2019). International insights into peer support in a neo-natal context: A mixed-methods study. *PLoS One, 14*(7), e0219743. https://doi.org/10.1371/journal.pone.0219743

Thomson, G., & Balaam, M.-C. (2021). Sharing and modifying stories in neonatal peer support: An international mixed-methods study. *Scandinavian Journal of Caring Sciences, 35*(3), 805–812. https://doi.org/https://doi.org/10.1111/scs.12895

Thomson, S., Michelson, D., & Day, C. (2015). From parent to "peer facilitator": A qualita-tive study of a peer-led parenting programme. *Child: Care, Health and Development, 41*(1), 76–83. https://doi.org/10.1111/cch.12132

Trickey, H. (2013). Peer support for breastfeeding continuation: An overview of re-search. *Perspective, 21*, 15–20. https://pdfs.semanticscholar.org/2def/6466c6d46 f2e6533c4cc18680697ffcc59bd.pdf?_ga=2.205735632.272560071.1597601033-155 2478630.1597601033

Voos, K., Miller, L., Park, N., & Olsen, S. (2015). Promoting family-centered care in the NICU through a parent-to-parent manager position. *Advances in Neonatal Care, 15*(2), 119–124. https://doi.org/10.1097/ANC.0000000000000136

Fetal Care Settings

18

SPECIALTY CARE SETTINGS

PERINATAL MANAGEMENT, FETAL THERAPY, AND THE FETAL THERAPY CENTER

CHRISTINA PAIDAS TEEFEY, SARAH ROBINSON, AND JULIE S. MOLDENHAUER ∎

FETAL DIAGNOSIS AND PERINATAL MANAGEMENT

The Role of the Obstetric Provider

The goal of any obstetric provider is to optimize the health and well-being of every pregnant woman and her unborn child under their care. The models for prenatal care and birthing vary considerably and are dependent on the underlying health of the woman and fetus, as well as the patient's desired birth experience. Prenatally diagnosed congenital anomalies are typically unanticipated and frequently require alterations in the patient's care plan. In most circumstances, the prenatal diagnosis of a congenital difference requires the pregnancy to be considered "high risk," which often involves an abrupt change in management. The impact of a prenatal diagnosis often takes a desired, highly anticipated pregnancy that is supposed to be a joyous situation and creates a burden of stress and anxiety for the woman and her family.

Primary obstetrical care providers include obstetricians, family practice physicians, advanced practice providers, and midwives who practice in settings with varying capabilities for the monitoring and intervention needs of a pregnancy affected by a prenatally diagnosed congenital anomaly. Referral to a maternal–fetal medicine (MFM) specialist is typically made by a primary obstetric provider who generally performs "routine" prenatal, delivery, and postpartum care. MFM specialists practice in various environments, ranging from smaller private consultative offices to large academic institutions and specialized fetal therapy centers (FTCs). Regardless of the type of practice, referral to an MFM can be requested for routine screening or diagnostic ultrasounds, abnormal laboratory screening results, family history, maternal obstetric or medical concerns, exposures, or a previously identified risk factor in the current or prior pregnancy, among other indications.

In the case of a prenatally diagnosed congenital anomaly, consultation with the MFM specialist provides a detailed discussion of the fetal abnormality and any associated findings, differential diagnosis, options for pregnancy management, and further recommendations for care. These recommendations often include further imaging, invasive diagnostic testing, or referral to an FTC for consultation and specialty care options that might include fetal intervention in certain cases. Serial imaging to monitor fetal status often provides multiple touchpoints for further counseling and discussion of expectations for the pregnancy and neonatal period. The anticipated neonatal outcome varies based on the fetal diagnosis, and it can include immediate complex newborn evaluation and care, surgical intervention, prolonged hospitalization, or palliative/comfort care in the most severe circumstances.

Providers in tertiary and quaternary care centers commonly have established multidisciplinary teams that include primary obstetric providers, MFM physicians, and neonatal specialists, allowing for streamlined care of the maternal–fetal dyad from the time of diagnosis until delivery. MFM specialists and primary obstetric providers collaborate to deliver ongoing care. This arrangement can look different in various settings, dependent on the individual needs of the patient. For example, in situations in which the pregnant patient is not in close proximity to a tertiary care center, accommodations might include co-management with local primary obstetric providers until the patient relocates for delivery near term. In short, the care team for pregnant patients carrying a fetus with a prenatally diagnosed congenital anomaly is multidimensional and is determined based on the needs of the individual and the fetal diagnosis.

THE FETAL THERAPY CENTER

Detection and assessment of congenital anomalies have continued to improve and open new avenues for diagnosis and intervention. Making this process easier to navigate and family centered has been the goal of the FTC. Advancements in imaging—specifically ultrasound, echocardiography, and magnetic resonance imaging—have allowed for earlier and more accurate diagnosis of fetal anomalies. In addition, the field of fetal therapy continues to evolve. Prior to the advent of the FTC, pregnant patients with a prenatally diagnosed congenital anomaly were shuttled between providers in various settings. The decentralized nature of this model resulted in the responsibility of care coordination falling on families, who were simultaneously required to process the fetal diagnosis and its impact on their unborn child, obtain specialized prenatal care and imaging, and seek subspecialty counseling to obtain further information. The FTC aims to assemble a multidisciplinary team in one location in order to streamline the process of diagnosis and care provision (Howell & Adzick, 2003). Some FTCs have further evolved to include birth options with the goal of keeping families together in one physical space and to better address the health needs of both the pregnant patient and the infant needing complex neonatal care.

Over time, FTCs have restructured the traditional fragmented approach to obstetric services with the goal of presenting an effective, multidisciplinary model to optimize outcomes for the mother and infant (Howell & Adzick, 2003). At the time of diagnosis, expectant parents receive unanticipated news about a physical anomaly in their unborn child that demands effective communication and a clear explanation. Additional consultation with genetic counselors, neonatologists, and other subspecialists can also provide additional support and aid in making an informed decision (Kemp et al., 1998; Metcalfe, 2018). In the setting of a prenatal diagnosis of an anomaly that is likely to require surgical management in the immediate neonatal period, prenatal consultation with a pediatric surgeon has been associated with decreased parental anxiety (Kemp et al., 1998).

FTCs attempt to individualize care by providing interdisciplinary care that can be tailored to the needs of the patient, family, and fetal diagnosis. The concept of the fetal center was first described in 1982 and has continued to evolve since that time (Harrison et al., 1982). In the present day, the goal of an FTC is to provide comprehensive care and expertise for the maternal–fetal patient with a focus on improving neonatal survival and quality of life in the setting of a congenital anomaly (Moon-Grady et al., 2017). Centers differ in that some offer solely diagnostic practice models, whereas others offer diagnosis and treatment with or without delivery units. Coordination of care is essential for families because continued care of the affected neonate often requires a specialized delivery plan or high-level subspecialty care immediately after birth. In order to obtain this level of care, families often temporarily relocate to an area closer to the specialized fetal center after being referred and remain away from home throughout their pregnancy and postpartum. Given the multiple layers of challenges faced by the expectant family, the degree of advanced care requires medical as well as psychosocial providers with expertise at every level.

The Multidisciplinary Fetal Care Team

The FTC is defined by its multidisciplinary team that provides a complete fetal assessment with in-depth counseling, as well as ongoing imaging, fetal therapy and surgery options, prenatal care, delivery services, postpartum care, and perinatal palliative care services. The multidisciplinary care team has changed over time and generally includes a combination of MFM physicians, radiologists, obstetricians, advanced practice nurses, certified nurse midwives, nurse coordinators, anesthesiologists, genetic counselors, neonatologists, pediatric surgeons, and pediatric subspecialists, as well as psychologists, psychiatrists, social workers, and other psychosocial support personnel (Harrison et al., 1982; Howell & Adzick, 2003; Moon-Grady et al., 2017). In addition, centers often establish fetal therapy oversight committees and maternal advocates that help provide further support and insight for providers and families. The collaborative efforts of the team work to provide continuity of care and a comprehensive approach beginning with the fetal assessment and ending with a transition to the postpartum period. Ease of access to each component of the multidisciplinary team is essential.

The role of psychosocial providers embedded within the multidisciplinary team is to assess the social, emotional, spiritual, and familial issues that patients and families may be experiencing. This aspect of the support team may consist of a clinical psychologist, perinatal psychiatrist, social worker, chaplain, and child life specialist. In order to adequately assess the patient's psychosocial needs and risk for psychological distress, providers should complete an initial mental health screening and perform ongoing assessments as clinically indicated. Clinical visits can be routinely incorporated into the patient plan of care or as needed throughout their pregnancy.

Maternal Fetal Evaluation

The FTC maternal fetal evaluation generally begins with confirmation of the fetal diagnosis through imaging, including ultrasound. Additional imaging using fetal echocardiogram and/or magnetic resonance imaging might also be employed to provide further details of the diagnosis. A thorough maternal history is obtained to determine any maternal risk factors associated with the pregnancy and fetal diagnosis. Genetic counselors meet with the patient to obtain a multigenerational family history and review the genetic implications of a fetal diagnosis, including testing options and recurrence risk in subsequent pregnancies. Social workers complete a detailed psychosocial history and identify any areas of concern related to the psychosocial needs of the patient and family. After the comprehensive assessment, the patient discusses the findings in depth with an MFM and pediatric subspecialists from various disciplines depending on the specific diagnosis. In this manner, parents receive counseling regarding the fetal diagnosis, associated prognostic implications, and pregnancy management options based on expert experience. Invasive testing such as amniocentesis is often discussed as an option to provide a definitive genetic or infectious diagnosis. Results from prior testing are also reviewed in depth with the patient in the context of the fetal findings. An outline of the plan for the remainder of the pregnancy is developed in conjunction with the patient and her family. Although the plan is fluid and can change based on new developments throughout the pregnancy, providers make an effort to discuss the most likely course for the pregnancy and the neonate. Psychosocial support and screening for perinatal mood and anxiety disorders begin at the time of the initial consultation. This plan is also individualized for the pregnancy based on identified stressors. Importantly, these challenges are identified by the physicians at the time of initial consultation, and ongoing developments throughout the pregnancy are relayed to the psychosocial team to optimize outcomes.

If the patient is deemed a candidate for fetal intervention, the procedure, risks, benefits, and alternatives, as well as the potential impact on future pregnancies, are discussed in depth. The family is able to speak with members of the team performing the procedure regarding the type of anesthesia used and its associated risks, postoperative hospital stay, medication management, recovery, and logistical planning for the remainder of the pregnancy. Supplemental resources are commonly given to the family for review after the consultation. Options for interruption or continuation of the pregnancy are discussed, and the family is provided with ample time to ask questions. If the decision is made to interrupt the pregnancy, the patient is offered support and assistance with planning. If there is no role for fetal intervention, ongoing pregnancy management and delivery planning are discussed. In the setting of a life-limiting anomaly, the option of perinatal palliative care is also reviewed (Howell & Adzick, 2003). The collaborative approach to the consultation helps facilitate complex decision-making in this difficult time, whether the decision is made to interrupt or continue the pregnancy. Team availability for continued planning and support is essential.

ONGOING PERINATAL CARE

Outpatient Care

After the initial fetal evaluation and consultation, ongoing care throughout the pregnancy can be continued locally in many circumstances, particularly if there is not a perceived risk for immediate neonatal intervention. However, if fetal intervention or complex neonatal care is anticipated, pregnancy management at the FTC may be necessary. In this setting, serial imaging guides the frequency of visits as well as timing and mode of delivery. Consultation with specialists such as lactation, neonatology, and anesthesia providers offers the patient the opportunity to gather further information, a feeling of empowerment and control, and allows for optimal planning. In the setting of open maternal–fetal surgery (OMFS) or need for immediate postnatal intervention, prenatal care is transitioned to the FTC and delivery is carefully timed (Howell & Adzick, 2003). In some cases, the FTC transitions patients back to their local providers for continued monitoring and delivery following fetal intervention. Certain fetal diagnoses (Table 18.1) pose a higher risk of rapid progression, growth restriction, alterations in amniotic fluid, or fetal decompensation that can lead to intrauterine fetal death. In these situations, very close fetal monitoring and antenatal testing are recommended in the third trimester, including serial growth scans, non-stress tests, biophysical profiles, and amniotic fluid evaluation. The frequency of visits can place increased strain and time commitments on the family, which can result in increased psychosocial stress.

Table 18.1 SUGGESTED ANTENATAL MONITORING IN THE SETTING OF A FETAL ANOMALY

Fetal Diagnosis	Interval Fetal Growth Ultrasound	Antenatal Surveillance
Congenital heart disease	Every 4 weeks throughout pregnancy	Initiated based on routine obstetric indication
Myelomeningocele/ open or closed neural tube defect	Every 4 weeks throughout pregnancy	Initiated based on routine obstetric indication
Growth restriction	Every 2 weeks throughout pregnancy	Weekly BPP or twice weekly mBPP beginning at 28–32 weeks or at time of diagnosis, whichever is earlier
Gastroschisis	Every 2–4 weeks throughout pregnancy	Twice weekly BPP and NST beginning at 32 weeks; begin at 28 weeks if growth restriction or abnormal amniotic fluid
Congenital diaphragmatic hernia	Every 4 weeks throughout pregnancy	Weekly BPP beginning at 34 weeks
Bowel obstruction	Every 4 weeks throughout pregnancy	Weekly BPP beginning at 32 weeks
Polyhydramnios	Every 4 weeks throughout pregnancy	Weekly BPP beginning at 32 weeks or at time of diagnosis
Post open maternal–fetal surgery (myelomeningocele, sacrococcygeal teratoma, lung lesion resection)	Every 2–4 weeks throughout pregnancy	Weekly ultrasound to monitor for postoperative complications and assess amniotic fluid; antenatal surveillance initiated depending on additional risk factors
Post minimally invasive intervention	Every 2–4 weeks throughout pregnancy	Weekly ultrasound for first 3–4 weeks to monitor for postoperative complications; antenatal surveillance initiated based on obstetric indication/additional risk factors
Multiple congenital anomalies, genetic syndrome	Every 2–4 weeks throughout pregnancy	Case specific; initiated based on routine obstetric indication

BPP, biophysical profile; mBPP, modified biophysical profile (includes fetal non-stress test and amniotic fluid index); NST, fetal non-stress test.

Delivery Units

Birth planning for a pregnancy diagnosed with a fetal anomaly involves the input and coordination of multiple subspecialists from a wide range of clinical services. The ultimate timing and route of delivery are influenced by both maternal and fetal factors, including pregnancy-related morbidity, acute change in fetal status, history of maternal–fetal surgery, fetal malpresentation, and the type of fetal anomaly. Certain anomalies, such as a giant omphalocele, sacrococcygeal teratoma, or unrepaired myelomeningocele, may benefit from a cesarean birth to avoid further neonatal complications. Spontaneous vaginal birth or vaginal birth with induced labor are safe options for most patients. Timing of birth depends on the fetal diagnosis and complications associated with this diagnosis. Delivery between 37 and 39 completed weeks of pregnancy is recommended for most patients. Anticipatory guidance about what to expect at the time of birth is provided during prenatal visits whenever possible.

Birth planning in the prenatal setting involves a discussion of the intrapartum and immediate postpartum periods and maintaining open lines of communication between the patient and the care team. Providing an opportunity for shared decision-making whenever possible allows the patient to exercise control in a seemingly uncontrollable situation (Cortezzo et al., 2019). For example, a discussion regarding patient preference for a support person at the time of birth or pain management plans can allow a patient-driven conversation about goals and personal expectations. Management of patient and family expectations is essential to establish. Explanations of routine practices such as continuous fetal monitoring may also be of help to the family. Given the anticipated need for immediate neonatal assessment or intervention, expectations immediately after birth are important to discuss. This includes immediate separation of the infant from their mother. Requests for skin-to-skin contact, delayed cord clamping, or immediately putting infants to breast may not be reasonable expectations for infants who have significant structural anomalies. Prenatal consultation with neonatologists or neonatal nurse practitioners can provide guidance about potential interventions, anticipated neonatal intensive care unit length of stay, and the unpredictable nature of newborn care when complicated by an anomaly. Neonatology may also add to the discussion of birth planning and expectations regarding neonatal medical intervention such as anticipated intubation or line placement. In addition, consultation with lactation specialists or nutritionists can guide discussions about optimal feeding methods for newborns and provide a framework for families to determine their own feeding goals for their infant. Assessing which aspects of these experiences are important to the parents and working with them to acknowledge the loss of those aspects of care while providing them with alternative methods of bonding may improve outcomes (Cole et al., 2017).

Postpartum Care

Care after the birth of an infant with a prenatal diagnosis of a congenital anomaly poses unique challenges. Most of these infants will require close monitoring and further evaluation in a neonatal intensive care or cardiac intensive care unit. The length of stay varies by diagnosis, but it is frequently weeks to months instead of the usual hours to days. Prenatal preparation includes establishing support networks both virtually and in person. These support networks can be composed of friends and family, or fellow parents who have infants or children with similar diagnoses. Each family works to find their balance in terms of forms of support that suit their needs. Screening for perinatal mood and anxiety disorders by nursing staff on the postpartum floor and in the intensive care setting should be an ongoing process. Before patients are discharged from the postpartum floor, a specific plan for follow-up should be made with each patient and family. This plan can be carried out by providers at the delivery center or by local providers based on the family situation and should consider the need for mental health and medical/postoperative evaluations. Postpartum care includes postoperative evaluations and routine postpartum care in addition to close monitoring for symptoms of perinatal mood disorders, which present frequently in these complicated circumstances. In the setting of a neonatal death, bereavement and grief counseling can be offered. Ongoing care with psychology or psychiatry providers may also be necessary. This communication is essential to ensure proper and thorough follow-up, which can also be difficult to coordinate in the setting of a long-term neonatal hospitalization. Communication between providers is essential to aid in a smooth transition for the patient who may be dealing with significant stressors related to the neonate at that time.

MATERNAL FETAL INTERVENTION AND MANAGEMENT

Historically, maternal–fetal intervention was limited to treating conditions that would lead to in utero or neonatal demise. However, the paradigm is shifting to include diagnoses that when treated in utero can improve quality of life. The option of maternal–fetal intervention requires the ability to confirm the diagnosis, extensive knowledge about the antenatal natural history of the disease, consultation with the appropriate specialists, and thorough compassionate and objective counseling regarding short- and long-term outcomes and procedure-specific risks and benefits for both the maternal and the fetal patient. The option of nonintervention and "routine" neonatal treatment should also be presented to the patient. The multidisciplinary team approach helps ensure understanding and provides psychosocial support and assessment of patient perception to ensure a truly informed consent process.

Generally, fetal therapy includes any intervention that aims to treat the fetus prior to birth. Treatment can include ultrasound-guided needle procedures, minimally invasive procedures, and OMFS. Needle procedures are generally performed under ultrasound guidance and include percutaneous umbilical cord blood sampling, intrauterine transfusion, and pharmacologic intervention. In general, needle procedures are deemed lower risk to the pregnant patient. These techniques are performed by an MFM and not necessarily in a FTC. More complex maternal fetal surgical interventions that impart a higher risk profile are generally performed at FTCs. These interventions include minimally invasive procedures typically performed using ultrasound guidance or a fetoscopic approach and OMFS that requires a maternal laparotomy and hysterotomy. Fetal surgery, whether minimally invasive or open, is associated with pregnancy risks including, but not limited to, chorioamniotic membrane separation, oligohydramnios, amniotic fluid leakage, preterm premature rupture of membranes, chorioamnionitis, preterm contractions, fetal distress, fetal demise, preterm delivery, and placental abruption (Teefey et al., 2020). In a systematic review, Sacco et al. (2019) reported a 20.9% (95% confidence interval [CI]: 15.22, 27.13) complication rate in more than 1,100 women undergoing OMFS. The majority of complications were considered minor (16%), defined as pulmonary edema that resolved with medication, chorioamnionitis, endometritis, blood transfusion, or bleeding during the procedure. Severe complications occurred in 4.5% of women undergoing OMFS and were defined as those requiring surgical or intensive care management. In contrast, 6.15% (95% CI: 4.93, 7.49) of more than 9,000 pregnant women undergoing fetoscopic procedures had associated maternal complications. Severe complications (placental abruption, hemorrhage requiring delivery, pulmonary edema, and amniotic fluid embolus) occurred in 1.7% of patients, whereas minor complications (bleeding during the procedure, chorioamnionitis, and need for transfusion) occurred in 4.3% (Sacco et al., 2019). It is imperative that patient counseling in the setting of congenital malformations involves an unbiased discussion of all available management options for the pregnancy, which should include termination of the pregnancy, fetal intervention, and, if indicated, expectant management and postnatal treatment. In the setting of a life-limiting diagnosis, the option of perinatal palliative care is also discussed. Potential diagnoses for which fetal intervention can be offered are shown in Table 18.2. The approach to fetal intervention depends on the specific fetal malformation and maternal risk assessment.

Open Maternal Fetal Surgery

The open surgical approach involves deep general anesthesia that additionally optimizes uterine relaxation. Often, a maternal epidural catheter is placed preoperatively to provide postoperative pain management. A large multidisciplinary team of MFM specialists, pediatric surgeons, pediatric cardiologists, maternal and pediatric anesthesiologists, sonographers, operating room nurses, and surgical support staff is present in the operating room to perform a maternal laparotomy, hysterotomy, and the designated fetal surgery. Additional surgical subspecialists are present depending

Table 18.2 EXAMPLES OF CONGENITAL ANOMALIES AND AMENABLE FETAL
INTERVENTION

Type of Intervention	Congenital Anomalies
Open maternal fetal surgery	Myelomeningocele, myeloschisis High-risk lung lesions: congenital cystic adenomatoid malformation, bronchopulmonary sequestration High-output vascular tumors: sacrococcygeal teratoma, mediastinal tumors
Ultrasound-guided	Shunt-based intervention for pleural effusion, macrocystic lung lesion, or obstructive uropathy Fetal blood transfusion and/or umbilical cord blood sampling Severe hypothyroidism and intra-amniotic administration of levothyroxine
Fetoscopic	Twin-to-twin transfusion syndrome Selective fetal growth restriction Twin anemia polycythemia sequence Severe aortic stenosis Amniotic band release Posterior urethral valves Congenital diaphragmatic hernia Myelomeningocele

on the fetal diagnosis. Postoperative recovery involves close maternal monitoring, inpatient pain control, tocolytic administration, follow-up ultrasound for viability, and bed rest. Oral tocolytic therapy is often continued throughout the pregnancy. Delivery via cesarean section is scheduled at 37 weeks if not indicated before that time. A 2-year time period is recommended prior to a subsequent pregnancy, and delivery by cesarean section is recommended for any future birth (Teefey et al., 2020).

Multiple psychosocial stressors can contribute to symptoms of depression, anxiety, and post-traumatic stress. Additional stressors include postoperative pain management, maternal activity restriction for the remainder of the pregnancy, relocation of the family in proximity to the FTC or a hospital with an adequate level of care that can respond to any postoperative or obstetric complications that may occur, weekly visits for ultrasound surveillance, long-term maternal hospital stay, delivery planning, and future family planning. The importance of ongoing comprehensive care is emphasized in these cases throughout the pregnancy and the postpartum transition. Integration of psychosocial providers is paramount for ongoing assistance with patient familial needs, screening for perinatal mood disorders, and management of symptoms as well as medication recommendations and management for mood disorders, if needed.

Over time, indications for OMFS have broadened to include lethal and nonlethal anomalies. Today, OMFS is performed with the goal of preventing further fetal decompensation or death and to improve long-term outcomes and quality of life. Once a fetal diagnosis has been confirmed and OMFS is deemed an option from the fetal perspective, extensive counseling and preoperative assessment take place. Maternal risks specific to OMFS include morbidity related to anesthesia, potential for acute blood loss requiring blood transfusion, need for tocolytic medication, wound complications, prolonged hospitalization, and placental dysfunction (Sacco et al., 2019; Teefey et al., 2020). Importantly, the hysterotomy in this type of surgery involves the contractile portion of the uterus, which increases the risk for uterine dehiscence or rupture in the index pregnancy and also in future pregnancies. The risk of uterine rupture is approximately 1% in the index pregnancy and approximately 10% in subsequent pregnancies (Goodnight et al., 2019; Moldenhauer et al., 2015).

MYELOMENINGOCELE

The prevalence of open neural tube defects in the United States is 3.5/10,000 live births (Parker et al., 2010). Myelomeningocele is the most severe form of neural tube defect and can be identified in the prenatal setting through serum screening and typical findings on ultrasound. These findings include cerebral ventriculomegaly, hindbrain herniation, lower extremity muscle wasting and/or talipes equinovarus, abnormalities in the vertebrae, and identification of a myelomeningocele sac. Clinical implications after birth depend on the lesion level and often involve lower extremity weakness and/or paralysis, sensory disturbances, bladder and bowel incontinence, sexual dysfunction, and significant hydrocephalus requiring ventriculoperitoneal shunt placement. During pregnancy, the neural placode is exposed to amniotic fluid, which results in ongoing damage to the spinal cord. The Management of Myelomeningocele Study (MOMS) was a multicenter randomized controlled trial that compared outcomes of prenatal closure to postnatal closure in cases of prenatally diagnosed myelomeningocele. The study found that children who underwent prenatal closure had a 50% decrease in need for shunt placement in the first year of life. In addition, these children were also likely to benefit from reversal of hindbrain herniation and functional improvement up to two levels, leading to a higher likelihood of independent ambulation (Adzick et al., 2011). Since publication of the MOMS trial, OMFS for myelomeningocele closure is considered a standard of care option for this nonlethal anomaly (Committee on Obstetric Practice Society for Maternal–Fetal Medicine, 2017).

LUNG LESIONS

The imaging diagnosis of fetal lung lesions is made based on the location and characteristics of the mass, including blood supply identified on ultrasound. The differential diagnosis of lung lesions in the fetus includes congenital cystic adenomatoid malformation (CCAM), bronchopulmonary sequestration, and bronchial atresia or stenosis. The CCAM volume ratio is used to monitor the size of the lesion and serves as a method to stratify fetuses into high-risk categories

(Crombleholme et al., 2002). Lesions can have significant growth throughout the second trimester, and serial ultrasound monitoring is performed to assess for mass effect, cardiac shift, and development of non-immune fetal hydrops. Fetal hydrops is diagnosed in the setting of fluid accumulation in two or more body cavities. Fetal hydrops is associated with increased risk of fetal demise and maternal mirror syndrome, which results in maternal hypertension, proteinuria, laboratory abnormalities, and pulmonary edema. Delivery is the sole treatment for maternal mirror syndrome, and OMFS is contraindicated. The majority of lesions do not result in hydrops and plateau in size by 30 weeks. These lesions are monitored throughout the pregnancy with the plan for postnatal management. In larger lesions, maternal betamethasone administration can result in stabilization or decrease in the size of the lesion and resolution of hydrops (Peranteau et al., 2016). OMFS with lobectomy of the affected fetal lung is offered in cases of predominantly solid (microcystic) masses prior to the development of overt hydrops given the high potential for fetal demise prior to the start of the third trimester. After 30 weeks of gestation, preterm delivery may be considered with multidisciplinary specialized planning (Teefey et al., 2020).

Vascular Tumors

Sacrococcygeal teratoma (SCT) is an example of a rare vascular tumor for which OMFS can be considered in the setting of evolving hydrops. Fetal SCT originates from the coccyx and is differentiated based on the predominant location within the fetal pelvis and abdomen. The large blood flow to the mass, along with arteriovenous shunting, creates a cardiovascular burden for the fetus and has the potential to result in high-output cardiac failure. In addition, hemorrhage within the SCT can lead to fetal anemia. After the diagnosis of fetal SCT is made, frequent ultrasounds and serial echocardiography are performed to monitor for any significant increase in tumor volume that can result in mass effect, increasing cardiac output, or for evidence of fetal anemia that can lead to hydrops. OMFS with the aim of debulking the tumor and decreasing the cardiac burden can be offered prior to 32 weeks, whereas preterm delivery is considered after this time with specialized delivery planning (Roybal et al., 2011).

Minimally Invasive Maternal Fetal Procedures

Ultrasound-guided minimally invasive techniques avoid the large hysterotomy and instead utilize small puncture sites through the uterine wall. This allows for vaginal delivery and minimizes the risk of uterine dehiscence and rupture associated with the large hysterotomy. Minimally invasive therapies include ultrasound-guided shunt placement and fetoscopic procedures, which are performed using maternal intravenous sedation and local or regional anesthesia with few exceptions.

PLEURAL EFFUSION AND MACROCYSTIC LUNG LESIONS

Ultrasound-guided shunt placement is performed in the setting of space-occupying lesions in the chest, such as a large pleural effusion or macrocystic CCAM. This can result in pulmonary hypoplasia or cardiac dysfunction leading to hydrops in the fetus. A primary pleural effusion is caused by a lymphatic malformation, whereas secondary effusions are associated with aneuploidy, cardiac anomaly, anemia, or infectious etiologies, among others. In the setting of early hydrops, a thoracoamniotic shunt can be placed to allow for chronic drainage of the fluid, resulting in resolution of hydrops and subsequent antenatal lung growth (Peranteau et al., 2015). Prior to offering a thoracoamniotic shunt, a thoracentesis or cyst aspiration is performed under ultrasound guidance to ensure chronic drainage could be beneficial. Cell studies from the pleural fluid as well as amniocentesis for genetic and infectious studies are recommended. Recurrence of the pleural effusion and review of these studies are necessary prior to offering a thoracoamniotic shunt. After shunt placement, serial ultrasounds are indicated, and a full-term vaginal delivery is anticipated. The most frequent complication is shunt displacement into the amniotic cavity (Peranteau et al., 2015).

OBSTRUCTIVE UROPATHY

Structural anomalies in the lower urinary tract can result in bladder outlet obstruction and pressure-related renal insufficiency in utero. Resulting oligohydramnios, specifically anhydramnios, if long term, causes severe pulmonary hypoplasia and neonatal death. Musculoskeletal development can also be affected. A vesicoamniotic shunt can be placed to allow chronic drainage of fetal urine and normalization of amniotic fluid, which allows for fetal lung development with the goal to improve survival. Serial vesicocentesis are performed to ensure functional fetal kidneys based on urinary electrolyte studies prior to offering vesicoamniotic shunting. It is important to understand that renal parenchymal damage that occurs prior to the shunt is unlikely to be reversed, and although lung development is facilitated, normal renal function is not necessarily anticipated (Morris et al., 2013). Complications specific to the procedure include shunt displacement or obstruction and potential for failure (Farrugia, 2020; Morris et al., 2013). Serial ultrasound monitoring after shunt placement is performed with anticipated term vaginal delivery and postnatal assessment and care by neonatology as well as pediatric urology and nephrology specialists.

MONOCHORIONIC TWIN COMPLICATIONS

The shared placenta is the source of increased risk in monochorionic twin pregnancies and results in unique complications compared to those associated with the dichorionic twin pair. Unequal placental sharing and the presence of intertwin vascular anastomoses within the placenta allow bidirectional blood flow between the fetuses that can result in a spectrum of pathology unique to monochorionic twins. These complications include twin-to-twin transfusion syndrome (TTTS), twin anemia polycythemia sequence (TAPS), and selective fetal growth restriction. The ability to detect these complications relies on accurate diagnosis of placentation, which is optimally assigned in the first trimester. The current recommendation is to begin monitoring for these complications at 16 weeks of gestation and continue throughout the pregnancy (Bahtiyar et al., 2015; Society for Maternal–Fetal Medicine & Simpson, 2013). Ultrasonographic findings are used to classify the development of TTTS based on the widely used five-stage Quintero classification system (Quintero et al., 1999). Due to the associated fetal morbidity of advanced stage TTTS (Stage 2 and higher), fetoscopic selective laser photocoagulation is the recommended first-line treatment prior to 28 weeks of gestation. Laser photocoagulation of the placental anastomoses at the chorionic plate is thought to correct the underlying imbalance and improve survival for at least one twin at 28 days of life (76% vs. 56%) compared to serial amnioreduction (Senat et al., 2004). As with other fetal diagnoses, all options are discussed, including continued observation, termination of the entire pregnancy, and selective fetal reduction. Risks specific to fetoscopic selective laser photocoagulation include septostomy and recurrence of TTTS and TAPS, and serial sonographic surveillance is required to monitor for their development throughout the pregnancy. Whereas spontaneous TAPS is extremely rare, postoperative TAPS complicates 10–15% of laser surgery procedures and is thought to occur secondary to a unidirectional shunting of blood from the former recipient fetus to the former donor fetus. A staging classification has also been described for TAPS and helps guide treatment options, which can include laser, intrauterine transfusion, or preterm delivery based on gestational age (Tollenaar et al., 2016). Fetoscopic laser photocoagulation of placental anastomoses in TTTS is associated with preterm delivery, with approximately 50% of fetuses being born prior to 34 weeks and 17% prior to 28 weeks (Malshe et al., 2017). Postoperatively, activity modification is recommended in an effort to allow healing and decrease the rate of these complications, which often occur within the first month after the procedure (Teefey et al., 2020).

ADDITIONAL MINIMALLY INVASIVE FETAL INTERVENTIONS
Development of minimally invasive techniques continues to be a major focus in the fetal intervention space. A fetoscopic approach to myelomeningocele closure is a minimally invasive alternative to OMFS, and it demonstrated a lower risk of uterine dehiscence at the hysterotomy site in a recently published series (Cortes et al., 2019). Ongoing work is being performed to determine the optimal technique that minimizes maternal risk and eliminates the need for cesarean birth in the index and subsequent pregnancies (Belfort et al., 2017). In fetuses with severe isolated left-sided congenital diaphragmatic hernia (CDH), fetal endoluminal tracheal occlusion (FETO) is associated with increased survival. This was not seen in moderate cases of left-sided CDH. Based on most recent protocols, in the most severe cases, as defined on ultrasound imaging, the endotracheal balloon is placed utilizing the fetoscopic technique at 27–29 weeks and is removed via fetoscopy or percutaneous needle puncture at 34 weeks. There is an increased risk of preterm birth, preterm rupture of membranes, and preterm labor associated with FETO (Deprest et al., 2021). Interestingly, the psychological impact of fetal therapy and maternal–fetal intervention is not yet known.

MATERNAL–FETAL MANAGEMENT
CONSIDERATIONS: THE PSYCHOSOCIAL PERSPECTIVE

Maternal Stressors Specific to Fetal Intervention

Patients may be admitted to the hospital for a prolonged period of time due to complications such as membrane separation, preterm premature rupture of membranes, or preterm contractions/preterm labor. Those who undergo fetal therapies may be required to observe bed rest at home or may be admitted for long-term inpatient hospitalization. These prolonged periods of rest should be addressed with the patient using a multifactorial approach. Physical therapy consultation may provide the patient with modified exercises to prevent deconditioning. Mental health assessment and follow-up are essential in the postoperative period because this time may incite new feelings, symptoms of depression due to isolated environment, anxiety, and trauma. Early consultation with psychology providers can allow for additional support, screening, and coping techniques. Medical management can also be considered based on recommendations. Participation in support groups may decrease some of the negative sequelae of prolonged isolation and limited activity. Virtual options can also help provide further support to patients for logistical reasons or in the time of the COVID-19 pandemic. In addition, social work can help families navigate the socioeconomic implications of a prolonged hospitalization, period of unemployment/leave of absence, and/or absence from the family unit and usual support network.

Perinatal Palliative Care

Counseling patients with an anticipated life-limiting fetal diagnosis should include the option of giving birth with the plan for perinatal palliative care. Perinatal palliative care and bereavement programs have been described in the literature, and these programs are instrumental in formulating a perinatal palliative care plan (Cole et al., 2017). This specialized approach focuses on helping a family understand what their child might face at the time of birth and what the parental wishes may be in various settings. An important aspect of the planning process is ensuring that these wishes are communicated to providers and to the delivery unit because the patient may present for an evaluation outside of the planned delivery time. Points of discussion that are critical for providers to communicate include parental goals for mode of delivery, how and when to monitor the fetus during labor, plans for neonatal resuscitation in the delivery room, additional testing that needs to be performed at the time of delivery, spiritual expectations, and how the family wishes to spend time with their infant after birth (Cortezzo et al., 2019).

Palliative care teams also assess risk for development of perinatal mood and anxiety disorders and create plans for follow-up with psychology and psychiatry as needed. Child life specialists help families with other children (either siblings or close relatives and friends) and have age-appropriate discussions about the fetal diagnosis and probability of neonatal death (Cole et al., 2017).

A perinatal palliative care consultation often begins with a discussion with a neonatologist and is followed by collaborative discussions with other members of the psychosocial team. These discussions include planning details after death (funeral and cremation services) as well as the emotional and financial aspects of these difficult decisions. Palliative care services available outside of the hospital setting are also discussed. MFM physicians continue to work with the family to provide ongoing obstetric input based on imaging assessments, which help guide timing and mode of delivery. Perinatal palliative care providers partner with expectant mothers and their families to develop individualized, seamless, and compassionate care plans that address their emotional, social, and familial needs (Cole et al., 2017).

IDEAS WORTH SHARING

- Accurate diagnosis and evaluation of a congenital anomaly allow for comprehensive counseling regarding pregnancy options.
- Fetal intervention via OMFS or a minimally invasive approach may be an option for certain congenital anomalies in specialized centers. This option involves extensive discussion about risks and benefits and often requires ongoing monitoring and specialized care.
- A multidisciplinary care team is essential to provide comprehensive care for this unique population of pregnant women and families.
- Ongoing psychosocial and medical support provides an infrastructure through which shared decision-making can take place.
- Integration of psychosocial services within a fetal center provides ongoing assessment and treatment of preexisting or perinatal mood disorders as well as support for families at high risk for depression, anxiety, and traumatic stress.

CONCLUSION

The psychosocial implications of a pregnancy affected by a congenital anomaly are significant, and successful navigation involves a multidisciplinary care team from the time of diagnosis through the postpartum period. Parental counseling in this context is complex, and management planning should involve shared decision-making whenever possible. The option of maternal–fetal intervention, when appropriate, is associated with additional maternal and fetal risks and can be an additional source of stress with unique challenges. The FTC aims to provide a collaborative environment that addresses these specific needs while working with families to give the most comprehensive care to this high-risk population.

REFERENCES

Adzick, N. S., Thom, E. A., Spong, C. Y., Brock, J. W., 3rd, Burrows, P. K., Johnson, M. P., Howell, L. J., Farrell, J. A., Dabrowiak, M. E., Sutton, L. N., Gupta, N., Tulipan, N. B., D'Alton, M. E., Farmer, D. L.; for the MOMS Investigators. (2011). A randomized trial of prenatal versus postnatal repair of myelomeningocele. *New England Journal of Medicine, 364*(11), 993–1004. https://doi.org/10.1056/NEJMoa1014379

Bahtiyar, M. O., Emery, S. P., Dashe, J. S., Wilkins-Haug, L. E., Johnson, A., Paek, B. W., Moon-Grady, A. J., Skupski, D. W., O'Brien, B. M., Harman, C. R., Simpson, L. L.; for the North American Fetal Therapy Network. (2015). The North American Fetal Therapy Network consensus statement: Prenatal surveillance of uncomplicated monochorionic gestations. *Obstetrics and Gynecology, 125*(1), 118–123. https://doi.org/10.1097/AOG.0000000000000599

Belfort, M. A., Whitehead, W. E., Shamshirsaz, A. A., Bateni, Z. H., Olutoye, O. O., Olutoye, O. A., Mann, D. G., Espinoza, J., Williams, E., Lee, T. C., Keswani, S. G., Ayres, N., Cassady, C. I., Mehollin-Ray, A. R., Sanz Cortes, M., Carreras, E., Peiro, J. L., Ruano, R., & Cass, D. L. (2017). Fetoscopic open neural tube defect repair: Development and refinement of a two-port, carbon dioxide insufflation technique. *Obstetrics and Gynecology, 129*(4), 734–743. https://doi.org/10.1097/AOG.0000000000001941

Cole, J. C. M., Moldenhauer, J. S., Jones, T. R., Shaughnessy, E. A., Zarrin, H. E., Coursey, A. L., & Munson, D. A. (2017). A proposed model for perinatal palliative care. *Journal of Obstetric, Gynecologic, and Neonatal Nursing, 46*(6), 904–911. https://doi.org/10.1016/j.jogn.2017.01.014

Committee on Obstetric Practice Society for Maternal–Fetal Medicine. (2017). Committee opinion No. 720: Maternal–fetal surgery for myelomeningocele. *Obstetrics and Gynecology, 130*(3), 672–673. https://doi.org/10.1097/AOG.0000000000002294

Cortes, M. S., Lapa, D. A., Acácio, G. L., Belfort, M., Carreras, E., Maiz, N., . . . & Nicolaides, K. H. (2019). Proceedings of the first annual meeting of the International Fetoscopic Myelomeningocele Repair Consortium. *Ultrasound in Obstetrics and Gynecology, 53*(6), 855–863.

Cortezzo, D. E., Bowers, K., & Cameron Meyer, M. (2019). Birth planning in uncertain or life-limiting fetal diagnoses: Perspectives of physicians and parents. *Journal of Palliative Medicine, 22*(11), 1337–1345. https://doi.org/10.1089/jpm.2018.0596

Crombleholme, T. M., Coleman, B., Hedrick, H., Liechty, K., Howell, L., Flake, A. W., . . . & Adzick, N. S. (2002). Cystic adenomatoid malformation volume ratio predicts outcome in prenatally diagnosed cystic adenomatoid malformation of the lung. *Journal of Pediatric Surgery, 37*(3), 331–338.

Deprest, J. A., Nicolaides, K. H., Benachi, A., Gratacos, E., Ryan, G., Persico, N., Sago, H., Johnson, A., Wielgos, M., Berg, C., Van Calster, B., Russo, F. M.; for the TOTAl Trial for Severe Hypoplasia Investigators. (2021). Randomized trial of fetal surgery for severe left diaphragmatic hernia. *New England Journal of Medicine, 385*(2), 107–118. https://doi.org/10.1056/NEJMoa2027030

Farrugia, M. K. (2020). Fetal bladder outflow obstruction: Interventions, outcomes and management uncertainties. *Early Human Development, 150*, 105189. https://doi.org/10.1016/j.earlhumdev.2020.105189

Goodnight, W. H., Bahtiyar, O., Bennett, K. A., Emery, S. P., Lillegard, J. B., Fisher, A., Goldstein, R., Jatres, J., Lim, F. Y., McCullough, L., Moehrlen, U., Moldenhauer, J. S., Moon-Grady, A. J., Ruano, R., Skupski, D. W., Thom, E., Treadwell, M. C., Tsao, K., Wagner, A. J., . . . Zaretsky, M.; for the fMMC Consortium sponsored by NAFTNet. (2019). Subsequent pregnancy outcomes after open maternal–fetal surgery for myelomeningocele. *American Journal of Obstetrics and Gynecology*, *220*(5), 494.e491–494.e497. https://doi.org/10.1016/j.ajog.2019.03.008

Harrison, M. R., Filly, R. A., Golbus, M. S., Berkowitz, R. L., Callen, P. W., Canty, T. G., Catz, C., Clewell, W. H., Depp, R., Edwards, M. S., Fletcher, J. C., Frigoletto, F. D., Garrett, W. J., Johnson, M. L., Jonsen, A., De Lorimier, A. A., Liley, W. A., Mahoney, M. J., Manning, F. D., . . . Schulman, J. D. (1982). Fetal treatment 1982. *New England Journal of Medicine*, *307*(26), 1651–1652. https://doi.org/10.1056/NEJM198212233072623

Howell, L. J., & Adzick, N. S. (2003). Establishing a fetal therapy center: Lessons learned. *Seminars in Pediatric Surgery*, *12*(3), 209–217. https://doi.org/10.1016/s1055-8586(03)00023-4

Kemp, J., Davenport, M., & Pernet, A. (1998). Antenatally diagnosed surgical anomalies: The psychological effect of parental antenatal counseling. *Journal of Pediatric Surgery*, *33*(9), 1376–1379. https://doi.org/10.1016/s0022-3468(98)90011-2

Malshe, A., Snowise, S., Mann, L. K., Boring, N., Johnson, A., Bebbington, M. W., Moise, K. J., Jr., & Papanna, R. (2017). Preterm delivery after fetoscopic laser surgery for twin–twin transfusion syndrome: Etiology and risk factors. *Ultrasounds in Obstetrics & Gynecology*, *49*(5), 612–616. https://doi.org/10.1002/uog.15972

Metcalfe, S. A. (2018). Genetic counselling, patient education, and informed decision-making in the genomic era. *Seminars in Fetal and Neonatal Medicine*, *23*(2), 142–149. https://doi.org/10.1016/j.siny.2017.11.010

Moldenhauer, J. S., Soni, S., Rintoul, N. E., Spinner, S. S., Khalek, N., Martinez-Poyer, J., Flake, A. W., Hedrick, H. L., Peranteau, W. H., Rendon, N., Koh, J., Howell, L. J., Heuer, G. G., Sutton, L. N., Johnson, M. P., & Adzick, N. S. (2015). Fetal myelomeningocele repair: The post-MOMS experience at the Children's Hospital of Philadelphia. *Fetal Diagnosis Therapy*, *37*(3), 235–240. https://doi.org/10.1159/000365353

Moon-Grady, A. J., Baschat, A., Cass, D., Choolani, M., Copel, J. A., Crombleholme, T. M., Deprest, J., Emery, S. P., Evans, M. I., Luks, F. I., Norton, M. E., Ryan, G., Tsao, K., Welch, R., & Harrison, M. (2017). Fetal treatment 2017: The evolution of fetal therapy centers—A joint opinion from the International Fetal Medicine and Surgical Society (IFMSS) and the North American Fetal Therapy Network (NAFTNet). *Fetal Diagnosis Therapy*, *42*(4), 241–248. https://doi.org/10.1159/000475929

Morris, R. K., Malin, G. L., Quinlan-Jones, E., Middleton, L. J., Hemming, K., Burke, D., Daniels, J. P., Khan, K. S., Deeks, J., Kilby, M. D.; for the Percutaneous Vesicoamniotic Shunting in Lower Urinary Tract Obstruction Collaborative Group. (2013). Percutaneous vesicoamniotic shunting versus conservative management for fetal lower urinary tract obstruction (PLUTO): A randomised trial. *Lancet*, *382*(9903), 1496–1506. https://doi.org/10.1016/S0140-6736(13)60992-7

Parker, S. E., Mai, C. T., Canfield, M. A., Rickard, R., Wang, Y., Meyer, R. E., Anderson, P., Mason, C. A., Collins, J. S., Kirby, R. S., Correa, A.; for the National Birth Defects Prevention Network. (2010). Updated national birth prevalence estimates for selected birth defects in the United States, 2004–2006. *Birth Defects Research Part A: Clinical and Molecular Teratology*, *88*(12), 1008–1016. https://doi.org/10.1002/bdra.20735

Peranteau, W. H., Adzick, N. S., Boelig, M. M., Flake, A. W., Hedrick, H. L., Howell, L. J., Moldenhauer, J. S., Khalek, N., Martinez-Poyer, J., & Johnson, M. P. (2015). Thoracoamniotic shunts for the management of fetal lung lesions and pleural effusions: A single-institution review and predictors of survival in 75 cases. *Journal of Pediatric Surgery*, *50*(2), 301–305. https://doi.org/10.1016/j.jpedsurg.2014.11.019

Peranteau, W. H., Boelig, M. M., Khalek, N., Moldenhauer, J. S., Martinez-Poyer, J., Hedrick, H. L., Flake, A. W., Johnson, M. P., & Adzick, N. S. (2016). Effect of single and multiple courses of maternal betamethasone on prenatal congenital lung lesion growth and fetal survival. *Journal of Pediatric Surgery*, *51*(1), 28–32. https://doi.org/10.1016/j.jpedsurg.2015.10.018

Quintero, R. A., Morales, W. J., Allen, M. H., Bornick, P. W., Johnson, P. K., & Kruger, M. (1999). Staging of twin–twin transfusion syndrome. *Journal of Perinatology*, *19*(8 Pt. 1), 550–555. https://doi.org/10.1038/sj.jp.7200292

Roybal, J. L., Moldenhauer, J. S., Khalek, N., Bebbington, M. W., Johnson, M. P., Hedrick, H. L., Adzick, N. S., & Flake, A. W. (2011). Early delivery as an alternative management strategy for selected high-risk fetal sacrococcygeal teratomas. *Journal of Pediatric Surgery*, *46*(7), 1325–1332. https://doi.org/10.1016/j.jpedsurg.2010.10.020

Sacco, A., Van der Veeken, L., Bagshaw, E., Ferguson, C., Van Mieghem, T., David, A. L., & Deprest, J. (2019). Maternal complications following open and fetoscopic fetal surgery: A systematic review and meta-analysis. *Prenatal Diagnosis*, *39*(4), 251–268. https://doi.org/10.1002/pd.5421

Senat, M. V., Deprest, J., Boulvain, M., Paupe, A., Winer, N., & Ville, Y. (2004). Endoscopic laser surgery versus serial amnioreduction for severe twin-to-twin transfusion syndrome. *New England Journal of Medicine*, *351*(2), 136–144. https://doi.org/10.1056/NEJMoa032597

Society for Maternal–Fetal Medicine, & Simpson, L. L. (2013). Twin–twin transfusion syndrome. *American Journal of Obstetrics & Gynecology*, *208*(1), 3–18. https://doi.org/10.1016/j.ajog.2012.10.880

Teefey, C. P., Soni, S., & Khalek, N. (2020). Maternal fetal surgery: Intervention and management. *Clinical Obstetrics and Gynecology*, *63*(2), 455–467. https://doi.org/10.1097/GRF.0000000000000534

Tollenaar, L. S., Slaghekke, F., Middeldorp, J. M., Klumper, F. J., Haak, M. C., Oepkes, D., & Lopriore, E. (2016). Twin anemia polycythemia sequence: Current views on pathogenesis, diagnostic criteria, perinatal management, and outcome. *Twin Research and Human Genetics*, *19*(3), 222–233. https://doi.org/10.1017/thg.2016.18

19

ROLE OF BEHAVIORAL HEALTH CLINICIANS IN FETAL CARE SETTINGS

LACY CHAVIS, SAKINA BUTT, AND ELIZABETH VAUGHT ■

In the United States, major structural or genetic birth defects affect approximately 3% of births each year (Centers for Disease Control and Prevention, 2018). Congenital anomalies have surpassed prematurity and are now the leading cause of infant mortality, representing approximately 20% of neonatal deaths (Matthews et al., 2015). Caring for the unique needs of a family and fetus with a congenital anomaly requires specialized care with clinical expertise. Fetal care centers (FCCs) have been established to provide comprehensive, coordinated, and multidisciplinary advanced care. Throughout the country, FCCs offer a wide spectrum of services. The majority of FCCs provide outpatient consultation and referrals, whereas a smaller number conduct fetal procedures and only a small percentage offer comprehensive services spanning the entire journey from fetal diagnosis to pregnancy management, labor and delivery with neonatal resuscitation, and neonatal intensive care unit (NICU) stay (Howell, 2013). Behavioral health clinicians (BHCs) often include psychologists, clinical social workers, psychiatrists, or fetal care nurse coordinators with subspecialty in perinatal and/or infant mental health. Each discipline has a unique training and skill set; although there may be some overlap among roles, there are also unique activities and clinical responsibilities for each of these behavioral health disciplines. BHCs in the FCC setting bring an additional level of expertise to the multidisciplinary team to support the multifaceted needs of pregnant women and their families. BHCs in FCC settings are positioned to provide screening and assessment, psychoeducation, and interventions to improve mental health and health behaviors during the perinatal period; consultation; staff and community training; and programmatic development (Dempsey et al., 2021).

PERINATAL MOOD AND ANXIETY DISORDERS IN FETAL CARE CENTERS

Perinatal mood and anxiety disorders (PMADs) are the most common medical complication during pregnancy and the postpartum period, affecting approximately 20–25% of women and their families (American College of Obstetricians and Gynecologists [ACOG], 2015). Population-based statistics show that 10% of fathers experience clinically significant symptoms of depression, anxiety, and/or traumatic stress in the perinatal period (Keesara & Kim, 2018; Singley & Edwards, 2015). Expectant parents who present in FCCs are at even greater risk for PMADs; however, the primary focus of the provider and family tends to be on the unborn child and the mother's physical health, resulting in missed symptoms of parental emotional functioning (Kett et al., 2017).

A diagnosis of a fetal anomaly in pregnancy can heighten the risk for perinatal depression, anxiety, and traumatic stress as expectant parents grieve the loss of their hoped-for healthy child and approach difficult options on how to proceed with care (Cole et al., 2016; Kaasen et al., 2010; Kingston et al., 2015). Learning of a fetal anomaly often increases the emotional vulnerability of expectant parents. Studies have shown that intrusive thoughts, anger, avoidance, grief, sadness, anxiety, and difficulties attaching to the fetus are commonly reported emotional reactions (Wool, 2011). Prevalence rates for maternal stress, anxiety, and depression in high-risk pregnancies have been shown to be as high as 40% (Kingston et al., 2015). Cole et al. (2016) conducted a retrospective study of 1,032 expectant mothers carrying fetuses with a confirmed anomaly and 788 expectant fathers. They found that 19.3% of women and 13.1% of men reported significant post-traumatic stress symptoms and scored positive for risk of a major depressive disorder on a common screening measure.

Maternal health concerns in the perinatal period are associated with increased risk for additional pregnancy complications, including miscarriage, gestational hypertension, preeclampsia, preterm birth, and infants born small for gestational age (Lenze, 2017). When considering perinatal mental health, mood concerns tend to receive greater attention than anxiety. However, both perinatal anxiety and mood issues have been linked to adverse neonatal and childhood outcomes. Adverse outcomes such as low birth weight, developmental challenges, as well as increased rates of attention-deficit/hyperactivity disorder and emotional/behavioral problems later in childhood have also been reported (Williams & Koleva, 2018).

BHCs working in FCCs provide expertise in integration of behavioral health within medical settings (Kaslow et al., 2008); PMADs; the parent–child relationship; and the integration of the overall health of the parent, infant, and family. The distinct activities they may engage in are described next.

SCREENING

Extensive evidence linking perinatal maternal mental health concerns to adverse outcomes during infancy and childhood has increased global awareness of the need for screening of PMADs. Consequently, the implementation of routine screening of women during pregnancy, especially those presenting with fetal complications, is advised to identify and intervene appropriately (Cole et al., 2016).

Routine screening for mental health disorders in pregnant women can help identify those who may need additional mental health support. However, due to variable insurance coverage and lack of a national health care mandate, the United States continues to lag behind in screening and caring for women at risk for PMADs. Indeed, more than 50% of women with PMADs go unrecognized and untreated (Lenze, 2017). Estimates from prior studies suggest the prevalence of major depression in partners is 9% or 10% and that of anxiety is between 4% and 18% (Lenze, 2017). Paternal postpartum depression rates are lowest during the 0–3 months postpartum period and highest during the 3–6 months period. Risk factors include past history of severe depression, prenatal depression, prenatal anxiety, lower educational status, having other children, and maternal prenatal depression (Ramchandani et al., 2008). Given the increased risk of PMADs among expectant parents with fetal anomalies, BHCs in FCC settings are positioned to implement systematic screening and response protocols to support patients and families.

SCREENING VERSUS ASSESSMENT

Before discussing optimal implementation of screening, it is important to highlight the purpose of screening and how it differs from assessment. A screening measure is defined as a tool that is used to identify a particular skill or ability that is highly predictive of a later outcome. With respect to perinatal mental health, screening measures serve to divide individuals into groups based on risk level (i.e., high and low risk) for mood and anxiety disorders. These measures are typically brief and narrow in scope to allow for quick identification of those who need more detailed assessment and/or intervention. Commonly used screening measures for depression and anxiety risk are listed in Table 19.1. Thus, although screening is helpful in identifying those at risk for PMADs, a positive screen does not equate to a diagnosis. Psychological assessment is typically needed following a positive screen to verify whether diagnostic criteria for a mental health disorder are met and to identify specific recommendations for treatment. Assessment is further discussed later in this chapter.

RECOMMENDED SCREENING PROTOCOLS AND TIME POINTS

Numerous national organizations have endorsed mental health screening during the perinatal period in an effort to improve pregnancy outcomes. ACOG (2015) recommends screening for perinatal mood at least once during the perinatal period, including pregnancy, and at least once in the postpartum period. The American Psychological Association (2018) recommends screening for depression twice during pregnancy—once in early pregnancy for preexisting psychiatric

Table 19.1 COMMONLY USED PERINATAL MENTAL HEALTH SCREENING MEASURES

Measure	Indication
Patient Health Questionnaire (PHQ-9)	General screening measure
Perinatal Anxiety Screening Scale (PASS)	General anxiety screening measure
Perinatal Obsessive–Compulsive Scale (PCOS)	Administer to women with a history of obsessive–compulsive disorder
Generalized Anxiety Disorder Scale (GADS)	Administer to women with anxiety symptoms or history of anxiety disorder
State–Trait Anxiety Inventory (STAI)	Commonly used measure of trait and state anxiety
Edinburgh Postpartum Depression Scale (EPDS)	Widely used postpartum depression measure
Center for Epidemiologic Studies Depression Scale (CES-D)	Commonly used self-report measure of depressive symptoms
Perceived Stress Scale (PSS)	Perception of stress
Perinatal Post-Traumatic Stress Disorder Questionnaire (PPQ)	Administer to women with a history of traumatic birth experiences, childhood trauma, and interpersonal violence
Impact of Events Scale–Revised (IES-R)	Traumatic stress events measure
Postpartum Depression Screening Scale (PDSS)	A measure of overall severity and seven specific symptoms

disorders and once in later pregnancy. Patients with medically complicated prenatal courses may need to be screened more frequently given the high-risk nature of the pregnancy and ongoing uncertainty, information about prognosis, and grief over a "typical" pregnancy and anticipated neonatal period.

Pregnant women are in increased contact with health care providers, thus providing multiple opportunities for screening that can better identify problems and initiate treatment for mental health needs (Lenze, 2017). Prior research has shown that women who are screened for maternal mental health concerns during pregnancy are more likely to access care compared to women who are screened in the postnatal period only (Venkatesh et al., 2016). This finding suggests that frequent contact with health care providers during pregnancy increases the ability to initiate appropriate treatment referrals.

Screening in FCCs has shown promising results in improving maternal mental health outcomes and reducing infant/child adverse outcomes (Lenze, 2017). However, the effectiveness of screening is reduced when follow-up services are not co-located or integrated into the setting. Similar to other medical populations, the rate of follow-through is less optimal if individuals have to venture outside of their typical care center to initiate and receive treatment (Yawn et al., 2012).

ASSESSMENT

Behavioral health clinicians in FCCs may also engage in assessment (either psychosocial or psychological, depending on the background discipline of the provider and purpose of the assessment). BHCs with social work backgrounds typically administer a psychosocial assessment. The psychosocial assessment differs from screening in that it involves obtaining a multidimensional picture of specific psychosocial factors. In other words, psychosocial assessment aims to identify risk factors for PMADs by examining several key areas outlined in Table 19.2 and psychological assessments. Assessments also have broader scope that typically involves providing psychoeducation to normalize commonly experienced symptoms as well as identifying appropriate referrals. BHCs should conduct screening measures to assess for health-promotion behaviors, anxiety, mood, traumatic stress symptoms, coping difficulties, and social supports because identification of those at highest risk is the first step in implementation of interventions (Rychik et al., 2013). Diagnostic assessments (typically administered by BHCs with a background in psychology or psychiatry) may be conducted to determine whether a patient meets criteria for a mental health disorder; these can involve a comprehensive interview, history of mental health disorders/symptoms, and often additional symptom measures. The purpose of the diagnostic assessment is to establish diagnosis/differential diagnosis and for treatment planning for mental health interventions.

Psychosocial and diagnostic assessments are typically performed by BHCs working in FCCs who have expertise in the integration of behavioral health care within the medical setting. Inclusion of BHCs in FCCs is extremely beneficial to ensure appropriate response to screening (including follow-up assessment)

Table 19.2 Risk Factors for Perinatal Mood and Anxiety Disorders

Personal history of anxiety/mood symptoms or disorder	Poor quality relationship with partner
Changes in hormones and sleep patterns	Family members who have experienced traumatic childbirth
Pregnancy ambivalence	History of perinatal loss
Maternal age	Fertility challenges
History of domestic violence	Family members with history of interpersonal violence
History of premenstrual dysphoric disorder	History of perinatal mood and anxiety disorders in family members
Lack of spousal/partner or familial support	Substance abuse
Adverse childhood experiences	Poverty
Psychosocial stressors (e.g., financial stress)	Personality vulnerabilities (e.g., low self-esteem)

and facilitation of treatment when needed. This is particularly necessary because many maternal–fetal medicine providers report believing they do not have the necessary training to implement these services (Lenze, 2017). The optimal approach for the FCC behavioral health clinician is to incorporate screening, assessment, and intervention services for individuals who are found to be at risk for or exhibit significant symptoms of PMADS (Keesara & Kim, 2018).

INTERVENTION

Medicine and health care in the United States have evolved and moved away from a provider-centered model to a patient-centered model characterized by multidisciplinary teams addressing both physical and psychological needs of patients (S. Johnson, 2013). This transformation in health care has carried over into specialty medicine, resulting in the rapid growth of FCCs and increased expertise in caring for pregnant women and fetuses. The BHCs in the FCCs address discontinuity in care that is often experienced when a congenital anomaly is detected by offering integrated diagnostic, obstetric, and neonatal care. As medicine has advanced, so too has the understanding of factors influencing perinatal health. Mood, stress level, physical health, geographic location, socioeconomic status, partner involvement, and perceived social supports have all been well documented to influence pregnancy and birth outcomes (Dunkel-Schetter & Glynn, 2010; Lenze, 2017). BHCs have made significant contributions in the development of interventions to improve mental and physical health during the perinatal period. Intervention services provided by BHCs in FCCs encompass consultation and group interventions as well as individual brief psychotherapy. Each of these is described in detail below.

CONSULTATION

One interventional role that BHCs can adopt in FCCs is to engage as a consultant to the team. In this model, the BHC may not have a prolonged relationship with the family that involves sustained intervention over time. Rather, the BHC may work with the team to facilitate communications, shared decision-making, and trauma-informed care in an indirect care model. Consultation provides the opportunity to discuss the family's understanding of the fetal diagnosis and overall health literacy, family concerns, communication preferences and styles, and potential pathways of care. Many FCCs adopt a multidisciplinary approach to offer integration and coordination of multiple medical specialists and BHCs to provide quality care and to facilitate joint decision-making on how best to manage the pregnancy (Cole et al., 2016; Kett et al., 2017). The incorporation of multiple individuals with differing fields of expertise, including BHCs, provides a forum for enriched information sharing and facilitates an open, shared dialogue in which parents' concerns and questions can be heard and addressed. In this way, integration of BHCs embraces a team approach affording time for parents to share their thoughts, beliefs, values, questions, and concerns. A BHC who consults with the medical team may be able to share information about the family's communication styles, values, and any psychological or psychosocial concerns that should be considered in developing a plan of care.

BHCs can also participate in team communications and team meetings with the patient and family. The initial fetal care consult meeting can inform the need for more in-depth or ongoing evaluation by the BHC and services that support cultural considerations and the family's expressed needs in the areas of mental, emotional, physical, and/or spiritual health during their pregnancy and perinatal/neonatal period. A family-centered care approach addresses all of these areas, promoting a greater sense of inclusivity and continuity of care (Howard, 2006). Establishing these provider–family relationships early on can lessen parental stress and anxiety that can be exacerbated by working with so many different care providers and by an uncertain future for their infant and family (Sanders & Hall, 2018). The inclusion of a BHC is vital to providing a holistic approach (Howard, 2006) and ensures that the parents' holistic needs are appropriately addressed. This is also a time for the BHC to identify parent and family strengths that can be reinforced during challenging times ahead, as well as identify areas that can benefit from additional intervention and support.

Parents with congenital anomalies who met with the multidisciplinary team in the FCC reported these meetings were highly beneficial (Kett et al., 2017). Parents expressed gratitude for the expert information provided, having their questions addressed, and the kindness and support offered by the fetal care providers and other team members. Concerns about the uncertainty for the future were expressed and acknowledged, giving parents a way to explore coping strategies along with the need for additional referrals for support. Most families do seek additional information through the internet, and follow-up discussion with a BHC can help illuminate what may or may not be true/applicable in their individual case.

BRIEF INTERVENTIONS

To reduce uncertainty surrounding the delivery experience and the NICU experience, BHCs may facilitate parental coping by setting up tours for families. A tour should include an overview of structural supports and the importance of the patient and parental role as an integral part of the care team. Parents need to be encouraged to ask questions and participate in their care and that of their infant. For NICU tours, while acknowledging the state-of-the-art highly technical environment, it is as important to help parents feel welcomed and empowered so they can envision themselves in their infant's room nurturing, loving, and parenting their infant. Regardless of the diagnosis, two universal parent questions must be discussed: "When can I hold my infant?" and "When can we expect to go home?"

Seeing the labor and delivery unit, operating room, and/or the NICU for the first time can be daunting and intimidating. The BHC can prepare parents ahead of time for what they may see and hear and ensure there is time to discuss any feelings that may have arisen during the tour(s); additional questions can be addressed then and/or through a follow-up phone call. Whether the mother is planning to breastfeed, pump, formula feed, or remains unsure, a subsequent lactation consultation should also be included. Most potential mothers have questions and need the reassurance that their feeding preferences will be supported. If electing to breastfeed/pump, mothers also need information on supplies and specifics on where and how their milk will be stored during their infant's NICU stay.

INDIVIDUAL PSYCHOTHERAPY

The effects of prenatal mental health support on maternal and infant well-being are well-documented. Women with greater prenatal mental health support experienced lower levels of stress during pregnancy, and they reported less substance abuse, better progress with labor, decrease in preterm births, improved birth outcomes (i.e., increased infant birth weight and APGAR scores), and increased satisfaction with prenatal care. Women with less mental health support were at greater risk for postpartum mood and anxiety concerns (Cunningham et al., 2019).

For those who are identified as being at increased risk for PMADs, there remains a significant gap in access to behavioral health services once a need has been identified. Integration of BHCs within an FCC helps reduce this barrier of access to treatment and further addresses the unique needs of each patient and family. BHCs work beyond the initial consultation, and supports can include brief individual therapy and/or group therapy services in an effort to promote resilience and decrease emotional stress in the prenatal and postpartum periods. Brief individualized therapy may involve the following:

- Use of evidence-based therapeutic strategies to address health behaviors (i.e., nutrition, physical activity, sleep hygiene, substance use and oral health, chronic disease prevention, and healthy weight) and medical adherence
- Use of evidenced-based, short-term treatment modalities to address a range of PMADs and trauma (i.e., cognitive–behavioral therapy [(CBT], interpersonal therapy [IPT], mindfulness, dialectical behavioral therapy, and eye movement desensitization and reprocessing)
- Behavioral health concerns (e.g., role transition, grief and bereavement, active problem-solving, and stress management)
- Interventions to support parent–infant attachment and foster parent engagement. Discussing fetal development during the last trimester in ways that reinforce and support the already developing connections and attachment process empowers the parents to know that they are contributing to the quality of their infant's experience (e.g., talking

to their infant, acknowledging movement with touch and words, and sharing feelings of love concern and caring).

GROUP THERAPY

There is a strong social process associated with pregnancy and birth. Expectant parents are naturally drawn to social connection to discuss uncertainties, compare symptoms, empathize with one another, and seek information. Innovative approaches to prenatal care have leveraged this naturally occurring desire for affiliation in formalizing group prenatal care. Group prenatal care was first pioneered by Sharon Schindler Rising (1998) with the Centering Pregnancy model. The Centering Pregnancy model incorporates prenatal care, risk assessment, education, and support in a cohort of expectant women of similar gestational ages. Typical groups comprise 8–12 women, with an established number of prenatal care sessions. Group members participate in self-care; receive brief individual medical checks; and engage in facilitated discussion on topics of pregnancy, childbirth, and parenting led by a prenatal care provider. Discussions aim to foster healthier behaviors, building new skills and giving/receiving social support (Ickovics et al., 2019; Rising, 1998, 2016). Such models are often not feasible in FCCs, but clinicians can still encourage patient/families to connect with other for support through referrals to support groups or therapy groups.

Evidence-based therapy groups include the CBT-based Mothers and Babies program (Tandon et al., 2014) and the IPT-based Reach Out, Stand Strong, Essentials for New Mothers (ROSE) program (J. Johnson et al., 2018). Mothers and Babies is a peer-to-peer support model with the goal of helping participants create healthy physical, social, and psychosocial environments. Typical intervention includes 6–12 weekly group sessions during pregnancy and 2–5 postpartum "booster sessions." The curriculum includes modules on the cognitive–behavioral theory of mood and health; physiological effects of stress; the importance of rewarding activities; reducing cognitive distortions and automatic thoughts; and the importance of social networks, positive mother–child attachment, and parenting strategies to promote child development and secure attachment in infants (Tandon et al., 2014). ROSE involves 4–6 prenatal group sessions lasting 60–90 minutes and 1 individual postpartum session. Program content covers topics of stress management, development of a social support system, role transitions, interpersonal conflicts common around childbirth, and role-playing exercises with group members (Zlotnick et al., 2016). Groups in the FCC setting offer a sense of community and support when many expectant parents of high-risk pregnancies feel a sense of isolation.

CONCLUSION

Behavioral health clinicians play a vital role in the provision of high-quality and holistic care during pregnancy by offering expertise in screening, assessment, and intervention. Both screening and assessments are crucial for identification and intervention of PMADs to prevent adverse outcomes. Screening and psychosocial assessments serve to identify individuals at risk and/or initiate intervention to mitigate the negative impact for the mother, father/partner, and infant. Collaborative care models encompassing mental health screening, diagnosis, and intervention embedded within the fetal care setting are recommended (Kaasen, et al., 2010; Lenze, 2017). A benefit to having BHCs embedded within the FCC is that these providers serve to reduce barriers to care and promote access to evidence-based services. Individual and group interventions have proven effective in the prevention and treatment of PMADs, leading to improved outcomes for the entire family unit (Lenze, 2017). An added benefit involves facilitation of a continuum of care starting in FCCs and extending to the NICU and beyond. BHCs also provide education, training, and support to other FCC providers.

REFERENCES

American College of Obstetricians and Gynecologists. (2015). Committee opinion No. 630: Screening for perinatal depression. *Obstetrics & Gynecology, 125*(5), 1268–1271. https://doi.org/10.1097/01.AOG.0000465192.34779.dc

American Psychological Association. (2018). *Position statement on screening and treatment of mood and anxiety disorders during pregnancy and postpartum.* https://psychnews.psychiatryonline.org/doi/10.1176/appi.pn.2019.3b19

Centers for Disease Control and Prevention. (2018). *Data & statistics on birth defects.* http://www.cdc.gov/ncbddd/birthdefects/data.html

Cole, J. C., Moldhenhauer, J. S., Berger, K., Cary, M. S., Smith, H., Martino, V., Rendon, N., & Howell, L. J. (2016). Identifying expectant parents at risk for psychological distress in response to a confirmed fetal abnormality. *Archives of Women's Mental Health, 19*(3), 443–453. https://doi.org/10.1007/s00737-015-0580-6

Cunningham, S. D., Lewis, J. B., Shebl, F. M., Boyd, L. M., Robinson, M. A., Grilo, S. A., Lewis, S. M., Pruett, A. L., & Ickovics, J. R. (2019). Group prenatal care reduces risk of preterm birth and low birth weight: A matched cohort study. *Journal of Women's Health, 28*(1), 17–22. https://doi.org/10.1089/jwh.2017.6817

Dempsey, A. G., Chavis, L., Willis, T., Zuk, J., & Cole, J. (2021). Addressing perinatal mental health risk within a fetal care center. *Journal of Clinical Psychology in Medical Settings, 28*(1), 125–136. https://doi.org/10.1007/s10880-020-09728-2

Dunkel-Schetter, C., & Glynn, L. (2010). Stress in pregnancy: Empirical evidence and theoretical issues to guide interdisciplinary researchers. In R. Contrada & A. Baum (Eds.), *The handbook of stress science* (pp. 321–343). Springer.

Howard, E. D. (2006). Family-centered care in the context of fetal abnormality. *Journal of Perinatology & Neonatal Nursing, 20*(3), 237–242. https://doi.org/10.1097/00005237-200607000-00011

Howell, L. J. (2013). The Garbose Family Special Delivery Unit: A new paradigm for maternal–fetal and neonatal care. *Seminars in Pediatric Surgery, 22*(1), 3–9. https://doi.org/10.1053/j.sempedsurg.2012.10.002

Ickovics, J. R., Lewis, J. B., Cunningham, S. D., Thomas, J., & Magriples, U. (2019). Transforming prenatal care: Multidisciplinary team science improves a broad range of maternal–child outcomes. *American Psychologist, 74*(3), 343–355. https://doi.org/10.1037/amp0000435

Johnson, J. E., Wiltsey-Striman, S., Sikorskii, A., Miller, T., King, A., Blume, J. L., Pham, X., Moore Simas, T. A., Poleshuck, E., Weinberg, R., & Zlotnick, C. (2018). Protocol for the ROSE sustainment (ROSES) study, a sequential multiple assignment randomized trial to determine the minimum necessary intervention to maintain a postpartum depression prevention program in prenatal clinics serving low-income women. *Implementation Science, 13*(1), 115. https://doi.org/10.1186/s13012-018-0807-9

Johnson S. B. (2013). Increasing psychology's role in health research and health care. *American Psychologist, 68*(5), 311–321. https://doi.org/10.1037/a0033591

Kaasen, A., Helbig, A., Malt, U. F., Naes, T., Skari, H., & Haugen, G. (2010). Acute maternal social dysfunction, health perception and psychological distress after ultrasonographic detection of fetal structural anomaly. *BJOG, 117*(9), 1127–1138. https://doi.org/10.1111/j.1471-0528.2010.02622.x

Kaslow, N. J., Dunn, S. E., & Smith, C. O. (2008). Competencies for psychologists in academic health centers (AHCs). *Journal of Clinical Psychology in Medical Settings, 15*(1), 18–27. https://doi.org/10.1007/s10880-008-9094-y

Keesara, S., & Kim, J. J. (2018). Outcomes of universal perinatal mood screening in the obstetric and pediatric setting. *NeoReviews, 19*(3), e152–e159.

Kett, J. C., Wolfe, E., Vernon, M. M., Woodrum, D., & Diekema, D. (2017). The multidisciplinary fetal center: Clinical expertise is only part of the experience. *Acta Paediatrica, 106*(6), 930–934. https://doi.org/10.1111/apa.13812

Kingston, D., James-Kelly, S., Tyrell, J., Clark, L., Hamza, D., Holmes, P., Parkes, C., Moyo, N., McDonald, S., & Austin, M. P. (2015). An integrated web-based mental health intervention of assessment-referral-care to reduce stress, anxiety, and depression in hospitalized pregnant women with medically high-risk pregnancies: A feasibility study protocol of hospital-based implementation. *JMIR Research Protocol, 4*(1), e9. https://doi.org/10.2196/resprot.4037

Lenze, S. N. (2017). Early childhood mental health: Starting early with the pregnant mother. *Child and Adolescent Psychiatric Clinics of North America, 26*(3), 411–426. https://doi.org/10.1016/j.chc.2017.02.001

Matthews, T. J., MacDorman, M. F., & Thorma, M. E. (2015). Infant mortality statistics from the 2013 period linked birth/infant death data set. *National Vital Statistics Reports, 64*(9), 1–30.

Ramchandani, P. G., Stein, A., O'Connor, T. G., Heron, J., Murray, L., & Evans, J. (2008). Depression in men in the postnatal period and later child psychopathology: A population cohort study. *Journal of the American Academy of Child & Adolescent Psychiatry, 47*(4): 390–398. https://doi.org/10.1097/CHI.0b013e31816429c2

Rising, S. S. (1998). Centering pregnancy: An interdisciplinary model of empowerment. *Journal of Nurse-Midwifery, 43*(1), 46–54. https://doi.org/10.1016/s0091-2182(97)00117-1

Rising, S. S. (2016). *The center pregnancy model: The power of group healthcare.* Springer.

Rychik, J., Donaghue, D. D., Levy, S., Fajardo, C., Combs, J., Zhang, X., Szwast, A., & Diamond, G. (2013). Maternal psychological stress after prenatal diagnosis of

congenital heart disease. *Journal of Pediatrics, 162*(2), 302–307.e1. https://doi.org/
10.1016/j.jpeds.2012.07.023

Sanders, M. R., & Hall, S. L. (2018). Trauma-informed care in the newborn intensive
care unit: Promoting safety, security and connectedness. *Journal of Perinatology,
38*(1), 3–10. https://doi.org/10.1038/jp.2017.124

Singley, D. B., & Edwards, L. M. (2015). Men's perinatal mental health in the transition to
fatherhood. *Professional Psychology: Research and Practice, 46*(5), 309–316. https://
doi.org/10.1037/pro0000032

Tandon, S. D., Leis, J. A., Mendelson, T., Perry, D. F., & Kemp, K. (2014). Six-month
outcomes from a randomized controlled trial to prevent perinatal depression in
low-income home visiting clients. *Maternal and Child Health Journal, 18*(4), 873–
881. doi:10.1007/s10995-013-1313-y

Venkatesh, K. K., Nadel, H., Blewett, D., Freeman, M. P., Kaimal, A. J., & Riley, L. E. (2016).
Implementation of universal screening for depression during pregnancy: Feasibility
and impact on obstetric care. *American Journal of Obstetrics & Gynecology, 215*(4),
517.e1–517.e5178. https://doi.org/10.1016/j.ajog.2016.05.024

Williams, K. E., & Koleva, H. (2018). Identification and treatment of peripartum anxiety disorders. *Obstetrics and Gynecology Clinics of North America, 45*(3), 469–481.
https://doi.org/10.1016/j.ogc.2018.04.001

Wool, C. (2011). Systematic review of the literature: Parental outcomes after diagnosis of
fetal anomaly. *Advances in Neonatal Care, 11*(3), 182–192. https://doi.org/10.1097/
ANC.0b013e31821bd92d

Yawn, B. P., Dietrich, A. J., Wollan, P., Bertram, S., Graham, D., Huff, J., Kuland, M.,
Madison, S., Pace, W. D.; in collaboration with the TRIPPD practices. (2012).
TRIPPD: A practice-based network effectiveness study of postpartum depression
screening and management. *Annals of Family Medicine, 10*(4), 320–329. https://doi.
org/10.1370/afm.1418

Zlotnick, C., Tzilos, G., Miller, I., Seifer, R., & Stout, R. (2016). Randomized controlled
trial to prevent postpartum depression in mothers on public assistance. *Journal of
Affective Disorders, 189*, 263–268. https://doi.org/10.1016/j.jad.2015.09.059

Neonatal Intensive Care Settings

20

NEONATAL INTENSIVE CARE SETTINGS

SARA C. HANDLEY AND DAVID A. MUNSON ■

Neonatology as a field had its origins in the 1940s as dedicated physicians shared their observations of diseases in newborns through early textbooks. There was little that could be done for infants born early or with congenital anomalies, but the 1960s saw the creation of the first intensive care units dedicated to infants. Even then, there was little more available than warmth, humidity, and supplemental oxygen. However, dedicated scientists, surgeons, cardiologists, anesthesiologists, and neonatologists rapidly improved the understanding of neonatal physiology and developed innovative interventions to expand what was available for the care of critically ill newborns (Philip, 2005). Now, a patient may survive when born as early as 22 weeks (Arzuaga & Cummings, 2019); an infant with severe congenital diaphragmatic hernia can have fetal intervention (Basurto et al., 2019); and patients with hypoplastic left heart syndrome, a once universally fatal condition, can expect a 67% long-term survival rate (Metcalf & Rychik, 2020).

All of these successes bring with them considerable risk. Congenital anomalies and extreme prematurity remain the leading causes of neonatal mortality. Both also can lead to long-term, life-changing morbidities. As the field of neonatology pushes the envelope of what is possible in neonatal intensive care units (NICUs), parents will continue to be confronted with heartbreaking events and decisions. This chapter provides a general overview of the NICU, preparing the reader to better provide psychosocial support to parents in this environment.

LEVELS OF NEONATAL INTENSIVE CARE

The Committee on the Fetus and Newborn at the American Academy of Pediatrics first published a classification of levels of neonatal care in 2004, which was most recently modified in 2012 (American Academy of Pediatrics, 2012). The statement describes NICUs ranging from Level I to Level IV, and the associated level-specific capabilities are summarized in Table 20.1.

The Level I designation describes the ability to provide initial resuscitation and stabilization. If an infant requires ongoing intensive care, the infant would be transferred to a higher level unit. Level I NICUs can be staffed by pediatricians, family practice physicians, or nurse practitioners. Level II NICUs are generally staffed by neonatologists and neonatal nurse practitioners and can support moderately premature infants (i.e., ≥32 weeks of gestation) and provide short-term mechanical ventilation and noninvasive respiratory support. Level III NICUs can provide resuscitation and ongoing intensive care for all infants, including the most preterm. Currently, the limits of viability include some surviving infants down to 22 weeks of gestation, which reflects the American College of Obstetricians and Gynecologists and the Society for Maternal–Fetal Medicine (2017) consensus stating that neonatal resuscitation at 22 to $23^{6/7}$ weeks can be considered. Level III NICUs have access to pediatric subspecialties and pediatric surgeons. However, some of this access may be met by relationships with a regional Level IV NICU within close proximity. Importantly, Level III NICUs must have the ability to provide ophthalmologic screening for retinopathy of prematurity (ROP). Many Level III NICUs are also high-volume delivery centers and set the standard of care for supporting premature infants. The neonatologists and other clinicians who work in high-volume Level III NICUs are experts in a variety of forms of mechanical ventilation and meeting the complex needs of extremely premature infants.

Level IV NICUs are based in pediatric hospitals or larger health systems. In addition to the capabilities of a Level III unit, Level IV units have broader access to pediatric and surgical subspecialists and can provide extracorporeal membrane oxygenation, a form of cardiopulmonary bypass provided at the bedside. Level IV NICUs have their origins in the post-surgical care of neonates and infants: The first modern NICU was started by Dr. C. Everett Koop at the Children's Hospital of Philadelphia in 1962 to improve the care of infants receiving ever more innovative surgical interventions. Level IV NICUs are referral centers, which admit premature infants with complications requiring specialized care, neonates of any gestational age requiring surgical interventions, and infants with congenital anomalies or primary genetic or metabolic disease. Due to their access to subspecialist pediatricians and surgeons, Level IV NICUs typically have multidisciplinary programs developed to support infants with specific syndromes.

Some Level IV NICUs provide care to infants born with congenital heart disease, but most large cardiac centers that repair and manage complex congenital heart disease have separate pediatric cardiac intensive care units (CICUs). Such units developed in response to the increasing complexity of cardiac surgery. In 1945, Alfred Blalock and his assistant, Vivien Thomas, performed the first subclavian to pulmonary artery shunt in a 15-month-old girl, opening the door to the possibility of survival for infants with complex congenital heart disease (Epstein & Brill, 2005). Cardiopulmonary bypass was developed in the 1950s, and soon thereafter neonates with congenital heart disease were having open-heart surgery.

Table 20.1 Neonatal Levels of Care

Level of Care	Capabilities	Provider Types
Level I: Well newborn nursery	Provide neonatal resuscitation (e.g., respiratory and cardiac support) at every delivery Care for well, term (>37 weeks of gestation) newborn infants after birth Care for infants born at 35–37 weeks of gestation who have stable respiratory and cardiac function Stabilize newborn infants who are ill and those born at <35 weeks of gestation until transferred to a higher level of care	Pediatricians, family physicians, nurse practitioners, and other advanced practice registered nurses
Level II: Special care nursery	Level I capabilities plus: Provide care for infants born at ≥32 weeks and weighing ≥1,500 g who have physiologic immaturity or who are moderately ill and are expected to improve rapidly and are not anticipated to urgently need subspecialty services Provide care for infants recovering after receiving intensive care Provide mechanical ventilation for a brief duration (<24 hr) or continuous positive pressure or both Stabilize infants born at <32 weeks of gestation and weighing <1,500 g until transfer to a neonatal intensive care facility	Level I health care providers plus: Pediatric hospitalists, neonatologists, and neonatal nurse practitioners
Level III: NICU	Level II capabilities plus: Provide sustained life support (e.g., mechanical ventilation beyond 24 hr) Provide comprehensive care for infants born at <32 weeks of gestation and weighing <1,500 g and infants born at all gestational ages and birth weights with critical illness Provide prompt access to a full range of pediatric medial subspecialists, pediatric surgical specialists, pediatric anesthesiologists, and pediatric ophthalmologists	Level II health care providers plus: Pediatric medical subspecialists, pediatric anesthesiologists, pediatric surgeons, and pediatrics ophthalmologists

(continued)

Table 20.1 CONTINUED

Level of Care	Capabilities	Provider Types
	Provide a full range of respiratory support that may include different types of mechanical ventilation (conventional and/or high-frequency ventilation) and inhaled nitric oxide Perform advanced imaging, with interpretation on an urgent basis, including CT, MRI, and echocardiography	
Level IV: Regional NICU	Level III capabilities plus: Located within an institution with the capability to provide surgical repair of complex congenital or acquired conditions Maintain a full range of pediatric medical subspecialists, pediatric surgical subspecialists, and pediatric anesthesiologists at the site Facilitate transport from hospitals with lower levels of neonatal care Provide outreach education to hospitals with lower levels of neonatal care	Level III health care providers plus: Pediatric surgical subspecialists (e.g., pediatric neurosurgeons and pediatric cardiothoracic surgeons)

CT, computed tomography; MRI, magnetic resonance imaging; NICU, neonatal intensive care unit.

Adapted from the American Academy of Pediatrics Committee on Fetus and Newborn (2012).

Pediatric CICUs arose out of the necessity to meet the needs of infants requiring complicated postoperative care (Epstein & Brill, 2005). CICUs provide care for children of all ages with severe heart disease; consequently, the physicians typically have training in pediatric critical care and cardiology, and only rarely in neonatology.

REGIONALIZATION

Regionalization is the concept that different levels of NICUs should be arranged across a geographic region in such a way that pregnant patients are directed to perinatal care most appropriate for their degree of risk. The goal has been for premature infants to be born in high-level (Level III) and high-volume NICUs with the most expertise and experience in their care, but the idea can also be applied to pregnant patients carrying a fetus with a known congenital anomaly. The March of Dimes and other organizations have advocated for the regionalization of NICU care since the 1970s (American Academy of Pediatrics, 2012). Neonates born prematurely between 23 and 37 weeks of gestation have a substantially lower mortality rate when born in a hospital with a higher level NICU, and rates of morbidities are similar among NICUs, even in the setting of increased survival of extremely premature infants, which should increase the incidence of morbidities. States vary considerably in their laws and policies pertaining to regionalization: Some require certification before opening NICU beds in a hospital with clearly defined definitions around levels of care, whereas others provide minimal guidance and no certification. The result is a wide variety of perinatal regionalization practices across states. Researchers have taken advantage of these variations to demonstrate a connection between level of unit and mortality (Lorch et al., 2012). Although this remains an area of some controversy, overall the evidence supports regionalization and efforts to cohort sicker patients in high-volume centers.

CLINICIANS IN THE NICU

Level III and IV NICUs are staffed by a large interprofessional team charged with the mission of caring for critically ill neonates and infants. As in other units in the hospital, nurses provide direct bedside care to the infants in the NICU, and many NICUs have layered in additional nursing experts with graduate degrees to provide leadership, develop programs, and support expert nursing practice at the bedside. These may include clinical nurse specialists and clinical nurse educators. Registered nurses and other master's-prepared nurses often fill additional roles in the NICU, including active participation in quality improvement initiatives, family education, vascular access, and leadership roles. The bedside nurse cares directly for the critically ill infant and provides emotional and psychological support to the infant's family. Senior nursing aids often provide a layer of support to complete nursing tasks and help make the unit run smoothly.

The medical team is led by a neonatologist, a pediatrician with fellowship training in neonatology. In hospitals with general pediatric and/or subspecialty pediatric training, residents and fellows may be a part of the medical team. Residents are physicians who are in training to become pediatricians, and fellows are pediatricians who are in training to become neonatologists. If present, fellows provide clinical leadership for the medical team, supported by the supervising neonatologist. Medical teams often also have advanced practice providers (APPs) who provide direct assessment and medical decision-making at the bedside. APPs often have considerable autonomy and are supported by a neonatologist. APPs may be nurse practitioners, physician assistants, or pediatricians.

The medical and nursing teams are supported by additional providers and staff, including clinical pharmacists, respiratory therapists, dieticians, child life specialists, physical therapists, occupational therapists, lactation consultants, speech therapists, case managers, social workers, and psychologists. It takes coordination and collaboration among all of these experts to maximize the chances of a good outcome in the critically ill neonate and, importantly, to help support a family through what is likely one of the most stressful experience of their lives (Kilpatrick et al, 2017).

COMMON DIAGNOSES IN HIGHER LEVEL NICUS

Level I and II NICUs may occasionally experience the birth of an infant with a life-threatening disease, immediate postnatal demise, or stillbirth, but in general this is an uncommon occurrence. For example, an obstetric emergency such as a uterine rupture can preclude transfer of the mother before birth and can cause profound illness in the newborn. High-risk pregnancies and pregnancies in which there is a known fetal anomaly are referred to hospitals with a Level III unit or plans are made for transport of the infant to a Level IV unit soon after birth. Some children's hospitals have delivery services for the purpose of delivering patients with known congenital diagnoses for immediate access to a Level IV unit. Consequently, Level III and IV units care for much higher risk infants than do Level I and II units, and they should have a robust psychosocial support system in place for families. It is helpful if the members of the psychosocial team have a general understanding of the diseases and complications with which their patient families will be coping, and so a description of the most common diagnoses follows.

Prematurity

The term *prematurity* refers to birth before 37 weeks of gestation, and prematurity is classified into categories depending on the degree of prematurity or by birth weight. Infants born between $34^{0/7}$ and $36^{6/7}$ weeks of gestation are considered *late preterm*, and these infants typically have a relatively benign course in the NICU or receive their care in a well-baby nursery. Many recent studies, however, have indicated that these relatively mature infants are at higher risk of complications, readmissions, and long-term developmental problems (Natarajan & Shankaran, 2016). *Moderate preterm* refers to infants born between $32^{0/7}$ and $33^{6/7}$ weeks, *very preterm* to those born between 28 and $31^{6/7}$ weeks, and *extreme preterm* to those born before 28 weeks of gestation. Note that the very preterm category is often described as less than 32 weeks and therefore may include extreme preterm infants as well. Birth weight is also used as a way to categorize the degree of prematurity and immaturity. The term *low birth weight* refers to infants born weighing less than 2,500 g, *very low birth weight* to those born weighing less than 1,500 g, and *extremely low birth weight* includes infants born weighing less than 1,000 g.

Extreme prematurity remains a life-threatening problem, with the highest risk of mortality occurring in the first week post-birth. In the past few years, enough

centers have reported survival at 22 weeks of gestation that some NICUs offer resuscitation at 22 weeks (Arzuaga & Cummings, 2019). However, because the risk
of mortality and morbidity remains extremely high between 22 and 23$^{6/7}$ weeks of
gestation, many NICUs practice with this window as a "gray zone," where families
and providers together may choose to forgo resuscitation to prevent the infant
from suffering secondary to a prolonged intensive care stay and a high risk of an
impaired quality of life among survivors. There is, however, considerable variation
in what is offered when delivery is occurring at this early gestation, and in practice
it is difficult to engage in truly informed and shared decision-making with a pregnant parent in labor (Arbour et al., 2020). Often, a team needs to discuss concerns
around survivability and morbidities after the infant has been born and resuscitation attempted. Once the infant is admitted to the NICU, psychosocial providers
play a critical role in providing emotional support; assessing the parents' understanding of the clinical road ahead; evaluating coping skills and resilience; and
eliciting the parents' values, hopes, and fears.

Complications of Prematurity

Every major organ system is at risk for disease in extremely preterm infants because they do not have the benefit of completing in utero development during the
third trimester. The risk of complications of prematurity increases as the degree of
prematurity increases. These complications are the primary reason that a patient's
course can feel like a roller coaster for parents. Psychosocial providers will need
to be able to support parents as the clinical status shifts from "everything is fine"
to acutely life-threatening or life-altering.

RESPIRATORY PROBLEMS

Respiratory distress syndrome refers to the lack of development of alveoli and
the inability of the premature lung to make surfactant. The surfactant deficiency
can be treated by giving exogenous surfactant, although many extremely preterm
infants also require mechanical ventilation to survive. Unfortunately, lung development does not proceed normally when an infant is no longer in utero, and when
this maldevelopment is combined with injury from both supplemental oxygen
and positive pressure from the ventilator, bronchopulmonary dysplasia (BPD) is
the result. BPD can range in severity from requiring some supplemental oxygen
via a nasal cannula at home to severe BPD requiring tracheostomy and years of
mechanical ventilation. Infants who develop BPD are also at risk for developing
pulmonary hypertension, which may need to be treated with pulmonary artery
vasodilators such as sildenafil, bosentan, nitric oxide, or treprostinil. Infants with
BPD will often also be treated with bronchodilators such as albuterol and with
diuretics such as furosemide or hydrochlorothiazide. Steroids such as dexamethasone are also often used to try to change the trajectory of disease in evolving BPD
(Abman et al, 2017).

INFECTIONS

Systemic infections are another potentially life-threatening and life-altering problem that patients confront in the NICU. In utero infection can be the cause of premature delivery, and some premature infants develop bacterial infections as a result. Such infections occurring within the first 72 hours after birth are referred to as early onset sepsis. Care of critically ill infants requires invasive support such as peripherally inserted central catheters, arterial lines, and breathing tubes. All of these may serve as a portal for bacterial or fungal infections. The medical and nursing teams use defined bundles of care to minimize the risk of hospital-acquired infections and are diligent in monitoring for the subtle first signs of infection (Shane et al., 2017). Consequently, extremely premature infants are often exposed to antibiotics during their NICU stay. These infections can be mild or can cause sepsis syndrome requiring medications to support blood pressure such as dopamine or epinephrine infusions. Hydrocortisone is also frequently used to help these drugs work more effectively. Sometimes sepsis is overwhelming and the patient dies in the face of maximum intensive care intervention.

NECROTIZING ENTEROCOLITIS

Necrotizing enterocolitis (NEC) is another disease that almost exclusively occurs in premature infants, although it can also be seen in term infants with congenital heart disease. The underlying pathophysiology of NEC remains incompletely understood, but it usually occurs at 2–6 weeks of age in a premature infant receiving enteral feeds, although the incidence is much lower if infants are exclusively receiving breast milk. NEC can be a relatively mild disease that responds to bowel rest and antibiotics, or it can come on quite suddenly and lead to death in a matter of hours. In fact, NEC continues to have a 30% mortality rate. Sometimes part of the bowel perforates, requiring surgery, and this is therefore referred to as surgical NEC. If a small segment is involved, recovery can be complete, but a more severely affected infant may lose most of their small bowel, and if they survive, they may require long-term intravenous nutrition (Rich & Dolgin, 2017). These patients with "short gut" are at risk for liver failure and other long-term complications.

INTRAVENTRICULAR HEMORRHAGE

Premature infants have a very fragile network of blood vessels in the germinal matrix within the ventricles of the brain, and these vessels may tear or rupture, resulting in a bleed called intraventricular hemorrhage (IVH). These bleeds may be small (i.e., grades I and II), may cause enlargement of the ventricles (i.e., grade III), or may extend into the tissue or parenchyma of the brain (i.e., grade IV). IVH may cause hydrocephalus requiring a ventriculoperitoneal (VP) shunt. A temporizing procedure called a reservoir can allow the intermittent removal of cerebral spinal fluid to relieve pressure on the brain related to hydrocephalus. Some NICU patients who have this procedure (or other temporizing cerebrospinal fluid diversions) avoid the need for placement of a VP shunt. The brain injury that accompanies the more severe forms of IVH typically impacts the motor tracks of the brain and is associated with an increased risk of motor impairment in childhood, including cerebral palsy (Ellenbogen et al., 2016).

Retinopathy of Prematurity

Premature infants also need to be monitored for the development of the eye disease ROP. In this disease, abnormal hormonal signals from the peripheral retina cause overproliferation of the developing blood vessels in the retina. If not found and managed, this can progress to a detached retina, resulting in loss of vision. Indeed, ROP remains a leading cause of blindness throughout the world; however, effective screening and management programs now largely prevent these most extreme outcomes in the United States. Currently, there are two ways to prevent progression if progressive disease is seen: laser ablation of the peripheral retina or injection of the medication bevacizumab (Hartnett, 2020). Nonetheless, the discovery of ROP requiring treatment can be yet another stressful event for parents of infants born prematurely.

Although there are certainly more diagnoses associated with prematurity, such as patent ductus arteriosus, apnea of prematurity, and anemia of prematurity, the problems described previously have the largest potential to alter an infant's life course. Not only are some of these diagnoses life-threatening but also the occurrence of these complications increases the risk of long-term developmental impairment and frequently prolongs the length of stay in the NICU. Families need to be updated regularly when these and other complications occur and they also need to be informed about problems they may face in the ensuing weeks of care. For example, IVH occurs in the first week after birth, so in the second week after birth as feeds are advanced, families need to learn about ongoing nutrition and the risks of infection and necrotizing enterocolitis. Furthermore, if an infant experiences multiple complications of prematurity, it is important to sensitively share what this means for their long-term outcome—the more problems an infant experiences in the NICU, the greater the risk of neurodevelopmental impairment (Schmidt et al., 2003).

Hypoxic–Ischemic Encephalopathy

When there is a perinatal event that impairs blood and oxygen delivery to the brain, the infant can present as critically ill. Causes may include shoulder dystocia, nuchal cord (when the cord is wrapped around the infant's neck), placental abruption (when the placenta pulls away from the wall of the uterus before the infant is born), or other less common events causing placental compromise. Most major organ systems can be impacted by such events. The infant may have respiratory failure requiring mechanical ventilation, heart failure requiring medications to support blood pressure, liver failure, acute kidney injury, and/or brain injury. The degree of encephalopathy is assessed on clinical exam and by brain wave monitoring with a full or partial montage electroencephalogram. If the perinatal event, clinical exam, and lab tests are all consistent with perinatal compromise of blood flow to the brain, then the infant may benefit from therapeutic hypo-thermia (i.e., "cooling") in addition to supportive intensive care for the other organ systems. By decreasing the infant's core temperature, the release of excitatory and potentially damaging neurotransmitters associated with reperfusion injury to the brain can be mitigated, decreasing the degree of brain injury. Although this therapy has been proven effective, especially in infants with moderate encephalopathy, it does not prevent all long-term morbidity, and the most severely impacted infants are still at high risk of death in the first hours to days after birth. For those severely encephalopathic infants who do survive, the impact can be profound, resulting in severe developmental delay (Wassink et al., 2019). It is critical for the multidisciplinary team to engage closely with families in discussing prognosis in order to support shared decision-making, including exploring the possibility of withdrawal of technology and end-of-life care.

Congenital Anomalies

Many congenital anomalies are considered primary surgical diseases because they require surgical intervention early in life. These include congenital diaphragmatic hernia, gastroschisis, omphalocele, intestinal atresias, tracheoesophageal fistula, congenital pulmonary adenomatoid malformations, lymphangiomas, and congenital heart disease. Many of these diagnoses are covered in considerable detail elsewhere in this book and are not discussed exhaustively here. However, they each can be life-threatening and often require a long stay in the NICU or CICU with exposure to many of the same interventions and complications described for premature infants—mechanical ventilation, central lines, risk for infection, and surgery—all of which may have long-term complications impacting quality of life. Psychosocial support for the parents of newborns with surgical disease is a critical element in optimizing outcomes for both the infant and the family.

Genetic Syndromes and Testing

The field of genetics is exploding with information as the cost and availability of sophisticated tests improve. The cheapest and most widely available test is the karyotype. In this test, a technician counts the numbers of paired chromosomes and can identify when there is an extra chromosome or can identify deletions when large pieces of chromosomes are missing. This test can identify the most common forms of triploidy—trisomy 21, 18, and 13. Trisomy 21 is commonly known as Down syndrome. The phenotype commonly includes congenital heart disease, intestinal malformations, a typical physical appearance, joint laxity, and intellectual disability. Trisomy 21 is rarely life-threatening in the newborn period, but patients may require surgery to address congenital heart disease or intestinal malformations. In contrast, trisomy 18 and 13 are commonly life-threatening syndromes in the days after birth, largely secondary to poor central nervous system control of breathing and heart rate. However, some patients with trisomy 18 and 13 will survive the neonatal period, and parents need to be supported through decisions regarding medical and surgical interventions. Infants with trisomy 13 and 18 have significant medical problems that may include congenital heart disease, bowel disease, cleft lip/palate, kidney disease, and brain malformations. Infants who grow into childhood will have significant developmental delay. There has been considerable debate in the medical literature about how much intervention should be offered to infants with trisomy 18 and 13, and parents are often aware that they may be counseled strongly for non-intervention. There is, however, a growing consensus that a transparent conversation in a shared decision-making model is appropriate for infants with trisomy 18 and 13, as with most other life-threatening diseases (Brosco & Feudtner, 2017).

Genetic testing now includes the ability to test for specific mutations, duplications, and deletions and, more recently, the ability to map the entire exome or genome of an individual patient. Whole exome and whole genome sequencing have solved many clinical mysteries by discovering a deletion or mutation in a gene that is known to cause a specific clinical syndrome. In these cases, the genetic characterization might provide clarity around prognosis and can help medical teams and families work through decisions ranging from palliative care to disease-specific therapies (Carroll et al., 2020). In contrast, a genetic difference seen on a test may be novel and have no clear connection to the problem seen in the patient. To further complicate matters, it can be safely concluded that the genetic difference is the cause of the problem seen in the infant, but there may only be a small number of similar cases described in the literature, making prognosis difficult to predict. The uncertainty created in these circumstances is often difficult for parents and clinicians alike to understand and process. Psychosocial team members and genetic counselors are critically important in helping a family navigate these questions of what is known and what remains uncertain. They can provide an outlet to process the emotional reaction to new information and help the family process their anxiety. When the genetic tests result in uncertainty, the team must base their discussions and collaborative decisions on the clinical findings rather than on genetic results.

SUPPORTING FAMILIES

Although all members of the NICU team provide essential support to the patient's family, a multidisciplinary psychosocial team made up of social work, psychologists, psychiatrists, chaplains, bereavement specialists, and/or child life specialists is critical to help a family navigate the ups and downs of a NICU course and process upsetting complications and diagnoses. Parents bring with them their own ideas of what it means to be a good parent along with their own views on what quality of life means to them based on their experiences, philosophies, religion, and other cultural influences. They may also have experienced trauma in their life or have pre-existing mental health issues, which may make coping with the stressors of their infant's clinical course more difficult. Psychosocial providers can assess families on admission for concerns that may make it more difficult for them to cope with events in the NICU and provide support and connect parents to resources to help with life stressors that do not disappear when an infant is admitted to the NICU. Throughout the NICU admission, the psychosocial team can continue to advocate for needed resources, provide direct support and counseling, and ensure that the parents' voices are heard when shared decisions are needed between the parents and the medical team. The psychosocial team often gets to know parents deeply, and their insights can in turn help the medical team navigate difficult news or challenging decisions more effectively. These ideas are explored in depth throughout the remainder of this book.

When there is significant concern that a disease or complication may be life-threatening or may impair future quality of life, a palliative care team can provide an additional layer of support. Such teams often have their own medical providers, chaplains, child life therapists, and social workers. A palliative care team can provide a safe and consistent space for families to explore their hopes and fears as they navigate difficult choices and challenging clinical events. By providing a separate team to navigate the emotions and meaning of a diagnosis with a challenging prognosis, the critical care team is then free to focus on the ongoing technical and medical care of the patient. Ultimately, the NICU and palliative care teams will need to collaborate with the parents to explore possible clinical paths and support parents in making decisions consistent with their values.

CONCLUSION

Infants in Level III and IV NICUs are confronted with a wide array of medical problems that may be life-threatening in the short term and may have long-term impact on their development and/or quality of life. Parents are rarely aware that such problems even exist, let alone that they could happen to their own infant. A NICU admission can represent a moment of profound crisis for families. Although all clinicians working in higher level NICUs need to be skilled in compassionate communication, an experienced and available psychosocial team—composed of social workers, psychologists, bereavement specialists, and/or child life therapists—is essential. Parents clearly need support if their infant dies, whether this is anticipated prenatally or the result of an unanticipated perinatal or neonatal event. But support is just as critical for the families of survivors of the NICU. Parents who have been effectively supported in building resilience and preparing themselves for future challenges will be empowered to provide the love and commitment that will give their infant the best chance to meet their potential. NICUs are therefore obligated to do everything possible to support and optimize parental emotional health.

REFERENCES

Abman, S. H., Collaco, J. M., Shepherd, E. G., Keszler, M., Cuevas-Guaman, M., Welty, S. E., Truog, W. E., McGrath-Morrow, S. A., Moore, P. E., Rhein, L. M., Kirpalani, H., Zhang, H., Gratny, L. L., Lynch, S. K., Curtiss, J., Stonestreet, B. S., McKinney, R. L., Dysart, K. C., Gien, J., . . . Nelin, L. D.; Bronchopulmonary Dysplasia Group. (2017). Interdisciplinary care of children with severe bronchopulmonary dysplasia. *Journal of Pediatrics, 181*, 12–28.

American Academy of Pediatrics Committee on Fetus and Newborn. (2012). Levels of neonatal care. *Pediatrics, 130*(3), 587–597.

American College of Obstetricians and Gynecologists and Society for Maternal–Fetal Medicine. (2017). Obstetric care consensus No. 6 summary: Periviable birth. *Obstetrics & Gynecology, 130*, 926–928.

Arbour, K., Lindsay, E., Laventhal, N., Myers, P., Andrews, B., Klar, A., & Dunbar, A. E. (2020). Shifting provider attitudes and institutional resources surrounding resuscitation at the limit of gestational viability. *American Journal of Perinatology*. Advance online publication.

Arzuaga, B. H., & Cummings, C. L. (2019). Deliveries at extreme prematurity: Outcomes, approaches, institutional variation, and uncertainty. *Current Opinion in Pediatrics, 31*(2), 182–187.

Basurto, D., Russo, F. M., Van der Veeken, L., Van der Merwe, J., Hooper, S., Benachi, A., De Bie, F., Gomez, O., & Deprest, J. (2019). Prenatal diagnosis and management of congenital diaphragmatic hernia. *Best Practice & Research: Clinical Obstetrics & Gynaecology, 58*, 93–106.

Brosco, J. P., & Feudtner, C. (2017). Shared decision making for children with trisomy 13 and 18. *JAMA Pediatrics, 171*(4), 324–325.

Carroll, J., Wigby, K., & Murray, S. (2020). Genetic testing strategies in the newborn. *Journal of Perinatology, 40*(7), 1007–1016.

Ellenbogen, J. R., Waqar, M., & Pettorini, B. (2016). Management of post-haemorrhagic hydrocephalus in premature infants. *Journal of Clinical Neuroscience, 31*, 30–34.

Epstein, D., & Brill, J. E. (2005). A history of pediatric critical care medicine. *Pediatric Research, 58*(5), 987–996.

Hartnett, M. E. (2020). Retinopathy of prematurity: Evolving treatment with anti-vascular endothelial growth factor. *American Journal of Ophthalmology, 218*, 208–213.

Kilpatrick, S. J., Papile, L. A., & Macones, G. A. (2017). *Guidelines for perinatal care.* American Academy of Pediatrics.

Lorch, S. A., Baiocchi, M., Ahlberg, C. E., & Small, D. S. (2012). The differential impact of delivery hospital on the outcomes of premature infants. *Pediatrics, 130*(2), 270–278.

Metcalf, M. K., & Rychik, J. (2020). Outcomes in hypoplastic left heart syndrome. *Pediatric Clinics, 67*(5), 945–962.

Natarajan, G., & Shankaran, S. (2016). Short- and long-term outcomes of moderate and late preterm infants. *American Journal of Perinatology, 33*(3), 305–317.

Philip, A. G. (2005). The evolution of neonatology. *Pediatric Research, 58*(4), 799–815.

Rich, B. S., & Dolgin, S. E. (2017). Necrotizing entercolitis. *Pediatrics I Review, 38*(12), 552–559. doi:https://doi.org/10.1542/pir.2017-0002

Schmidt, B., Asztalos, E. V., Roberts, R. S., Robertson, C. M., Sauve, R. S., Whitfield, M. F.; Trial of Indomethacin Prophylaxis in Preterms (TIPP) Investigators. (2003). Impact of bronchopulmonary dysplasia, brain injury, and severe retinopathy on the outcome of extremely low-birth-weight infants at 18 months: Results from the Trial of Indomethacin Prophylaxis in Preterms. *JAMA, 289*(9), 1124–1129.

Shane, A. L., Sánchez, P. J., & Stoll, B. J. (2017). Neonatal sepsis. *Lancet, 390*(10104), 1770–1780.

Wassink, G., Davidson, J. O., Dhillon, S. K., Zhou, K., Bennet, L., Thoresen, M., & Gunn, A. J. (2019). Therapeutic hypothermia in neonatal hypoxic–ischemic encephalopathy. *Current Neurology and Neuroscience Reports, 19*(1), 2.

21

ROLE OF BEHAVIORAL HEALTH CLINICIANS IN THE NICU SETTING

ROCHELLE STEINWURTZEL, SANDHYA S. BRACHIO, SHEAU-YAN HO, AND SOLIMAR SANTIAGO-WARNER ■

The behavioral health clinician (BHC) in the neonatal intensive care unit (NICU) covers a vast scope of practice that incorporates pediatric/developmental, clinical, clinical health, family systems, cultural, and counseling psychology. As an active member of a large interdisciplinary team, the BHC must integrate into the fast-paced team culture of the NICU and simultaneously maintain a macro perspective of the working systems in place. This chapter discusses the importance of screening, assessment, interventions, staff support, and interprofessional collaboration within the NICU and the hospital system and also with external organizations and resources.

PROVIDING CULTURALLY INFORMED CARE

As a prologue to understanding best practices in the NICU, the BHC must first take the lens of providing culturally informed care. Clinical training for BHCs historically has a Western philosophy approach that is not culturally congruent and applicable to all populations (Nader et al., 2013). Theories and diagnoses are socially constructed, and therefore as a culturally centered BHC, one must be able to modify interventions in order to help alleviate symptoms and, at the same time, empower the patient. BHCs must practice from a culturally informed care approach and offer interventions that are culturally congruent based on the uniqueness of each family unit (Nader et al., 2013). It is also imperative that BHCs recognize their own implicit and explicit biases and how they impact the quality of patient care.

Communication is essential to establishing a therapeutic alliance with each family. BHCs must assess comprehension capacity, whether the family speaks another language, or if there are challenges due to low health literacy. BHCs should also be open to learning from the family and their unique approaches to communicating and coping with life challenges. BHCs need to understand that families' experiences in the NICU have a sociocultural backdrop. Issues of oppression, race, class, political, and ecological disruptions are stressors that are chronic and historically rooted (Nader et al., 2013). Therefore, failing to put these factors into context can lead to misinterpretation of the actions and communication styles of the family. Asking the family, "What do I need to know about you, your family, and your child to best support you?" begins the conversation of an open dialogue. Using a cultural humility informed lens, the BHC can determine what resources make sense for a given family. If there is a need, the BHC can create a collaborative partnership with community agencies, religious organizations, and local establishments to create a comprehensive network of resources for patients' families and the hospital (Craig et al., 2020).

PERINATAL MENTAL HEALTH SCREENING IN THE NICU

The BHC serves as an important leader in the establishment and implementation of mental health screening of parents in the NICU. Raising staff awareness regarding the importance of parental mental health and its impact on infant health and development is pivotal to the success of programmatic initiatives and for systematic screening to identify parents at greatest risk. Moreover, the BHC is critical in creating a culture of awareness, sensitivity, and empathic care.

Infants born to mothers struggling with perinatal mood and anxiety disorders (PMADs) are at risk for adverse neurodevelopmental outcomes (Earls et al., 2019). Infants admitted to the NICU are at even higher risk because their need for developmentally appropriate interaction and, often, decreased responsiveness at baseline can be exacerbated by their mother's struggle to connect emotionally secondary to PMADs (Lefkowitz et al., 2010). Mothers of premature infants are 40% more likely to develop PMADs in comparison to the general population due to increased burden of family and financial stress (Vigod et al., 2010). Anxiety, depression, and post-traumatic stress have been reported in mothers and fathers following the birth of a preterm infant, with symptoms persisting for months to years after birth and discharge from the NICU (Hynan et al., 2013; Roque et al., 2017). Furthermore, maternal perinatal depression is associated with increased odds of adolescent and adulthood depression in offspring (Tirumalaraju et al., 2020), and untreated PMADs have an estimated societal cost of $14 billion, with a per mother–child dyad cost of approximately $31,800, from conception to 5 years (Luca et al., 2020).

Given the short- and long-term toll of PMADs on public health, it is imperative to establish appropriate screening within the NICU and to appropriately assess and intervene to better help families and society (Earls et al., 2019). Successful screening for PMADs requires collaboration among a team of maternal and pediatric providers, psychologists, social workers, frontline clinicians, and nurses. Several institutions have highlighted their experiences in establishing a postpartum depression screening program in the NICU (Cherry et al., 2016; Mounts, 2009). Because there is no universal screening protocol for the NICU setting and there are multiple well-validated measures, it is helpful to use quality improvement methodology, through iterative trial and review of small tests of change, to establish a workflow for screening that functions best within the context of each individual institution. For example, at one institution, the Patient Health Questionnaire-2 (PHQ-2) was chosen as a bilingual screening tool due to ease of administration and its established utilization in pediatric outpatient clinics within the hospital system. A process map was developed for screening parents of admitted infants at 2 weeks, 1 month, 2 months, and 4 months of age. Nurses were educated on how to administer the PHQ-2 to families at these set time points, and the medical team was encouraged to incorporate discussion of PHQ-2 data into the care plan during daily rounds. Parents or caregivers with a positive screen were discussed at the divisional weekly interdisciplinary rounds and approached by BHCs for further assessment and disposition planning for NICU-based clinical interventions or referral to outpatient mental health providers. Informational sessions were provided for nurses, physicians, and other frontline providers, linking the timing of screening to common milestones in the NICU.

Although the utility of mental health screening has been well established, there are still many barriers to successful implementation. The success of a PMAD screening program relies heavily on buy-in and collaborative teamwork. Not only do multiple stakeholders have to agree on the importance of such an initiative, but also they have to be active participants in the workflow (Cherry et al., 2016). BHCs and other NICU providers are essential facilitators to promote collaboration among various stakeholders to implement a process to effectively screen parents and caregivers involved in the infant's care.

PSYCHOSOCIAL ASSESSMENT

In addition to participating in the standardized screening program for all parents, NICU BHCs, often social workers, assess how the family functions and the types of support needed to help cope with the NICU environment. The initial psychosocial assessment is multimodal and consists of obtaining information from the parents, reviewing medical charts, speaking with the medical team, and observing family dynamics and functioning within the medical setting. The assessment can occur either in the NICU or in the mother's postpartum recovery room. The assessment questions are classified into nine general categories: (a) parental physical and functional status; (b) parental emotional and mental health; (c) knowledge of illness and preferences; (d) family coping and bereavement risk; (e) family/ caregiver health and functional status; (f) family and relationship issues; (g) cultural, spiritual, religious, and traditional beliefs; (h) communication and literacy issues; and (i) resource needs and safety (Cagle et al., 2017). When discussing perinatal issues, the assessment should include a detailed history of challenges with infertility, maternal medical complications in pregnancy, and pregnancy or infant loss. The BHC must be careful about how this information is documented in the infant's medical chart and keep in mind the parents' protection and privacy, especially when there are concerns about intimate partner violence or sensitive legal matters. The psychosocial assessment can be a therapeutic tool that helps families engage and create a therapeutic alliance with the BHC as well as with the rest of the interdisciplinary team. Through the BHC's assessment, the NICU team may gain a better understanding of the family's narrative and the support needed. When parents feel trust and support from the team, they feel empowered to be an active participant in their infant's medical care.

Psychosocial assessment is ongoing and is based on the stepped transitions faced by NICU families. A theoretical framework outlined by Bachman and Lind (1997) includes three phases characterized by a particular milestone and/or crisis that NICU families go through in succession: the entry phase, connecting phase, and launching phase. The entry phase is the family's initial emotional impact of dealing with a crisis. On admission to the NICU, the family deals with many uncertainties, sometimes including difficult life and death discussions. During this phase, the BHC should conduct a thorough assessment of the family's needs, risks, resources, and coping. Information from these assessments is used to guide interventions, frequency of parent presence, care planning, referrals to other interdisciplinary team members, and community resources. In the connecting phase, parents utilize coping mechanisms such as establishing a NICU schedule or routine, identifying supportive helpers in their social circle and within the hospital, and initiating practical self-care routines within the context to deal with stress and trauma as they assimilate and adjust to their new "normal." Here, families learn to make sense of their infant's medical needs and status, navigate their identity as parents, and provide care under these challenging circumstances. In the launching phase, parents begin to accept their infant for who they are and less as a critically ill infant. Parents also begin the task of accepting that they likely have a child with special needs who may require additional support. With infant development, medical stability, and proper support and encouragement, parents assume a more active role in their infant's care and ideally make decisions related to support services and discharge.

The partnership between BHCs and NICU staff allows for a holistic holding environment for the family during an often intense period. The BHC can assess and determine when in the continuum a family would benefit from additional psychosocial support by the NICU psychologist. The NICU psychologist can also receive referrals from various team members, ranging from the bedside nurse to the front desk staff. Similar to the assessments conducted by the social worker, the NICU psychologist uses a biopsychosocial framework to better understand the medical, psychological, and social variables affecting the family and incorporates information gathered from the parent(s) self-report, chart information, and clinical and staff observations and reports (Hoffman et al., 2020). Attending interdisciplinary rounds is valuable for ongoing clinical assessment; the psychologist learns information about infants' medical situations, hears the team's perceptions of the infants' and families' needs, and also gains a global perspective of the NICU. The information gathered on the micro and macro levels helps guide an understanding of the system in the moment and how this may be impacting interactions between parents and staff and between staff members.

Often, follow-up assessments with the parent or caregiver are conducted in a conversational way, keeping diagnostics, dynamics, and systems issues in mind. Diagnostic questions and information gathering are integrated fluidly to gather personal perceptions of experiences related to pregnancy, birth, the infant's health and functioning, and maternal/infant hospital courses. The BHC listens and assesses for the following caregiver/parent variables: real versus perceived supports; coping resources and needs; estimated level of cognitive functioning; educational and occupational history; legal history; past and current relational styles; perception and interpretation of information; current and past mental health, trauma, interpersonal history, and PMAD symptoms; history of medical illnesses and interactions with medical and/or social institutions; housing and food security; perceptions of parenting roles; and current and past emotional concerns for siblings and other household members.

Identifying and addressing the psychosocial needs of NICU families in an ongoing manner allows for effective communication between the family and the interdisciplinary team. The BHC continuously gathers information from parents and staff about the psychosocial circumstances while trying to understand earlier life experiences that may be relevant to current behavioral responses and coping capacities. There is a constant interplay between assessment and interventions that further enhances the BHC's case formulation and treatment planning.

INTERVENTIONS

The BHC in the NICU must practice cognitive and emotional flexibility, tolerance of the unknown, and a willingness to shift from intensive psychotherapist in one moment to consultant in another (Hoffman et al., 2020). In more traditional psychological practice, the frame of the interaction is bolstered by the physical boundary of a private room. Patients also typically come in for an identified reason. In the NICU, even though the identified patient is the infant, much of the intervention is typically conducted with the adults surrounding the infant—parents and other family members, as well as the NICU staff who are working tirelessly to provide critical medical care. Interventions require knowledge about infant development and infant mental health; family systems; attachment and dyadic work; adult psychopathology; and health as the confluence of psychological, societal, and medical variables. This background knowledge allows BHCs to promote coping, parental identity development, and also address underlying interpersonal and intrapsychic challenges as they arise in the context of trauma.

At the heart of psychosocial interventions lie the essential qualities of compassion, empathy, and nonjudgmental curiosity that help provide validation for parents' emotional experiences, information in the service of empowerment, and the relational connections that can help reduce the impact of toxic stress. Interventions in the NICU can broadly address underlying fear, trauma, and loss by supporting parents in decision-making and empowering them to assume the role of expert on their child and providers of emotional and physical support (Sanders & Hall, 2018). Parenting ideology develops long before an infant is born, although much of the parental identity gains comfort and security in the rituals of parenting (Flacking et al., 2012). A critical component of promoting resiliency and acceptance of reality is to balance an acknowledgment of grief for what is lost (i.e., the ideal birth experience or imagined parenthood) with recognition of what is still possible. It is essential to help parents and staff understand the important link between acts of parenting, parental identity, and bonding on physiological and emotional levels, for both parents and infants.

From an emotional perspective, parents, and mothers in particular, often express feelings of guilt, shame, mourning, and anxiety about their NICU experience (Roque et al., 2017). In the aftermath of a traumatic birth experience, parents may experience physical and emotional separation and detachment from their infants (Flacking et al., 2012). These challenges of attachment often lead to a struggle in the development of a parental identity, even for parents who have already parented other children. Similarly, parents often express worry about "breaking" or "damaging" their infant and feel uncertain how to tend to their infant's needs. The combination of stressful circumstances enhances risk for poor parental mental health functioning, the dyadic relationship in the NICU and after discharge, and in the longer term developmental outcomes for the child and family (Sanders & Hall, 2018). The BHC plays a critical role in helping parents downregulate their own stress responses so they can buffer their infant's physiological response to the stress of prematurity and the NICU. Buffering relationships in the NICU are essential to protecting the infant, parent, dyad, and staff in the context of multiple layers of potentially absorbed toxic stress and trauma impact on infants, parents, and staff.

The Pediatric Psychosocial Preventative Health Model is a helpful framework used to stratify prevention and intervention based on family psychosocial risk level (Kazak et al., 2015). Universal interventions in the NICU setting are largely preventive and involve psychoeducation, family-centered support, and screening for psychosocial risk factors. They serve to orient and ground families as they navigate unique NICU stressors. Psychoeducational resources may include a letter of introduction from the BHC with information about availability, general education about the normal emotional aspects of becoming a parent in the NICU, and other available resources such as NICU orientation groups or parent support groups within the NICU. NICU orientation groups, ideally developed in conjunction with an interdisciplinary team and co-led by various NICU team members, help provide general information about the NICU system, model effective patient–provider communication, and introduce general strategies to establish self-care routines while developing parenting and bonding behaviors with the infant. Parent support groups offer an opportunity for NICU parents to build community in the unit, visit more frequently, and actively engage in their child's care and care team (Hall et al., 2015). Parent support groups can focus more on assessing parents' emotional and practical needs, offering psychological support; fostering capacities to understand their emotional struggles; tolerating ambiguity and uncertainty; developing coping skills and seeking additional supports from friends, family, and professionals; and encouraging peer-to-peer support in order to enhance a sense of community among parents in the NICU. Internet support groups and communities can also be useful for families (Hunt et al., 2018), although it is important for the BHC to research these groups for legitimacy and whether there is opportunity to collaborate with their facilitators.

The screening protocol and assessment process discussed previously in this chapter help identify families that require targeted and clinical interventions. Close working relationships with the medical and nursing teams allow for discussions to identify families who raise concern based on behavioral observations at the bedside (e.g., under- or overstimulation of the infant, anxiety, avoidance, sadness, anger, and lack of joy in interactions with the infant). Parental absence from the NICU and lack of consistent contact between the parent and the NICU caregiving team are other important signals for more targeted interventions (Hynan et al., 2015).

Targeted interventions can include bedside or private room psychotherapy and can incorporate phone or video platforms. A virtual visit program is a targeted intervention that can facilitate bonding between parents and siblings who are not able to visit the infant in person or with sufficient regularity. These virtual visits require a team to facilitate and can help with family bonding, infant development, and reducing disparities in access to the infant and the team for parents who cannot be in the hospital as frequently due to other responsibilities. The BHC can be instrumental in developing a virtual visit program as an advocate for parental and infant mental health. These interventions not only help facilitate connection between the family and infant but also create opportunities for staff to connect with the family and with the infant. This, in turn, enhances trust between the NICU staff and the family.

Specific clinical interventions are implemented at the individual level and also require close liaison work with interdisciplinary members of the NICU team. The BHC works to educate parents and staff about the important role of the "rituals of parenting" and can liaise between the parents and staff to discern appropriate caregiving behaviors based on the infant's medical status. Incorporating skin-to-skin care, supportive touch, and participation in routine care such as diaper changes, taking temperature, and feedings can help facilitate bonding and mitigate anxiety and depression (Hoffman et al., 2020). Helping parents and staff "understand" the infant's cues, brainstorming opportunities for parent–child bonding, and using reflective listening and empathic understanding to deeply hear the family's needs allow for understanding this potentially traumatic event in the narrative of new-found NICU parenthood and identity development. Although much focus is on mothers, part of the BHC's role is to assess the needs of the other primary care-giver or parent and to hold space in the minds of the staff for the entire family's roles and needs. Many of these concepts are presented in a pilot study that mod-ified child–parent psychotherapy to address the specific needs of infants and families in the NICU (Lakatos et al., 2019).

Family presence during emergencies (e.g., witnessing resuscitation efforts) can provide a form of support and protection and may help in coping with loss. Clinical guidelines for family-centered care include an institutional standardiza-tion of inclusion of psychosocial support (e.g., social worker, nurse, chaplain, and trained staff member) in emergency responses (Davidson et al., 2017). Perinatal and neonatal palliative care interventions are also interdisciplinary and place an emphasis on pain management, spiritual support, grief and bereavement, and honoring cultural practices. Offering support to parents may include framing dif-ficult decisions as acts of care and encouraging them to participate in their child's care. The BHC can be instrumental in helping parents understand their feelings related to potential end-of-life situations and helping them formulate multiple plans depending on their infant's changing medical status. Helping the parents explore and express their needs based on cultural, religious, and/or personal meaning making can facilitate how the team, including parents, proceeds during these difficult times.

Sometimes, the most challenging situations present as dynamic challenges in the NICU in which the team becomes "split," with some staff feeling angry as a result of a parent's perceived micromanagement and criticism, whereas other staff members feel more understanding and sympathetic toward the parent(s). In these cases, the BHC needs to collect data from multiple staff and the parent(s) to create an effective case conceptualization, develop an alliance with the parent(s) and staff, and then guide the overarching strategy to enhance the experiences of safety and trust among all members of the interpersonal and systemic dynamics at play. In addition, the BHC should facilitate referrals for parents with clinical diagnoses that require longer term formal mental health treatment and/or addi-tional resources.

CASE EXAMPLE

Jane Smith was born at 24 weeks and weighed 450 g at birth. Ms. Smith gave birth to Jane early as a result of developing preeclampsia and delivered in triage. The NICU psychologist met Ms. Smith while rounding the unit to leave a welcome letter at the bedside (universal intervention).

Ms. Smith began to attend the parent support group facilitated by the BHC (universal intervention) and eagerly accepted suggestions for helpful apps, par-enting rituals such as reading to her infant, developing a routine that allowed for self-care days, and managing "well-meaning" family members. In group, she shared about her birth trauma and the experience of observing Jane during a resuscitation (targeted intervention).

Individual sessions at bedside addressed sources of stress and support, her long commute to the hospital, household chores and finances, self-care needs, the demands of breast pumping, and ways to cope and problem-solve challenges (targeted intervention). Over time, it became clear that despite Jane's eligibility for skin-to-skin care, Ms. Smith remained terrified of holding her daughter or even introducing a scent cloth for fear of "further damaging" Jane. Difficulty pumping added to her feelings of shame and guilt associated with the perceived "failings" of her body. The BHC consulted with the bedside nurses and lactation consultants helping Ms. Smith. Together they developed plans with Ms. Smith that helped her begin to process her trauma and fears of "damaging" her baby and to begin bringing her physically and emotionally closer to Jane (clinical intervention).

Years later, Ms. Smith returned to speak at the NICU parent support group. She shared that she often felt conflicted about wanting to be with her infant and also dreamt of "running away and never coming back to the hospital again." She told the parents at the group that she felt ashamed of these feelings in the past but had come to understand that having mixed feelings does not make one a bad parent; it makes one a human being.

STAFF INTERVENTIONS

The NICU's acuity and intensity can lead to stress, burnout, vicarious traumatization, and compassion fatigue if the staff is not supported accordingly (Hall et al., 2015). As such, it is important that NICU staff members at all levels are included and considered in staff interventions; this includes nonclinical staff such as facilities workers and unit clerks. BHCs play an essential, albeit sometimes informal, role in supporting the well-being of all staff who are affected by the intensity and stress of the NICU setting.

Several factors may contribute to staff distress, including miscommunication, lack of understanding of psychosocial issues and dynamics, physical work environment, interpersonal relationships with other team members, and neonatal and infant death. In order to help staff with the many challenges they face as part of the NICU team, the BHC must first develop the team members' respect and trust. Much of this work involves being visible and available for parents and staff as much as possible. As described previously, toxic stress overwhelms the neurological system, shifting into a fight-or-flight response (Sanders & Hall, 2018). NICU staff, who chronically endure various degrees of stress under the most trying situations, need to have a trusting relationship based on the compassion, nonjudgment, and competence of a BHC. They need to feel safe and secure in order to seek guidance and share vulnerability.

BHCs can help support NICU staff by acting as a liaison between staff members and the family, helping facilitate discussion and understanding of the family stressors, dynamics, and ways of coping (Hall et al., 2015). These interventions can involve integrating various sources of information and working with staff to identify ways to approach the family in order to enhance feelings of safety and trust. Behaviors that indicate lack of trust in the team or others must be examined as signals that BHCs may not know the whole picture. The BHC can help enhance openness in the staff by learning more about the parent's source of stress and mistrust and approaching any tensions with compassion and understanding. BHCs are instrumental in helping staff identify signs of burnout, compassion fatigue, distress, and other concerns that directly impact quality of work, provider and patient satisfaction, and patient outcomes (Hall et al., 2015).

BHCs can formally and informally engage staff in psychoeducation on various topics, such as normal responses to the infant's hospitalization, PMADs, family-centered care, perinatal grief and bereavement care, and culturally responsive care. When staff are educated about these topics, they feel empowered to support families, which builds a positive relationship and experience despite the medical outcome (Hall et al., 2015). The BHC also plays an important role in helping staff understand trauma and how chronic stress affects the brain and behavior in infants, parents, and staff. The BHC can work with staff to create compassion and empathy for themselves as well as their patients' families. The BHC's role often entails helping the staff understand their critical role in downregulating or "holding" the parents (by recognizing the trauma and stress reactions) so that parents can provide the loving care their infants need to experience the world as safe and comforting (Sanders & Hall, 2018). Trauma-informed care education modules have been developed using evidence-based practices. Online education modules draw upon these trauma-informed practices to help NICU providers address common psychosocial challenges in the NICU (see https://www.nationalpe rinatal.org/staff-education).

Dissociation and compartmentalization are normative and sometimes functional forms of coping with medical trauma; however, relying solely on dissociation to cope can be detrimental and ultimately lead to increased distress or burnout. Although clinical event debriefing is standard practice across medical units, this process typically focuses on what went wrong (e.g., skills deficit and timeliness) rather than what went well. In addition to offering one-on-one support for staff, BHCs can bolster staff support by facilitating group debriefing sessions. These sessions allow the staff to process their emotions and review the events after a challenging case, integrating medical and psychosocial perspectives (Hall et al., 2015). These meetings can be structured by first stating the problem but also discussing how the team can improve for similar cases in the future. Debriefing usually happens around difficult ethical and moral cases or following the death of a patient. However, debriefing sessions are encouraged to process any challenging case. At times, there are challenges with staff attending these meetings due to time restrictions or lack of encouragement from senior leadership. In the latter case, the BHC may need to partner with nursing and medical leadership to encourage staff participation.

Complex care conferences can create a space to discuss some of the most challenging medical and emotional cases. These conferences allow the team to discuss various medical and psychosocial issues in depth in a holistic way. Patients are usually discussed in shorter segments throughout the day and week. Reserving an hour once or twice per month allows team members to reflect on a complicated case from multiple perspectives. The team can create a consistent and coherent plan that incorporates ways to address medical challenges while integrating how to better meet staff and family emotional needs. Often, discussion may address why moral distress may be arising among staff, sources of parental and staff miscommunication and dissatisfaction, and how to improve the infant's and family's experience of life in the NICU while acknowledging staff needs as well. The conference goals are often created with an eye toward enhancing development, providing comfort and palliation while tending to full medical interventions and improving daily experiences.

Offering this interdisciplinary time in reflective discussion can provide opportunities for understanding team members' perspectives and challenges. This type of perspective-taking can potentially enhance capacities for empathy and compassion toward each other, the family, the infant, and themselves. The BHC's presence and activity in these meetings can address psychosocial needs of the staff and families.

In partnership with the chaplaincy service, BHCs may also provide bereavement interventions to staff after an infant has died; this can serve as a forum for collective healing for both NICU staff and families (Levick et al., 2017). Some of these interventions may include conducting a remembrance ceremony, creating a memorial space within the NICU, offering a meeting room for reflection and writing, and lighting a battery-operated candle as a symbol of acknowledgment next to a card for staff to sign. Another creative staff intervention is inviting staff to write down thoughts, wishes, and hopes onto dissolving paper and putting it in a water bowl; the water can then be used to nourish a tree planted in remembrance of the infant's life.

Some programs have found that the integration of a BHC in the NICU, support groups, mentorship programs, and bereavement and grief-focused team debriefs help curtail burnout by facilitating opportunity to share stories, create meaning, and connect to feelings around witnessing chronic loss and stress (Hynan et al., 2015). Reflective peer consultation, consisting of psychoeducation and supervision, may result in more effective staff and improved morale, stronger boundaries, less hierarchical structure, decreased stress levels among staff, higher satisfaction in work and personal relationships, enhancement in trauma-informed care of patients, and earlier identification of parent/patient stress. (Lorrain, 2016). Investing in the wellness of NICU staff is undoubtedly a critical and integral component of caring for NICU patients and their families.

LIAISON AND PARTNERSHIPS

Behavioral health support, both in the hospital and in the community, is vital to the reduction of parental PMADs; impaired parent–infant bonding; and child developmental, behavioral, and/or cognitive delays. In addition to the formal support of BHCs, lactation consultants, chaplains, child life specialists, bereavement coordinators, and others may provide unique perspectives and skill sets that can help support parental and family well-being. It is wise to be aware of and to collaborate with other team members to address families' multifaceted needs.

Within the hospital, team partnership can be fostered by providing a structure and vision for interdisciplinary rounds. Discussing psychosocial needs with the interdisciplinary team is integral to providing well-rounded care for infants and their families. For example, assessment for postpartum depression and its relation to maternal milk supply would allow the medical team to be cognizant of these overarching factors influencing medical care. It would also allow the psychologist, the lactation consultant, and the social worker to partner to support the family.

Some families may not want or need hospital-based support and instead prefer connecting with other families and resources in their community. Research has demonstrated that peer support networks improve mental health outcomes (Hunt et al., 2018). Connecting families with the institutional family advisory council or larger organizations such as the March of Dimes, National Perinatal Association, Hand to Hold, Vermont Oxford Network, and Postpartum Support International can help offer comfort, increase acceptance, and empower parents to become advocates for their families. Another way BHCs can act as a liaison is to create peer support networks for parents. Current NICU parents can learn about the process and experiences from alumni parents who have experienced the NICU first-hand. In addition, the peer support network creates a community of shared experiences and reduces feelings of isolation, anxiety, and depression (Hunt et al., 2018). The sense of an in-person or virtual community of a peer-to-peer support network can be nurturing and empowering for parents (Hall et al., 2015), particularly for those from collectivistic cultures. When offering support to families, it is important to consider the family's cultural context and social location and to maintain a trauma-informed perspective. These approaches are congruent with family-centered development care (Hall et al., 2017), which outlines better practices in neonatal intensive care and encourages providers to meet families where they are and to provide holistic, culturally centered care.

IDEAS WORTH SHARING

- The BHC is an outsider entering at a particularly stressful point in the family's journey. Each family is an expert in their experience and process. It is important to respect, honor, and be open to learning from each family what they have been through and what they need.
- BHCs need to be aware of their own biases, misconceptions, and stereotypes. They should also consider how presenting issues may be connected to systemic and structural issues of poverty, racism, and injustice. Adopting a lens of cultural humility may help with building

trust. Modifying interventions in a culturally congruent manner may also help the team better meet the family's needs.

- Integrating discussion of psychosocial needs into interdisciplinary rounds and partnering with other members of the interprofessional team can enhance patient care.
- When creating programs in the NICU, BHCs should conduct a needs-based assessment and pay attention to the community being served, getting input from current and former NICU families. For example, instead of a traditional support group process, some NICUs use a "coffee and conversations" approach.
- Collaborate with local community resources that are culturally congruent with the identified family. Peer support networks and organizations can help with overall adjustment to the NICU.

CONCLUSION

To support families in their journey in the NICU, BHCs must work holistically and collaboratively. They need to understand the interconnectedness of the micro, mezzo, and macro systems and incorporate them into their screening, assessment, and treatment approach (Nader et al., 2013). Through meaningful dialogue with families and their providers, BHCs can be more conscious of their unique role and contribution to shaping the patient–provider experience in the NICU.

REFERENCES

Bachman, D. H., & Lind, R. F. (1997). Perinatal social work and the family of the newborn intensive care infant. In *Fundamentals of perinatal social work: A guide for clinical practice* (pp. 21–37). Routledge.

Cagle, J. G., Osteen, P., Sacco, P., & Frey, J. J. (2017). Psychosocial assessment by hospice social workers: A content review of instruments from a national sample. *Journal of Pain and Symptom Management*, 53(1), 40–48.

Cherry, A. S., Blucker, R. T., Thornberry, T. S., Hetherington, C., McCaffree, M. A., & Gillaspy, S. R. (2016). Postpartum depression screening in the neonatal intensive care unit: Program development, implementation, and lessons learned. *Journal of Multidisciplinary Healthcare*, 9, 59–67.

Craig, S. L., Eaton, A. D., Belitzky, M., Kates, L. E., Dimitropoulos, G., & Tobin, J. (2020). Empowering the team: A social work model of interprofessional collaboration in hospitals. *Journal of Interprofessional Education & Practice*, 19, 100327.

Davidson, J. E., Aslakson, R. A., Long, A. C., Puntillo, K. A., Kross, E. K., Hart, J., Cox, C. E., Wunsch, H., Wickline, M. A., Nunnally, M. E., Netzer, G., Barnes, N. K., Sprung, C. L., Hartog, C. S., Coombs, M., Gerritsen, R. T., Hopkins, R. O., Franck, L. S., Skrobik, Y., . . . Curtis, J. R. (2017). Guidelines for family-centered care in the neonatal, pediatric, and adult ICU. *Critical Care Medicine*, 45(1), 103–128.

Earls, M. F., Yogman, M. W., Mattson, G., Rafferty, J.; Committee on Psychosocial Aspects of Child and Family Health. (2019). Incorporating recognition and management of perinatal depression into pediatric practice. *Pediatrics, 143*(1), e20183259.

Flacking, R., Lehtonen, L., Thomson, G., Axelin, A., Ahlqvist, S., Moran, V. H., Ewald, U., Dykes, F.; SCENE group. (2012). Closeness and separation in neonatal intensive care. *Acta Paediatrica, 101*(10), 1032–1037.

Hall, S. L., Cross, J., Selix, N. W., Patterson, C., Segre, L., Chuffo-Siewert, R., Geller, P. A., & Martin, M. L. (2015). Recommendations for enhancing psychosocial support of NICU parents through staff education and support. *Journal of Perinatology, 35*(Suppl. 1), S29–S36.

Hall, S. L., Hynan, M., Phillips, R., Lassen, S., Craig, J. W., Goyer, E., Hatfield, R. F., & Cohen, H. (2017). The neonatal intensive parenting unit: An introduction. *Journal of Perinatology, 37*, 1259–1264.

Hoffman, C. C., Greene, M., & Baughcum, A. E. (2020). Neonatal intensive care. In B. D. Carter & K. A. Kullgren (Eds.), *Clinical handbook of consultation in pediatric medical settings* (pp. 277–294). Springer.

Hunt, H., Whear, R., Boddy, K., Wakely, L., Bethel, A., Morris, C., Abbott, R., Prosser, S., Collinson, A., Kurinczuk, J., & Thompson-Coon, J. (2018). Parent-to-parent support interventions for parents of babies cared for in a neonatal unit: Protocol of a systematic review of qualitative and quantitative evidence. *Systematic Reviews, 7*(1), 179.

Hynan, M. T., Mounts, K., & Vanderbilt, D. (2013). Screening parents of high-risk infants for emotional distress: Rationale and recommendations. *Journal of Perinatology, 33*, 748–753.

Hynan, M. T., Steinberg, Z., Baker, L., Cicco, R., Geller, P. A., Lassen, S., Milford, C., Mounts, K. O., Patterson, C., Saxton, S., Segre, L., & Stuebe, A. (2015). Recommendations for mental health professionals in the NICU. *Journal of Perinatology, 35*, S14–S18.

Kazak, A. E., Schneider, S., Didonato, S., & Pai, A. L. (2015). Family psychosocial risk screening guided by the Pediatric Psychosocial Preventative Health Model (PPPHM) using the Psychosocial Assessment Tool (PAT). *Acta Oncologica, 54*(5), 574–580.

Lakatos, P. P., Matic, T., Carson, M., & Williams, M. E. (2019). Child–parent psychotherapy with infants hospitalized in the neonatal intensive care unit. *Journal of Clinical Psychology in Medical Settings, 26*(4), 584–596.

Lefkowitz, D. S., Baxt, C., & Evans, J. R. (2010). Prevalence and correlates of posttraumatic stress and postpartum depression in parents of infants in the neonatal intensive care unit (NICU). *Journal of Clinical Psychology in Medical Settings, 17*(3), 230–237.

Levick, J., Fannon, J., Bodemann, J., Munch, S., & Ahern, K. (2017). NICU bereavement care and follow-up support for families and staff. *Advances in Neonatal Care, 17*(6), 451–460.

Lorrain, B. (2016). Reflective peer consultation as an intervention for staff support in the NICU. *Newborn and Infant Nursing Reviews, 16*(4), 289–292.

Luca, D. L., Margiotta, C., Staatz, C., Garlow, E., Christensen, A., & Zivin, K. (2020). Financial toll of untreated perinatal mood and anxiety disorders among 2017 births in the United States. *American Journal of Public Health, 110*(6), 888–896.

Mounts, K. O. (2009). Screening for maternal depression in the neonatal ICU. *Clinics in Perinatology, 36*(1), 137–152.

Nader, K., Dubrow, N., & Stamm, B. H. (2013). *Honoring differences: Cultural issues in the treatment of trauma and loss.* Routledge.

Roque, A. T. F., Lasiuk, G. C., Radünz, V., & Hegadoren, K. (2017). Scoping review of the mental health of parents of infants in the NICU. *Journal of Obstetric, Gynecologic & Neonatal Nursing, 46*(4), 576–587.

Sanders, M. R., & Hall, M. L. (2018). Trauma-informed care in the newborn intensive care unit: Promoting safety, security and connectedness. *Journal of Perinatology, 38*(1), 3–10.

Tirumalaraju, V., Suchting, R., Evans, J., Goetzl, L., Refuerzo, J., Neumann, A., Anand, D., Ravikumar, R., Green, C. E., Cowen, P. J., & Selvaraj, S. (2020). Risk of depression in the adolescent and adult offspring of mothers with perinatal depression: A systematic review and meta-analysis. *JAMA Network Open, 3*(6), e208783.

Vigod, S. N., Villegas, L., Dennis, C. L., & Ross, L. E. (2010). Prevalence and risk factors for postpartum depression among women with preterm and low-birth-weight infants: A systematic review. *BJOG: An International Journal of Obstetrics & Gynaecology, 117*(5), 540–550.

22

REGULATION, RELATIONSHIPS, AND REFLECTION

DEVELOPMENTAL CARE IN THE NICU

AYELET TALMI AND JOY V. BROWNE ∎

The mental health needs of both fragile infants with special health care and developmental needs and their families are central to the work of integrated behavioral health providers in neonatal intensive care units (NICUs). Using an infant mental health (IMH) approach, behavioral health providers focus on optimizing relationships between fragile infants and their families, fragile infants and medical professionals, families and medical professionals, and among medical professionals working in NICUs. IMH services that promote infant–parent relationships and socioemotional competence through the provision of developmentally supportive care, in combination with the growing focus on identifying and addressing parental mental health needs, form the core of behavioral health interventions in the NICU. *Regulation* of fragile infants occurs through developmentally supportive interventions, in the context of relationships with caregivers, and by optimizing self-regulation opportunities. *Reflection* and *reflective practice* are the mechanisms by which behavioral health providers address and support relationships among fragile infants, their families, and the professionals with whom they work (Browne, 2020).

Behavioral health providers working in the NICU and community settings are, by necessity, IMH providers charged with promoting healthy early relationships, addressing the impact of adverse and stressful experiences and environments, and supporting well-being and long-term developmental and relational outcomes. Core concepts in IMH involve considering the infant, the caregivers, the relationships, and the caregiving context; delivering services that help keep the infant in focus and in the caregiver's mind; and utilizing reflective practice and reflective supervision to guide behavioral health care and build professional capacity (Weatherston & Browne, 2016).

Best practices for behavioral health providers in NICU settings include implementing specialized and evidence-based approaches spanning identification, evaluation, and intervention to enhance developmental, relational, and health outcomes. Behavioral health providers who work in intensive care settings provide intervention services to fragile infants and their families along the continuum from universal and preventive services to focused services for at-risk populations and, finally, tertiary services (Zeanah et al., 2005). *Universal and preventive* interventions in the form of developmentally supportive care are applied at the NICU level and for individual infants and their families. Prevention of long-term neurodevelopmental problems happens through recognizing behavioral communication of the infant and verbal and nonverbal communication from the family members; minimizing stressful occurrences; enhancing neuroprotective experiences; and promoting regulation during procedures, caregiving, and hospitalization. *Focused* services for at-risk infants and families include identification of potentially stressful events, conditions, relationships, and environments and providing supports that buffer the stressful experiences. Finally, *tertiary* intervention includes provision of individualized environmental and caregiving interventions and evidence-based therapeutic strategies to address existing pathology and/or refer/collaborate with intensive care developmental specialists and other mental health interventionists to deliver these services.

In addition to a continuum of intervention levels from universal and preventative to focused to tertiary, a continuum of ports of entry for behavioral health exists. For infants, the effects of early stressful experiences in the absence of buffering and regulating relationships, referred to as "toxic stress," may result in long-term disruptions in socioemotional and physiological regulation, development, and long-term outcomes (Shonkoff, 2016). The impact of adverse experiences and environments stemming from being in the NICU (e.g., medical treatments, disease progression, and relationship disruptions) must be considered in the context of situational and familial circumstances that influence developing relationships and directly impact infant, caregiver, and staff well-being.

REGULATION AND DEVELOPMENTALLY SUPPORTIVE, NEUROPROTECTIVE CARE

Developmental care is a neuroprotective approach designed to optimize the physical (distal) environment of intensive care as well as the caregiving (proximal) environment that is individualized to the infant's behavioral communication. Infant- and family-centered developmental care ensures that services and supports are responsive to infant regulatory needs. Universal and preventive interventions during hospitalization promote a neuroprotective environment, sensitive individualized caregiving, and inclusion of the family in all aspects of care. Focused interventions are provided when risk factors and adversity are identified.

What About the Infant?

As the viability of infants born early has increased due to improved medical interventions and caregiving, lingering morbidities have been identified using more sophisticated research methodologies and with renewed focus on this population of infants and families. Whereas self-regulatory skills typically emerge in the first few months of life as external regulation from primary caregivers decreases and infant self-regulatory capacity increases, fragile infants are more likely to struggle with regulation, demonstrating difficulties with feeding, sleeping, and soothing during this time. Research shows that fragile infants are at risk of experiencing significant behavioral, social–emotional, and mental health issues that persist into adulthood as a result of their prenatal and postnatal experiences and environments (Sammallahti et al., 2017).

In the 1970s and 1980s, the impact of the environment and caregiving on infants' organization and outcomes was identified as critical to understanding neurodevelopment and designing neuroprotective interventions. In addition, there was a recognition that the impact of these two aspects of early hospitalization on infants' brains was significant and long-lasting. Dr. Heidelise Als was an early scholar and researcher on infant behavioral communication and interventions. She developed an approach to identify infant responses to stressful events and provided individualized strategies to ameliorate those responses and promote better neurobehavioral outcomes (Als, 1991, 1998). Dr. Stanley Graven also recognized the impact of intrusive sensory environments for infants and families in NICUs and brought together professionals to explore the science underlying the impact on infant and family outcomes, resulting in the development of nationally recognized NICU environmental design standards (Graven, 1997; White, 2020). In addition, a number of developmental psychobiologists have provided translational insights into the impact of early birth and hospitalization, which has further enhanced the understanding of the need for developmentally appropriate neuroprotective care (Browne &White, 2011). Current research into aspects of developmental care in NICUs owes a great deal to these pioneering efforts to improve brain protection and enhance neurodevelopmental outcomes.

Evidence-Based Neuroprotective Models

A number of infant neurodevelopmental protective approaches are used in the United States to enhance infant outcomes and provide parental support (see Table 22.1 for an overview of several evidence-based interventions currently practiced in NICUs). Some approaches offer direct interventions with the infant and some with the parents. Several of the individualized intervention programs provide integrated

Table 22.1 Developmental Care Training Programs Typically Used in the United States

Program	Main Construct	Content	Training
Newborn Individualized Developmental Care and Assessment Program (NIDCAP; https://nidcap.org)	Synactive theory including defined systems of autonomic, state, motor, and self-regulation	Teaches individualized assessment of infant behavioral communication, inferred developmental goals, and recommendations for intervention	Two-day basic didactic and bedside assessment and extended (1–2 years) mentored application resulting in reliability and certification
Family and Infant Neurodevelopmental Education (FINE): Foundational pathway to NIDCAP (https://nidcap.org)	Based on synactive theory, brain development, and evidence-based practices	Neurodevelopmental foundational information and application to NICU clinical work	FINE 1: Two-day introduction FINE 2: Mentored application of content FINE 3: Special clinical application
Newborn Behavioral Observation (NBO; https://www.newbornbehaviorinternational.org)	Newborn and young infant behavioral organization and relationship building	Demonstrates and discusses infant behavior with parents	Three partial days of didactic
Family Nurture Intervention (FNI; https://nurturescienceprogram.org/family-nurture-intervention)	Calming cycle theory; autonomic conditioning	Encourages parent–infant emotional connection with odor, touch, and voice during skin-to-skin care	Individualized to train family nurture specialists in NICUs
Creating Opportunities for Parent Empowerment (COPE for HOPE; https://copeforhope.com/nicu.php)	Stress reduction and coping through education and behavioral intervention	Parent education to reduce stress/anxiety and engage with their infant using CDs and/or audiotaped information, workbook, and bedside support	On-site NICU educational and behavioral approaches and consultation; use of COPE NICU Program Implementation Training Manual
Family Integrated Care (FI; http://familyintegratedcare.com)	Family-centered care	Creates professional–parent partnership in NICU to care for their infant	Program development using online toolkit includes four "pillars" of staff education and support, parent education, NICU environment, and psychosocial support

approaches that include a number of evidence-based strategies and thus are multi-modal and individualized (e.g., Newborn Individualized Developmental Care and Assessment Program [NIDCAP]). Some programs emphasize just one modality (e.g., kangaroo mother care), and some focus on an intervention for the family system.

A Consensus Panel of Interprofessionals performed systematic reviews of the best available evidence for strategies common to neurodevelopmental care, and this resulted in the publication of *Standards, Competencies and Recommended Best Practices for Infant and Family Centered Developmental Care* for infants in intensive care (Browne et al., 2020), which should be considered when practicing in intensive care units with infants. Similarly, in Europe, the European Foundation for the Care of Newborn Infants' *European Standards of Care for Newborn Health* (https://www.efcni.org/activities/projects-2/escnh) have been developed.

As an extension of the application of recommended standards and intervention strategies for infants, attention to the psychosocial needs, not only those of families (Hynan & Hall, 2015) but also those of staff members and the systems they work in, must be considered. Behavioral health providers who work in NICU settings also have published guidelines to identify competencies guiding practice and training. These competencies include essential knowledge and skills in the six areas of science, systems, professionalism, relationships, application, and education (Saxton et al., 2020).

Two evidence-based, *focused* interventions that provide neurodevelopmental care for all infants in intensive care are described here. Considered to be the "gold standard" for neurodevelopmental care, the NIDCAP model (https://nidcap.org) has shown evidence for improved short- and long-term neurodevelopmental outcomes for infants who were at birth very low birth weight, into school age (McAnulty et al., 2013). This approach provides a defined theory, a strategy for structured observation, and individualized interventions to ameliorate stressful experiences and thus improve neurodevelopmental outcomes for infants. Because the training to certification is complex and lengthy, an introductory program of Family and Infant Neurodevelopmental Education (FINE) is designed for all NICU professionals providing care to infants and families in intensive care. The FINE program provides a beginning pathway to becoming a NIDCAP professional. In addition, to provide continuity as the infant and family transition to the community, programs with similar theoretical and observational approaches are now being implemented. The BABIES and PreSTEPS model (Browne & Talmi, 2012) and the Infant Behavior Assessment and Intervention Program (Van Hus et al., 2013) provide continuity through the transition home and to community-based services.

Developmentally Supportive Care Screening, Assessment, and Evaluation

With appropriate training, behavioral health professionals can conduct neurodevelopmental evaluations with fragile infants to determine neurodevelopmental status and design individualized neuroprotective interventions. Noble and Boyd (2012) describe some of the most commonly utilized, valid exams for infants in intensive care settings, including the Assessment of Preterm Infants' Behavior (APIB), the Brazelton Neonatal Behavioral Assessment Scale (NBAS), the Neurobehavioral Assessment of the Preterm Infant, the Neuromotor Behavioral Assessment, the Neonatal Intensive Care Unit Network Neurobehavioral Scale (NNNS), and the Test for Infant Motor Performance. Selected assessments are described here.

The APIB (Als et al., 2005) is a hands-on neurodevelopmental exam that was derived from the NBAS (Brazelton, 1978) specifically for preterm and high-risk neonates. It includes an evaluation of the infant's systems—autonomic, motor, state, interaction, and regulation—and scores for examiner facilitation, responses to reflex elicitation, and summary scales. The NNNS (Lester et al., 2004) was designed to examine stress and withdrawal of the at-risk and drug-exposed infant and is currently used for research and clinical neurobehavioral assessment in infants from approximately 34 weeks gestational age to 4 or 5 weeks post term (i.e., 45 weeks gestational age). It is derived from the NBAS and the APIB, among other newborn examinations, and includes evaluation of the neurobehavioral organization, reflexes, motor development, and tone of the infant.

The Newborn Behavioral Observation (NBO; McManus & Nugent, 2014) is not an evaluation per se but, rather, is used with families of newborns, including hospitalized infants, to observe the behavioral capacities and develop recommendations for support for successful development. As an inherently family-centered approach, families are included as partners in the NBO sessions.

Other examinations more specific to individual systems such as motor development or feeding can be administered by qualified therapists but are typically not utilized by behavioral health professionals. However, knowledge of different therapeutic evaluations may be helpful in supporting families to understand results of the exams and implement individualized interventions.

RELATIONSHIPS AND FAMILY-LEVEL INTERVENTIONS

Unfortunately, many of the documented long-term difficulties faced by preterm and fragile infants involve emotional, behavioral, and cognitive problems that may stem from relationship disruptions. Whereas NICUs provide technological and pharmacological interventions to address the complex medical needs of preterm and fragile infants, relatively little emphasis is placed on interventions that support infants' relationships with their families. Due to the heightened vulnerability to relationship disruptions that infants and families experience in the NICU, along with the long-term consequences of poor early relationships, supporting infant–caregiver interactions should be one of the main goals for both NICU and community-based behavioral health professionals working with fragile infants and their families.

Infant–caregiver relationships, particularly very early in development, depend on a caregiver's ability to notice, interpret, and respond appropriately to infants' behavioral communication. The infant–caregiver relationship emerges through repeated interactions that are supportive and nurturing. Well-timed interactions with parents and consistent caregivers help regulate infants' physiological responses (e.g., heart rate, breathing rate, and body temperature), social and emotional responses (e.g., reactions to distress), and nutritional needs (e.g., successful feeding experiences). Infant–caregiver relationships also provide the foundation for the emergence of self-regulation and self-comforting capacities (Browne & Talmi, 2012).

What About the Family?

The pregnancy and newborn period is often a time of tremendous physical, psychological, and emotional upheaval and change. Behavioral health providers frequently address multiple facets of these transitions with caregivers whose infants are hospitalized in the NICU. Considering the well-being of the whole family as well as individual members is essential to providing behavioral health supports in the NICU (Browne et al., 2016). Behavioral health providers are often called upon to identify and address critical issues related to parental mental health and family circumstances that may impact their caregiving capacity. Parental mental health issues, including depression, anxiety, substance use, and trauma, may exist prior to the birth of their infant or have new onsets subsequent to the birth and hospitalization of their infant (Del Fabbro & Cain, 2016). High-risk circumstances may require *tertiary* interventions to address behavioral health needs. For example, mothers with a history of substance use, young mothers, mothers experiencing perinatal mood or anxiety disorders during pregnancy and after delivery, and mothers with a history of trauma benefit from behavioral health services in pregnancy, the NICU, and after their infants transition home (Ashby & Bromberg, 2016).

The stressful experience of having an infant hospitalized in the NICU may impact both caregiver well-being and the caregiver's capacity to interact and develop a relationship with the infant. Identifying and addressing caregiver mental health concerns in NICUs is essential to supporting caregiver well-being and infant–parent relationship development. Some hospital settings universally screen for mental health concerns such as depression and anxiety, whereas others rely on referrals to external mental health services when caregivers request support or when concerns arise from the NICU team. Universal screening reduces the likelihood that parental struggles will be overlooked and increases the likelihood that behavioral health services will be delivered when needed.

Evidence-Based Interventions to Support Relationships Between Fragile Infants and Their Families

The recently developed Family Nurture Intervention (FNI) program has been implemented in NICUs with significant positive behavioral and neurodevelopmental outcomes for both mothers' and infants' mental health and physiology. Based on calming cycle theory (Welch, 2016), the FNI utilizes nurture specialists to support NICU mothers as they hold their infants skin-to-skin (kangaroo mother care) and focuses on the emotional connection between the dyad. Significant positive outcomes are documented for infant behavior, social–emotional, and neurodevelopmental outcomes that endure into childhood (Welch et al., 2015, 2020).

Other evidence-based programs providing support to families include educational components provided during hospitalization in the NICU. The Creating Opportunities for Parent Empowerment (COPE) program employs both audio CD and workbook education with behavioral support strategies in the NICU to enhance the parent's understanding of their infant's behavior and how to parent a preterm infant (Melnyk et al., 2001). Results have shown lower maternal anxiety and depression, greater confidence in their parental role, greater ability to care for their infant, and enhanced parent–infant interaction (Askary Kachoosangy et al., 2020).

Technology to Promote Relationships

Emerging technological applications that allow electronic observations and support communication in intensive care units have been increasingly utilized to alleviate the challenges when parents and family members have difficulty being with their hospitalized infants in person. Hello Baby (https://hellobaby.us) is one such application of electronic communication. Separations due to psychosocial and environmental factors (e.g., family distance from the NICU, financial barriers, and restrictions related to mitigating exposure to diseases) have necessitated innovations in electronic communication and connection when infants are hospitalized in the NICU. Similarly, behavioral health providers have successfully utilized telehealth modalities to deliver interventions to families of fragile infants.

Preparing for the Transition Home and Providing Continuity for Community-Based Services

Behavioral health providers in the NICU are frequently involved in supporting families as they prepare for transition home and establish connections to community resources. Targeted referrals to the family's medical home (i.e., primary care), specialty services including mental health, therapeutic services, and public health support services can be facilitated by behavioral health providers, with a particular emphasis on connecting families with early intervention services and IMH supports (Murch & Smith, 2016). In the United States, the Individuals with Disabilities Education Act (Part C) provides developmental evaluation and supports in a family's local community. Often, infants can be identified in the intensive care unit as categorically eligible for Part C services, and an Individual Family Service Plan can be initiated. Referrals to qualified early interventionists should be a priority, particularly those who have had training in relationship-based and family-centered developmental approaches appropriate for the med-ically fragile newborn and young infant, such as the BABIES and PreSTEPS models (Browne & Talmi, 2012). The BABIES and PreSTEPS models focus on evidence-based relationship-building approaches to assessment and intervention for an infant's *B*ody function, *A*rousal and sleep, *B*ody movement, *I*nteraction with others, *E*ating, and *S*elf-soothing (BABIES). Support for families will focus on best practices of *P*redictability and continuity, *S*leep and arousal organization, *T*iming and pacing, *E*nvironmental modifications, *P*ositioning and handling, and *S*elf-soothing supports (PreSTEPS).

What About the Context?

Family circumstances may also impact infant–parent relationships and create additional complexity in meeting the needs of fragile infants and their families. Social determinants of health account for a greater percentage of health outcomes than interventions intended to address issues such as mental health concerns. All infants and families have basic needs that include sufficient food, safe shelter, financial stability, healthy relationships, and access to health care resources. Unfortunately, when families lack access to adequate, safe, and stable resources and supports, their ability to develop and nurture relationships with their fragile infants may be compromised because of stress, dangerous environments, and deprivation. Poverty, homelessness and housing instability, family and community violence, and food insecurity are among the many contextual factors that directly impact infant–parent relationships and well-being. Importantly, systemic racism and discrimination cause undue burden and create barriers for families of color that can exacerbate the already complicated circumstances of parenting a fragile infant. In addition, significant disparities exist in rates of preterm birth and in maternal and infant mortality and morbidity rates for African American and Latino families compared to White families (Keating et al., 2020).

What About the NICU?

NICU professional staff strive to integrate their medical, technological, and pharmacological skills with the interpersonal and psychosocial aspects of their work with infants and families. Challenges for staff include demanding assignments and responsibilities in combination with increased complexity in cases and the type of medical and developmental care provided. As part of the routine care they provide, NICU professionals are often required to administer invasive and painful, albeit necessary, procedures and/or engage in caregiving that disrupts infant regulation. Inherent to the NICU environment is staff involvement in cases in which infants die and families are grieving. The toll of unrecognized trauma resulting from these aspects of care weighs heavily on the professional and personal lives of NICU staff.

NICU professionals working with fragile infants and their families need support from behavioral health providers and training in IMH approaches in order to enhance their ability to provide optimal services and expand their reflective capacity. Behavioral health providers with appropriate training and mentorship are uniquely suited to identify fragile infant neurodevelopmental status, complex relationship dynamics, and environmental effects on well-being. In addition, in light of their focus on the interaction between regulation and relationships, they are well positioned to contribute to the creation of physical and psychological spaces that promote optimal proximal and distal environments and support the development of nurturing relationships between infants and their families. As such, the availability of behavioral health providers enables NICU staff to better identify the impact of hospitalization on infants and families and communicate this to care teams and families.

Reflection and Reflective Practice: Promoting Regulation and Relationships

Reflection and reflective practice are core components of behavioral health professionals' engagement with infants and their families. *Reflection* involves a person's capacity to organize experiences and make sense out of the words and actions of others. With reflection, professionals think more carefully about their own and others' behaviors. Reflection also helps one understand what motivates people to do what they do and why people are the way they are (Smith & Wollesen, 2004). *Self-reflection* is a person's ability to look inward and consider the reasons for their own actions and reactions to events and relationships.

Reflective Practice Interacting with Infants

Behavioral health professionals in NICU settings operate from the assumption that all infants and families have strengths, and they help caregivers both identify those strengths and reflect on how to use them to enhance relationships. Caregivers promote optimal relationship development and IMH by being available—physically, psychologically, and emotionally—for their infants. Caregivers also foster mental health when they are aware of and sensitive to infants' patterns, behavioral communication, states, emotions, and communication efforts, as well as the effect of the environment on infants. Using reflective questions to promote *reflective functioning* (i.e., the capacity to be reflective) in parents ultimately leads to behavior changes that support infant development and the infant–caregiver relationship and increase the infant's and family's overall well-being. For example, asking a parent what would help them be ready for their infant's surgery creates an opportunity for the parent to identify their thoughts and feelings and what might be helpful to them so that they can best support their infant's recovery.

By enhancing reflective functioning, behavioral health providers can increase their awareness of an infant's efforts to communicate and of the meaning of an infant's behavioral communication. As parents become more reflective, they respond more appropriately and become more attuned to their infant's signals and behavioral communication (Kelly & Barnard, 2000). This includes structuring the environment to match their infant's needs. Reflective functioning also leads to an increased ability to evaluate situations, choose alternatives, and implement action plans. Finally, depending on feedback from their infants, caregivers flexibly adapt their behaviors to optimize their infants' responses, engaging in co-regulation that leads to optimal mental health and infant self-regulation skills.

Reflective Practice with Families

A *reflective stance*, in which professionals consider what is happening in the moment from the perspective of those involved and in the context of relationships, helps professionals better understand what they see and assists parents in interpreting and responding to their infant's behaviors. By using a reflective stance to examine their own interactions with infants and their families, professionals can better support parents and caregivers to function more reflectively themselves. When behavioral health professionals identify the reactions, thoughts, and feelings that arise in their work with families through reflective practice, they are able to use this awareness when engaging with infants and their families. These reflections help promote understanding of parental experiences that can, in turn, be used in the context of therapeutic relationships.

By promoting caregivers' and family members' reflective functioning skills, behavioral health professionals strengthen the caregiver–infant relationship. These reflective skills help caregivers interact with their infants in ways that further support the relationship; foster the development of co-regulation and self-regulation skills; and promote cognitive, physical, and social–emotional development. Importantly, when reflective functioning is cultivated, behavioral health professionals' strengths are simultaneously promoted. Reflective functioning enhances professionals' ability to provide sensitive care for fragile families, improve their own social interaction skills, highlight their program's effectiveness, and foster community collaboration.

When using a reflective practice approach, behavioral health providers working with fragile infants and their families help parents and family members

- reflect on their personal experiences, thoughts, and feelings—reflect on what the infant's emotional world might be like;
- make connections between parents' hopes, dreams, and expectations and the realities of having an infant who was hospitalized in the NICU;
- obtain the information they need to understand their infant;
- understand their infant's behavioral communication and respond appropriately; and
- advocate for their infant, parent their infant, develop plans for their infant, and put those plans into action.

Reflective Practice in Context

Reflective practice requires both intentionality and practice. Reflective practice can be effectively used across a wide array of situations. In daily communication and interactions, reflection can help enhance interactions, facilitate communication, and clarify misunderstandings. During difficult conversations, when emotions escalate, or in challenging situations that raise concerns, considering reactions to people and circumstances provides an opportunity to examine others' perspectives, open communication channels, and deescalate tensions. Reflection is helpful in cultivating relationships and addressing emotional states, needs, and reactions. It is also a helpful tool in professional development and can be used effectively in supervision to help cultivate behavioral health provider capacity to engage in challenging work with fragile infants and their families.

In addition to engaging in reflective work with families, behavioral health providers can support and facilitate reflective functioning and reflective practice with NICU professionals. Cultivating a reflective stance allows NICU professionals to understand and integrate the challenging experiences and complex circumstances that fragile infants and their families face during hospitalization and after the transition home. Reflective practice and behavioral health supports mitigate the cumulative stress of working in intensive care settings, reducing burnout, fatigue, and turnover by building provider capacity to address challenging cases and situations. Consequently, reflective practice promotes the formation of strong relationships among professionals, infants, and families, ultimately leading to improved relational and health outcomes.

IDEAS WORTH SHARING

The Gift of the Question

Behavioral health professionals working with infants with special health care needs and their families are often in roles in which they are expected to provide "the" answer because of their specialized training and tools to evaluate infants and make recommendations about next steps. In fact, consultations often occur because a "problem" has already been identified and behavioral health professionals are called upon to find the solution and implement it. This process is challenging, particularly when there are no easy answers or solutions or when the answers are difficult to hear (e.g., a poor prognosis or bad news).

An alternative to giving answers involves asking questions. Reflective questions provide families with a framework in which to consider their situation. Questions also help families describe their infant's and their own experiences and use their resources to formulate solutions. Asking reflective questions can strengthen relationships, clarify issues, provide a focus on particular topics, promote observational skills, identify information gaps, generate alternatives, and foster confidence. Behavioral health providers can select the appropriate types of questions to meet the goals of the interaction (Table 22.2).

By asking reflective questions, behavioral health providers can cultivate strong relationships with family members while supporting their role as the experts and capable caregivers of their infants. Reflection can be a powerful way of helping caregivers solve problems using their own capabilities, thus promoting

Table 22.2 Reflective Questions and Suggested Stems

Type of Question	Example Question Stems
Miracle	"If you woke up and things were different, what would it look like?"
Exception	"Can you think of a time when . . . ?" "Tell me about a time when it worked well for you."
Clarification of resources	"Who helps you . . . when you need them to?" "What have you tried that has worked well before?" "What would help you be ready for . . . ?"
Coping	"How have you been able to . . . so well?" "What did you notice when . . . ?" "How have you handled similar things in the past?"
Presumptive	"When . . . happened, what was it like for you?" "How are you feeling about . . . ?"
Action	"What happens when you . . . ?" "When do you want to . . . ?" "What do you think about . . . ?"
Relationship	"How would (person) feel?" "What is it like for (person)?"
Scaling	"On a scale of 1 to 10, what is this experience like for you?" "What would it take to move you from a [number] to a [number]?"

Source: Copyright Talmi, Browne, and Smith-Sharp (2004).

self-confidence and coping skills. At the same time, asking reflective questions in the course of an intervention models a problem-solving process that enhances a family's ability to be aware of and responsive to their infant's behavioral communication and needs.

CONCLUSION

For fragile infants, long-term difficulties include emotional, behavioral, and cognitive problems that may stem from difficulties with regulation and relationship disruptions. Fragile infants who are born at risk for lingering developmental concerns often require specialized assessment and intervention services based on their unique developmental needs to promote regulation and provide neuroprotective care. Programs such as NIDCAP, FNI (Welch, 2016), kangaroo care (Boundy et al., 2016), and other family-level interventions (e.g., COPE) allow behavioral health, medical, and allied health providers to simultaneously promote well-being and enhance optimal neurodevelopmental and relational outcomes.

The sophisticated technological, environmental, interventional, and pharmacological strategies employed in NICUs to address the complex medical needs of fragile infants often lack evidence-based behavioral health interventions intended to support early relationships. Promoting optimal early relationships among fragile infants, their caregivers, and NICU professionals is a priority for behavioral health providers because of the heightened vulnerability that infants and families experience in intensive care settings in conjunction with the long-term consequences of regulatory and relationship difficulties. Providing relationship-based evaluations, preventive interventions, and relationship-based family support services for fragile newborns and their families is complex and requires area specialization and appropriate mentoring.

Supporting early relationships for high-risk infants will have long-term effects on infants and families. Behavioral health providers need to utilize commonly practiced developmental care and evidence-based standards when advocating for infant- and family-centered developmental care (Box 22.1). They should be essential members of the developmental care team, providing informed mental health supports to both families and professionals in intensive care. A collaborative coordinated effort among hospital and community professionals and families is necessary to appropriately assess and provide therapeutic intervention to support optimal caregiver–infant relationship development.

Ultimately, fragile infants and their families can be optimally supported both in the NICU and after they transition home when the principles of reflective practice are incorporated into behavioral health and NICU interventions. As such, behavioral health providers are uniquely positioned to provide sensitive, supportive, and reflective interactions with fragile infants, their families, and the professionals who serve them to foster optimal growth and development and healthy relationships long after the infants leave the NICU (Table 22.3).

Box 22.1

ROLES OF THE BEHAVIORAL HEALTH PROVIDER IN THE NICU

1. Ensure that infants, families, and staff have access to behavioral health providers, supports, and services along the continuum from universal/preventive to targeted to tertiary in the NICU and after the transition home.

2. Recognize and support efforts to create intensive care environments that promote individualized, developmentally supportive neuroprotective care to optimize infant regulation.

3. Support parents in promoting infant regulation by responding to infant behavioral communication in the context of their relationship with their infant.

4. Identify positive and negative environmental and psychosocial factors and address barriers that interfere with supporting nurturing relationships.

5. Develop and implement supportive interventions for NICU staff and families to mitigate the impact of stressful and adverse experiences, including regulatory and relationship disruptions.

6. Monitor infant regulation and parent and staff well-being and provide support, interventions, and referrals as needed to optimize both development and relationships.

7. Build workforce capacity for delivering behavioral health services in the NICU through training in evidence-based approaches, promoting reflective practice, and cultivating reflective functioning in professionals and family members.

8. Advocate for policies that advance equitable access to high-quality behavioral health services for fragile infants and their families.

9. Develop, implement, and sustain integrated behavioral health services as the standard of care for fragile infants, their families, and the professionals who serve them.

Adapted from Browne and Talmi (2016) and Browne et al. (2016).

Table 22.3 ACTIONS OF PROFESSIONALS AND CORRESPONDING REACTIONS AND EXPERIENCES OF PARENTS AND FAMILY MEMBERS

When Professionals . . .	Parents and Caregivers . . .
Indicate that it matters what a parent knows	Feel respected and validated as being able to care for their infant
Build parents' confidence	Feel confident
Create teachable moments	Observe and assess their experiences, values, knowledge, and feelings
Suggest ways to consider a situation or challenge without offering "the" answer	Develop the skills to critically assess and select possible solutions on their own
Provide parents with the opportunity to recognize and apply their knowledge	Feel knowledgeable and experienced, like they are the experts about their infants
Provide parents with the opportunity to identify need for more information	Recognize gaps in knowledge and identify what information they need
Supply information that is based on the parents' request or a parent-identified need	See themselves as collaborators, rather than recipients of services; feel listened to and validated
Create meaningful moments	Experience meaningful connection with their infant
Offer to be on the journey with parents, walk beside them and provide support	Feel supported and not alone

Adapted from Smith and Wollesen (2004); copyright 2004 Center for Family & Infant Interaction, University of Colorado School of Medicine.

REFERENCES

Als, H. (1991). Neurobehavioral organization of the newborn: Opportunity for assessment and intervention. *NIDA Research Monograph*, *114*, 106–116. http://www.ncbi.nlm.nih.gov/pubmed/1754009

Als, H. (1998). Developmental care in the newborn intensive care unit. *Current Opinion in Pediatrics*, *10*(2), 138–142. http://www.ncbi.nlm.nih.gov/pubmed/9608890

Als, H., Butler, S., Kosta, S., & McAnulty, G. (2005). The Assessment of Preterm Infants' Behavior (APIB): Furthering the understanding and measurement of neurodevelopmental competence in preterm and full-term infants. *Mental Retardation and Developmental Disabilities Research Review*, *11*(1), 94–102. https://doi.org/10.1002/mrdd.20053

Ashby, B., & Bromberg, S. R. (2016). Infant mental health with high risk populations. *Newborn and Infant Nursing Reviews*, *16*(4), 269–273. https://doi.org/10.1053/j.nainr.2016.09.016

Askary Kachoosangy, R., Shafaroodi, N., Heidarzadeh, M., Qorbani, M., Bordbbr, A., Hejazi Shirmard, M., & Daneshjoo, F. (2020). Increasing mothers' confidence and ability by Creating Opportunities for Parent Empowerment (COPE): A randomized,

controlled trial. *Iranian Journal of Child Neurology, 14*(1), 77–83. https://www.ncbi.
   nlm.nih.gov/pmc/articles/PMC6956963/pdf/jcn-14-077.pdf

Boundy, E. O., Dastjerdi, R., Spiegelman, D., Fawzi, W. W., Missmer, S. A., Lieberman,
   E., & Chan, G. J. (2016). Kangaroo mother care and neonatal outcomes: A meta-
   analysis. *Pediatrics, 137*(1), e20152238. https://doi.org/10.1542/peds.2015-2238

Brazelton, T. B. (1978). The Brazelton Neonatal Behavior Assessment Scale: Introduction.
   Monographs of the Society for Research in Child Development, 43(5–6), 1–13.

Browne, J. V. (2020). Infant mental health in intensive care: Laying a foundation for
   social, emotional and mental health outcomes through regulation, relationships
   and reflection. *Journal of Neonatal Nursing, 27*(1), 33–39. https://doi.org/10.1016/
   j.jnn.2020.11.011

Browne, J. V., Jaeger, C. B., & Kenner, C. (2020). Executive summary: Standards,
   competencies, and recommended best practices for infant- and family-centered developmental care in the intensive care unit. *Journal of Perinatology, 40*(Suppl. 1),
   5–10. https://doi.org/10.1038/s41372-020-0767-1

Browne, J. V., Martinez, D., & Talmi, A. (2016). Infant mental health in the intensive
   care unit: Considerations for the infant, the family and the staff. *Newborn and Infant
   Nursing Reviews, 16*(4), 274–280. http://dx.doi.org/10.1053/j.nainr.2016.09.018

Browne, J. V., & Talmi, A. (2012). Developmental supports for newborns and young
   infants with special health and developmental needs and their families: The BABIES
   model. *Newborn and Infant Nursing Reviews, 12*(4), 239–247.

Browne, J. V., & Talmi, A. (2016). Reflections on infant mental health practice,
   policy, settings, and systems for fragile infants and their families from prenatal
   and intensive care through the transition home and to community. *Newborn
   and Infant Nursing Reviews, 16*(4), 255–257. http://dx.doi.org/10.1053/
   j.nainr.2016.09.014

Browne, J. V., & White, R. D. (2011). Foundations of developmental care. *Clinics in
   Perinatology, 38*(4), xv–xvii. https://doi.org/10.1016/j.clp.2011.09.001

Del Fabbro, A., & Cain, K. (2016). Infant mental health and family mental health issues. *Newborn and Infant Nursing Review, 16* (4), 281–284. https://doi.org/10.1053/
   j.nainr.2016.09.020

Graven, S. N. (1997). Clinical research data illuminating the relationship between the
   physical environment and patient medical outcomes. *Journal of Healthcare Design,
   9*, 15–19.

Hynan, M. T., & Hall, S. L. (2015). Psychosocial program standards for NICU parents.
   Journal of Perinatology, 35(Suppl. 1), S1–S4. https://doi.org/10.1038/jp.2015.141

Keating, K., Murphey, D., Daily, S., Ryberg, R., & Laurore, J. (2020). *Maternal and
   child health inequities emerge even before birth. State of Babies Yearbook 2020.* Zero
   To Three.

Kelly, J. F., & Barnard, K. E. (2000). Assessment of parent–child interaction: Implications
   for early intervention. In J. P. Shonkoff & S. J. Meisels (Eds.), *Handbook of early
   childhood intervention* (pp. 258–289). Cambridge University Press.

Lester, B. M., Tronick, E. Z., & Brazelton, T. B. (2004). The Neonatal Intensive Care
   Unit Network Neurobehavioral Scale procedures. *Pediatrics, 113*(3 Pt. 2), 641–667.
   http://www.ncbi.nlm.nih.gov/pubmed/14993524

McAnulty, G., Duffy, F. H., Kosta, S., Weisenfeld, N. I., Warfield, S. K., Butler, S. C., &
   Als, H. (2013). School-age effects of the Newborn Individualized Developmental

Care and Assessment Program for preterm infants with intrauterine growth restriction: Preliminary findings. *BMC Pediatrics, 13*, 25. https://doi.org/10.1186/1471-2431-13-25

McManus, B. M., & Nugent, J. K. (2014). A neurobehavioral intervention incorporated into a state early intervention program is associated with higher perceived quality of care among parents of high-risk newborns. *Journal of Behavioral Health Science & Research, 41*(3), 381–389. https://doi.org/10.1007/s11414-012-9283-1

Melnyk, B. M., Alpert-Gillis, L., Feinstein, N. F., Fairbanks, E., Schultz-Czarniak, J., Hust, D., Sherman, L., LeMoine, C., Moldenhauer, Z., Small, L., Bender, N., & Sinkin, R. A. (2001). Improving cognitive development of low-birth-weight premature infants with the COPE program: A pilot study of the benefit of early NICU intervention with mothers. *Research in Nursing & Health, 24*(5), 373–389. https://doi.org/10.1002/nur.1038

Murch, T. N., & Smith, V. C. (2016). Supporting families as they transition home. *Newborn and Infant Nursing Reviews, 16*(4), 298–302. https://doi.org/10.1053/j.nainr.2016.09.024

Noble, Y., & Boyd, R. (2012). Neonatal assessments for the preterm infant up to 4 months corrected age: A systematic review. *Developmental Medicine & Child Neurology, 54*(2), 129–139. https://doi.org/10.1111/j.1469-8749.2010.03903.x

Sammallahti, S., Heinonen, K., Andersson, S., Lahti, M., Pirkola, S., Lahti, J., & Raikkonen, K. (2017). Growth after late-preterm birth and adult cognitive, academic, and mental health outcomes. *Pediatric Research, 81*(5), 767–774. https://doi.org/10.1038/pr.2016.276

Saxton, S. N., Dempsey, A. G., Willis, T., Baughcum, A. E., Chavis, L., Hoffman, C., & Steinberg, Z. (2020). Essential knowledge and competencies for psychologists working in neonatal intensive care units. *Journal of Clinical Psychology in Medical Settings, 27*(4), 830–841. https://doi.org/10.1007/s10880-019-09682-8

Shonkoff, J. P. (2016). Capitalizing on advances in science to reduce the health consequences of early childhood adversity. *JAMA Pediatrics, 170*(10), 1003–1007. https://doi.org/10.1001/jamapediatrics.2016.1559

Smith, S., & Wollesen, L. (2004). *The new beginnings life skills development curriculum home visitors handbook* (2nd ed.). Brookes.

Talmi, A., Browne, J. V., & Smith-Sharp, S. (2004). *A professional's guide for reflective practice*. Center for Family & Infant Interaction, University of Colorado School of Medicine, Aurora, CO.

Van Hus, J. W., Jeukens-Visser, M., Koldewijn, K., Geldof, C. J., Kok, J. H., Nollet, F., & Van Wassenaer-Leemhuis, A. G. (2013). Sustained developmental effects of the infant behavioral assessment and intervention program in very low birth weight infants at 5.5 years corrected age. *Journal of Pediatrics, 162*(6), 1112–1119. https://doi.org/10.1016/j.jpeds.2012.11.078

Weatherston, D., & Browne, J. V. (2016). What is infant mental health and why is it important for high-risk infants and their families? *Newborn and Infant Nursing Reviews, 16*(4), 259–263.

Welch, M. G. (2016). Calming cycle theory: The role of visceral/autonomic learning in early mother and infant/child behaviour and development. *Acta Paediatrica, 105*(11), 1266–1274. https://doi.org/10.1111/apa.13547

Welch, M. G., Barone, J. L., Porges, S. W., Hane, A. A., Kwon, K. Y., Ludwig, R. J., &
    Myers, M. M. (2020). Family nurture intervention in the NICU increases autonomic
    regulation in mothers and children at 4–5 years of age: Follow-up results from a
    randomized controlled trial. *PLoS One*, *15*(8), e0236930. https://doi.org/10.1371/
    journal.pone.0236930

Welch, M. G., Firestein, M. R., Austin, J., Hane, A. A., Stark, R. I., Hofer, M. A., Garland,
    M., Glickstein, S. B., Brunelli, S. A., Ludwig, R. J., & Myers, M. M. (2015). Family
    nurture intervention in the neonatal intensive care unit improves social-relatedness,
    attention, and neurodevelopment of preterm infants at 18 months in a randomized
    controlled trial. *Journal of Child Psychology and Psychiatry*, *56*(11), 1202–1211.
    https://doi.org/10.1111/jcpp.12405

White, R. D. (2020). Recommended standards for newborn ICU design, 9th edi-
    tion. *Journal of Perinatology Supplement*, *40*, 2–4. https://doi.org/10.1038/s41
    372-020-0766-2

Zeanah, P. D., Stafford, B., & Zeanah, C. H. (2005). *Clinical interventions to enhance
    infant mental health: A selective review*. National Center for Infant and Early
    Childhood Health Policy at UCLA.

23

UNCERTAINTY AND COPING IN THE NICU

RELATIONSHIPS MATTER

ZINA STEINBERG AND SUSAN KRAEMER ■

The core predicament of medicine—the thing that makes being a patient so wrenching . . . —is uncertainty. . . . Medicine's ground state is uncertainty. And wisdom—for both the patients and doctors—is defined by how one copes with it.

—ATUL GAWANDE (2002, p. 229)

CASE EXAMPLE

It all started with the 20-week ultrasound. We got to the doctor's office filled with anticipation. We had tried so hard to have this baby: five rounds of IVF [in vitro fertilization], injections, drugs. There were miscarriages—one really late at 15 weeks. We would go through times of hope and then we would tumble into darkness. Finally, we let ourselves believe that we were actually going to have a baby. Never did we imagine that the ultrasound would tell us this! We were now thrown into a scary world of neonatal intensive care and newborn heart surgery! So many decisions and once again, so much that we won't know. I'm worn out. I guess you could say that I am just holding on.

—*NICU parent*

Elevated levels of emotional distress in neonatal intensive care unit (NICU) parents are now widely and uniformly reported (Davis et al., 2003; Staver et al., 2021).

Parents' instincts to hold, cuddle, caress, and bounce their infant are thwarted because their infant is often connected to machines with tubes, wires, and monitors that often restrict parental access. Nurses and doctors demonstrate expertise and exude confidence; some parents are befuddled and silenced; some are terrified, challenged, and challenging.

An infant may enter the NICU for several reasons—preterm birth, peripartum complications, or congenital abnormalities. Indeed, preterm birth is a leading cause of infant mortality and morbidity. Mild, moderate, and severe disability and congenital anomalies often require immediate and subsequent surgeries or complicated treatment protocols. Parents of preterm and full-term infants needing intensive care face uncertain futures. The taken-for-granted expectations of parenthood have been shattered, and parents are catapulted into the alien and medicalized world of the NICU, where uncertainty is a given and even small changes in an infant's health can trigger a crisis (Lasiuk et al., 2013). In addition, racial and ethnic disparities are evidenced in the NICU, as they are in medical care in general (Givrad et al., 2021). Becoming a parent in the NICU thus presents great challenges to mental health.

This chapter focuses on how the shock of upended expectations along with sustained uncertainty challenge parents as they work valiantly to cope with fetal abnormality diagnoses and/or giving birth to an infant in need of intensive care. Central importance is placed on enhancing the relationships in the NICU that form an intersecting and resilience fostering web supporting the parent–infant dyad. Additional focus is on the role of the mental health professional in encouraging and guiding these relationships. Helping parents experience their daily value to their infant mitigates parents' vulnerability, helplessness, and powerlessness. Providing parents with a relationship with a mental health worker who is not involved in medical decision-making frees parents to voice feelings of ambivalence and even regret. Supporting parents in their relationship with staff (and encouraging and bolstering staff in turn) counters parental feelings of isolation and leads to greater confidence and competence.

Uncertainty is worse than all.

—A. DUMAS (1894/1922, p. 105)

Uncertainty is woven into the fabric of life, yet it is mostly pushed out of consciousness. Neurobiologists and neuroendocrinologists have begun to assert that the theoretical underpinning of stress is uncertainty. When the brain cannot reduce uncertainty, the individual's "allostatic load" is burdened, leading to such symptoms as impaired memory and cognition, lack of control, and cardiovascular and cerebrovascular events (Peters et al., 2017). Emotional responses (heightened anxiety and depression) are activated that further damage the individual's ability to cope with uncertainty. Birth is often accompanied by some uncertainty and preoccupation, but most parents are filled with expectant anticipation and fantasies of a hopeful future. Donald Winnicott (1956), in theorizing about normal maternal development, understood this postpartum time to entail a psychic shift that he called "primary maternal preoccupation," in which the new mother exhibits an intense protectiveness and vigilance. At times, this normative state shifts to a level of worry that can become all-consuming. When this newborn period has been preceded by difficulties getting pregnant followed by rounds of assisted reproductive technology in which each trial yields only an approximate 39% chance of pregnancy for women younger than age 35 years and 11% for women older than age 40 years (Centers for Disease Control and Prevention, 2013), or by perinatal loss (Campbell-Jackson & Horsch, 2014; Robertson Blackmore et al., 2011), confidence about a certain imagined future is elusive. Similarly, when genetic testing or a 20-week ultrasound has revealed congenital abnormalities that signal a more complex medical picture or an uncertain future, finding a way to and through this normal maternal preoccupation can be treacherous. Preoccupation with one's ill newborn means continually re-engaging with the possible trauma as well as feelings of helplessness, inadequacy, and vulnerability. These may lead a parent to feel anxiety, depression, guilt, and shame. Postpartum depression (PPD), anxiety, and acute stress disorder (precursors of post-traumatic stress) are documented at worrisome levels; for some, this can extend well into and even beyond the first postpartum year. Lefkowitz et al. (2010) found acute stress disorder in 35% of mothers and 24% of fathers at 3–5 days post NICU admission, and the percentage was higher if subclinical acute stress disorder symptoms was considered. Post-traumatic stress disorder (PTSD) at 30 days post admission was found in 15% of mothers and 8% of fathers, and again, the percentage increased when subclinical levels were recognized. PPD (including subsyndromal PPD) at 30 days post admission was found in approximately 56% of mothers, and one-third of mothers reported suicidal thoughts and 16% of mothers met the criteria for both PPD and PTSD. Some studies have followed parents post discharge. For example, Gerstein et al. (2019) found that at 5 years post discharge, 14% of mothers were depressed and NICU stress and depression independently predicted negative and intrusive parenting behaviors when the child was 5 years old. This confirms results of other studies that demonstrate that early maternal depression has a negative impact on early parent–child relationships (Field, 2010).

The sustained uncertainty that can cloak many families in the NICU may have begun much earlier with struggles around infertility and may continue for months or years after discharge to home (Lasiuk et al., 2013). There may be ongoing questions of neurological status, respiratory fragility, developmental delays, and levels of chronic care that can be emotionally and financially draining, all disrupting the parents' fundamental assumptions and expectations about themselves and their futures. The concept of "ambiguous loss," first described by Boss (1999) as the limbo state of loss experienced by families of Vietnam missing-in-action soldiers, has also been used to capture the state of prolonged uncertainty experienced by some NICU parents (Golish & Powell, 2003). It describes a state of grief in which there is a significant loss, but the person is alive. In the NICU, the parents have a live child and are encouraged to focus on the infant's care, but this may leave them feeling unseen in the grief they may experience in not being able to take their infant home and also alone with all the uncertainty and anxiety surrounding the hospitalization.

Research has demonstrated that uncertainty in illness can lead to an inability to determine the meaning of illness-related events and occurs in situations in which medical providers and patients are unable to assign definite values to events and/or are unable to accurately predict outcomes (Mishel & Braden, 1988). In more complex NICU stays, there are long periods of uncertainty about both the course of treatment and the overall outcome. Parents talk about the NICU experience as riding a roller coaster that rarely stops. Ambiguity regarding the illness, complex treatment protocols, inadequate information, and unpredictability about the course of the illness are dimensions of this uncertainty. Prognostic uncertainty is particularly destabilizing. When this uncertainty is foregrounded, parents' expectations and confidence can be severely challenged. In the case example at the beginning of this chapter, after multiple trials of in vitro fertilization and several miscarriages, an ambiguous finding on a 20-week scan suggests that the fetus may need neonatal stabilization and cardiac surgery soon after birth. The parents in this example, already shaped by the ordeal of multiple losses, now brace for more. Will their infant survive to term? Will their infant need the neonatal surgery? Survive the surgery? Will their infant fully recover? And how long will it be before they will be able to hold him, feed him? Once home, how will they manage that first winter season of common colds? Home nursing or medical daycare may need to be incorporated and managed. Financial considerations might become paramount. Parents may experience a lack of agency, a heightened state of arousal, and a feeling of constant threat. In addition, parents may begin to feel increasingly alienated, even exiled, from their friends and families as the trajectories of their lives propel them in new and unwanted directions (Wilson & Cook, 2018).

CASE EXAMPLE: BED REST—A STILL BODY, AN AGITATED MIND

"Babies come easily in my family," whispered Patty, a 36-year-old exhausted new mom,

> But not for me. So, we began rounds of IVF. Two rounds, nothing, then I got pregnant, but I miscarried at 19 weeks. Then finally, I was pregnant with triplets. The doctors, armed with data, strongly encouraged us to reduce to two embryos. We struggled with that—after all, we had such a hard time getting pregnant. But they told us about the potential problems of multiple births, and we followed their guidance. The horrible part is that we couldn't tell my parents—to them this was an abortion—so I had to keep the reduction a secret. But now, these two little babies born at 27 weeks are so fragile

and hooked up to machines. One of them is really sick and I don't know if he'll make it. At 24 weeks I started to have labor pains and was put on hospital bed rest. That really sucked. We were scared. I thought endlessly about the baby that we reduced and the miscarriage at 19 weeks, those "almost" babies. I was racked with jealousy towards women that were complaining about their baby's colic. On bed rest, I incessantly wondered if God is punishing me, you know, that reduction. Nurses, while on bed rest and now, tell me to take it one day at a time. But for years I have felt at the edge of a cliff. I wonder what's wrong with me, with my body, why I am failing as a female and no one can tell me what will happen next.

Patty was 24 weeks pregnant when she was put on hospital bed rest. She brings a particularly challenging, though not unique, story to bed rest: multiples trials of IVF, miscarriage, fetal reduction. But even women with far less complicated courses who are placed on bed rest find themselves with anxious minds googling about all the things that might go wrong; they are grappling with uncertainty. In addition, some might be leaving at home other children. This unborn child, she might secretly think, is pulling her away from her known and loved children. And then financial worries might erupt. For many families in the United States, each day of leave from work taken prenatally is a family-leave day taken away from being home with the baby post-birth. Bed rest is not stress-free.

Pregnant mothers and the soon-to-be fathers—those on bed rest and those easily carrying to term—have already started to build a relationship in their thoughts with their unborn children. Reveries and fantasies, hopes, dreams, expectations, and fears become more elaborated from between 4 and 7 months of gestation (Benoit et al., 1997). When the pregnancy ends prematurely, this crucial process of psychological preparation for infants is often short-circuited.

Attachment between mother and infant begins even before birth. Attachment representations that help shape the dyadic relationship between the infant and the mother are affected by the mother's perceptions of her infant's personality and behaviors, and her perception of her relationship with her infant, all of which begin prenatally. Mothers of preterm infants are less likely than mothers of term infants to have "balanced/integrated" attachment representations entailing a well-organized sense of the fetus (Forcada-Guex et al., 2011). In mother–infant interaction studies, many of these mothers may show less positive affective involvement and communication. The infants, neurologically immature, appear more withdrawn and "low-keyed" and are less able to effectively communicate their needs compared to full-term infants (Clark et al., 2008). Mothers, to compensate, may become more intrusive and controlling (Crawford & Benoit, 2009, Hall et al., 2015). Mothers with high PTSD and depressive symptoms are also more likely to have distorted/ambivalent representations of their infant, which are associated with less positive behavioral outcomes (Forcada-Guex et al., 2011; Hall et al., 2015).

INFORMED CONSENT IN THE FACE OF UNCERTAINTY

Often under conditions of grave uncertainty and heightened anxiety, parents are asked to share in medical decision-making. When premature labor begins at 24 weeks (considered the edge of viability) or a profound fetal diagnosis presents earlier on, the medical team meets with the parents to present its findings, to offer recommendations, and to invite parents to participate in shared decision-making (Haward et al., 2017). Parents may be confronted with complex information, probability-filled statistics and medical terminology, which in the context of heightened stress may make these conversations quite fraught. To enable parents to cope with what is asked of them, this communication of risks needs to be built on a foundation of trust, which in turn depends on a genuine interest in the past experiences and current feelings of the parents, including their subjective interpretations of decisional outcomes, their tolerance of risk and uncertainty, and other personal factors. A prenatal consult needs to attend to the capacity of the parent(s) to digest information and ask questions and needs to be scanning for the parent's emotional state. Dissociative features such as numbness, flatness, and/or staring off are signals for the medical provider to talk less and to ask and listen more. Or, as Karkowsky (2020), a maternal fetal medicine physician, writes, "Sometimes . . . more information doesn't enrich us; it can beggar us. I had to learn the hard way" (p. 54), "Informed consent is a relationship" (p. 176). With probabilities and statistical risks weighing on them, parents-to-be may be susceptible to misinterpreting off-hand comments, and tensions can build with family and friends and even hospital staff. Ideally, a NICU psychologist or other qualified behavioral health clinician can be available to help the parent at this vulnerable time.

The NICU: A World Apart

> My wife got pregnant with our 6- and 8-year-olds and I never thought much about it. We were a family. This time with IVF . . . not so easy. Now I've passed through a secret wall—you know those walls that you touch and they magically open and another world appears. This is a "not real" but "so real" world and suddenly we are in it. I'm trying to be strong, but man, this is hard.
>
> —*NICU father*

There is no doubt that uncertainty stalks the corridors of the NICU. Parents may be told that it can be an "unsettling" experience—a roller coaster of feelings—but few feel prepared for what they will find. They are not prepared after the birth to leave the hospital without an infant or to know what to say to friends and family, who in turn may not know what to say to them. And if this is their first child, they really do not recognize themselves with a transformed identity as new parents: "I heard the nurse say 'Mommy,' and I looked around to see who she may have been talking to. Mommy? When did that happen? It was so jarring" (NICU mom). The daily uncertainties make coping a challenge. New problems occur without warning. New acronyms must be mastered—PVL, IVH, NEC, ROP—and feelings about these diagnoses contained. Even when an infant is a "feeder and grower," there are bad days, and going home can feel far away.

Offering anticipatory guidance to help emotionally prepare expectant parents for the NICU and psychoeducation once parents are in the NICU is of great value. Examples include the following:

- Preparing parents for what it might feel like to go home after birth without their infant. Said one parent, "I felt so empty; so hollowed out. What happened, I cried. Who am I?"
- Coping with the uncomfortable feelings and statements of family and friends. For example, "My friend didn't know whether to say 'Congratulations' or 'I'm sorry' and I didn't know what to say to her."
- Acknowledging with parents that the learning curve is steep: "They talk in this medical jargon. At first, I got dizzy and words seemed garbled. It was as if I was underwater."
- Educating parents on how the NICU is staffed: nurses, attendings, residents, and fellows. It is especially important to help parents understand the rotations of staff and that even when primary nurses and advanced practice providers are assigned, there will still be multiple people, each with a distinct personality, to interact with and adjust to. "I feel flooded. So many people speaking to me quickly and in a lingo that goes over my head. And when there is always a new nurse, I am afraid to leave my baby and go home."
- Recognizing with parents that the NICU roller coaster is not just a good day and then a bad day; it can feel devastating: "I choose to go on a roller coaster. I didn't choose this and that makes a world of difference."
- Explaining the importance of regular visiting, even when difficult: "I felt empty, tired, and depressed sitting by the isolette. The nurse seemed so busy and competent, and I was all thumbs. Then she came over and showed me the best ways to touch my baby. And she said that maybe soon, I would be able to hold him! She made me feel like there was something important that I could do."
- Alerting parents that the bed side nurse is a valuable team member: "I walked in, and no one said hello. I gulped and made myself go over to the isolette. Finally, I smiled and asked her how her morning was—like in a friendly way—and she seemed relieved to chat. What a difference that made. I never imagined that she would be shy and even afraid of me! That was the beginning of being a team."

- Educating parents about the powerful intervention of skin-to-skin (kangaroo care) for both infant and parent and their relationship: "I was scared to let the nurse put him on my chest; he is so tiny. But she encouraged me. It was magic. I cried but it was with an enormous smile. For the first time I felt like a mom."

- Forewarning parents about how uncertainty and its attendant stresses often yield miscommunication and misunderstandings: "After this meeting with the doctor about the brain bleed, I called my husband and he shot one question after another at me. The doctor didn't know what would happen next, but my husband kept thinking that I hadn't asked the right questions, or I hadn't understood, or I hadn't listened. It was horrible."

- Encouraging parents to ask for help: "Friends ask, 'What can I do?' and at first it got me angry. You mean I have to tell you what you can do? Then desperate, I asked a friend to pick up my 3-year-old. I was surprised that she was relieved to know what I needed."

It is important to normalize any encounters with a mental health professional, especially a psychologist. Psychologists can introduce themselves saying that they meet *all* the new parents and are happy to meet them and their infant, perhaps taking the moment to join with the parent in noticing and admiring their infant. A psychologist should let parents know that the hospital recognizes that the NICU is a difficult place to be, how they can be contacted, and that they look forward to getting to know the parents.

In the NICU, the relationships with the medical and nursing providers matter mightily, and the psychologist can support these providers in developing their relationships with the parent.

Nurses, in particular, can sustain a parent through the weeks of roller-coaster medical crises and prolonged uncertainty. Steinberg and Patterson (2017) describe the nurse as an "emotional umbilical cord," maintaining the lifeline between mother and NICU infant. Davis and colleagues (2003) identified an inverse relationship between depressive symptoms among NICU mothers and experiencing support from nursing staff. A 1-point decrease in nursing support as perceived by the parent increased the risk of depression by 6%.

The psychologist can play a vital role keeping the history of each family in mind through the rotating shifts of medical providers. When the psychologist can make connections for the medical staff, particularly the nurse, the staff is better able to help the parents. A psychologist might notice a father watching the nurse, new to this family, as if waiting for the nurse to make a mistake and even hurt his infant, who is a surviving twin. By talking about the family's loss, the psychologist helps the nurse appreciate, understand, and be less reactive to the father's mistrust, fear, and vigilance.

Often, however, staff rotations make trusting relationships between parents and NICU medical and nursing staff difficult. There are also indications that racial and class inequities play out in nursing assignments (Sigurdson et al., 2020).

Even when the culture of the NICU prioritizes team consistency, parents may find themselves trying to get to know several different staff each week. Steinberg and Patterson (2017) documented that in one Level IV NICU, infants and families interacted with between 27 and 53 nurses and 15 doctors in 1 month. Six years later, after primary nursing was instituted, these numbers were still high, with an average of 18–37 nurses and 15 doctors monthly, which can be quite daunting for parents. The rotation of neonatologists can particularly affect the consistency of information, which can be another major hurdle to a parent's comfort.

Going Home: The Third Crisis

Everyone says I should be happy now, that I should stop worrying. But going home is scary. Is she really ready? She did turn blue last week. Remember?

—NICU parent

It is said that giving birth early or learning of a prenatal diagnosis is the first crisis, admission to the NICU is the second, and going home is the third. This comes as a great surprise to NICU parents who have watched other parents say tearful goodbyes to medical and nursing staff and wondered when they would be able to carry their infant in the car seat out of the hospital. Many are shocked to discover their fear as the day of discharge approaches.

The emotions that accompany uncertainty are fully aroused again when parents leave the NICU with their infant (White et al., 2017). No doctors and nurses at the ready. No monitors and alarms to alert them to difficulty. Only themselves. It is wished-for, lonely, and frightening. Parents are already emotionally depleted and now find themselves preoccupied about their ability to keep their infant safe and about rehospitalizations, cognitive and motor delays, and long-term sequelae. Questions that they were too afraid to ask before now take hold in their minds—fearful questions about the future. The anxiety and depression that burdened parents during the NICU stay now shadow the joyous homecoming. These emotions and preoccupations surrounding all the uncertainties can interfere with the relationship they build with their infant. Parents may find themselves alert to every ache and wheeze, convinced that their infant is urgently ill.

Research on children with previous medical ailments showed that parents of these once ill children tend to view them as vulnerable even when there is no longer a medical need. Termed "parental perception of child vulnerability," this tendency correlates with compromised developmental outcomes at 1 year and is associated with behavior problems and more somatic and internalizing symptoms at age 3 years (de Ocampo et al., 2003). In addition, research documents that these families are frequent users of medical emergency departments (Chambers et al., 2011). A NICU psychologist can prepare parents for this probable upsurge in focus on all the uncertainties and can alert them to the likelihood of anniversary reactions and viewing the child as more vulnerable than the child is in reality.

MITIGATING CHALLENGES TO COPING ACROSS SETTINGS

Although the omnipresent fact of uncertainty can neither be underestimated nor swept away, parents' coping skills can be increased and their resilience enhanced. By paying particular attention to the issues discussed in this section, psychologists can help mitigate the challenges to coping.

Focus on Relationships

Relationships are a bulwark against the potential trauma that lurks as parents receive jarring results of genetic tests or anatomical ultrasounds or as they sit by the isolette in the NICU (National Scientific Council on the Developing Child, 2004). NICU care needs to be relationship-based, with the parent–infant relationship at its core. This relationship focus is in tension with the practice of many critical care units in which infants, some say of necessity, are separated from their mothers (Flacking et al., 2012).

As noted previously, postpartum mood and anxiety disorders can have a negative effect on the mother–infant and mother–child relationship going forward. Toxic stress occurs in the absence of protective parental support, and parents who are depressed or highly anxious may need help to be the nurturing parent that they so wish to be. Focusing on the parent–infant relationship in the NICU and on the central bolstering relationships in the parents' lives can have a long-lasting effect on the child's development. The psychologist keeps a laser focus on the parent's relationship to the staff—particularly the nurse—noting the ways in which this vital relationship can be stabilizing or derailing. Paying close attention to the intersecting webs of relationships encircling the parent–infant relationship helps counteract the strong forces of fragmentation that exist in medical intensive care settings.

Kangaroo Care

One of the main ways to focus on both the parent–infant relationship and the physiological needs of the infant is by insistently and consistently advocating for kangaroo care (i.e., skin-to-skin). The evidence is ample that kangaroo care offers multiple benefits to the growing NICU infant and to the relationship between the parent and the infant (Boundy et al., 2016; Feldman et al., 2014). Parents report "finally feeling like a mom" and they cry tears of joy. Yet, the encouraging of kangaroo care can be uneven despite the evidence for its efficacy (Morelius & Anderson, 2015; Penn, 2015). In addition, kangaroo care may suffer the fault lines of racial bias, with Black and Hispanic families less encouraged to provide this for their infants (Sigurdson et al., 2020). The psychologist working with the parent and the nurse can help each feel more comfortable and rewarded by kangaroo care.

SILENT CRISIS

Some parents rarely visit their infant in the NICU; some do not visit at all. Some question doctors and nurses endlessly and challengingly; some never ask anything. Psychologists can pay attention to what is not there—the silent crisis. A parent may live too far away to visit or have other children to care for, but it also may be something more difficult to notice. Perhaps the family has experienced unconscious bias in the NICU, making them feel unwelcome (Givrad et al., 2021), or perhaps the parent is too depressed or anxious. She may feel that she is bad for the infant, that the infant's prematurity is her fault and she better stay away. Or others may be telling her—verbally or nonverbally—that she is "in the way" when she visits. Perhaps the infant turned blue while she was last holding him and she has not visited since. Avoidance is a symptom of PTSD. Although it is difficult to keep in mind the parents who are rarely in the NICU or, for example, are reluctant to hold their infant, research suggests the importance of reaching out to these parents and being curious about their experience. Lower maternal visitation rate predicts higher maternal depression at infants' 4-month corrected age (Greene et al., 2015). Increased visiting leads to defined neurobehavioral differences between the infants visited and held more often and those who were not, with better quality of movement, less arousal, and less stress for the infants visited and held more (Reynolds et al., 2013).

Assessing the Family: Bear Witness to a Traumatic Reproductive History

> Doesn't anyone care what I went through? Won't anyone listen?
> —*NICU parent*

Each encounter a psychologist has with parents is a relationship-building moment, even when the psychologist is assessing the family and their social supports. The initial assessment and subsequent encounters represent opportunities for parents to begin to review the history of their reproductive trials, their dashed hopes, their losses, and their tentative joys; it is a way to begin to heal the ruptures, create coherence out of chaos, and author a new narrative. Making meaning of this period of their lives is an essential step in moving forward and finding enhanced strength for the uncertain future ahead. The psychologist is performing the vital function of bearing witness to parents' experiences, giving them meaning. To this end, the assessment might include the following questions:

- Are there family members that you are not telling about the NICU admission?

- Have there been other NICU infants in your family?
- What do you know about how that infant fared?
- Are there stories or hints of stories in your family of ill infants? Stories of neonatal losses? Children with significant developmental delays?
- Have there been recent medical crises in your family?
- Are there stories of medical errors that haunt your family?
- How was your pregnancy, emotionally?
- How did you react when you first saw your baby?
- Do you feel that your baby knows you? Do you or did you feel that your baby did not really belong to you?
- How has this been for your partner? Your children? Others in your family?

Attend to the Medical and Nursing Providers

Emotionally aroused families can act in ways that may be misunderstood by staff. Psychologists can help the nurse feel more comfortable "chatting" (Fenwick et al., 2001) and developing a team relationship with the parents. Some nurses do this naturally, some need more coaching, and still others have their own past experiences that make this difficult. Psychologists can be curious about nurses' and doctors' perceptions and observations and listen to their stories with the goal of helping them reflect on their own reactivity (Steinberg & Kraemer, 2010). In addition, doctors and nurses are also vulnerable to the traumatic tensions of the NICU and are at risk of compassion fatigue and/or burnout if needed structural and psychological support is absent (Cricco-Lizza, 2014).

IDEAS WORTH SHARING

- Meet, whenever possible, with both parents, or the mother and her support person. Ongoing communication reduces parental stress and anxiety, and it increases confidence and sense of agency.
- Help parents find ways to support each other, even if their current ways of coping seem discordant. Validate each person's coping style. Help parents tolerate the confused feelings of the other.
- Allow room for and bear witness to parents' grief—the shattered expectations of a "perfect pregnancy" and "perfect" infant.
- Allow for and normalize shifting emotional states—for example, grief/joy, acceptance/denial, control/helplessness, and hopefulness/despair.
- Educate parents about the prevalence, risk factors, and symptoms of postpartum mood and anxiety disorders and why getting help matters.
- Help parents understand that their self-identities are undergoing profound disruption—that events have overturned their fundamental assumptions about themselves and the world.

- Pay close attention to parents' stories of infertility and assisted reproductive technology. Ask about former pregnancies, abortions, miscarriages, stillbirths, and medically recommended reductions.
- Be interested and willing to meet with other family members, particularly the infant's grandparents.
- Learn about other medical crises and experiences with chronic illness and disability in families.
- Ask about their other children.
- Encourage parents to find ways to connect with friends and family, recognizing that guilt, self-blame, shame, and jealousy may be barriers.
- Pay attention to what is *not* there, the "silent crisis"—parents not being present or asking few questions. Be curious as to why.
- Help medical staff understand the social and emotional context of this particular family, especially their reproductive history and traumatic events involving loss/disability and possible past medical errors.
- Keep in mind that there is a complex intersection of race, gender, immigration status, poverty, and health care, and this can be seen in obstetrical care and in the NICU, adding to the uncertainties that families face.
- Recognize that non-heteronormative family configurations (e.g., two moms, two dads, surrogates, and donor eggs) can heighten sensitivities that may breed communication difficulties, undermining relationships with staff.
- Help nurses appreciate their vital role as an "emotional umbilical cord"— a lifeline between infant and mother.
- Be prepared to answer forthrightly questions about the NICU and tailor information to the specific family. If feasible, have the expectant parents tour the NICU prior to birth or provide an orientation upon admission.

CONCLUSION

The mental health challenges surrounding the uncertainties of prenatal diagnoses, maternal complications (e.g., bed rest), prematurity, the NICU, and beyond are serious. And for some, it is proceeded by a rocky reproductive course, leaving the parent highly vulnerable. Yet, the primal need to protect and love one's newborn prevails, and the continual striving to be a good parent makes the role of a NICU psychologist endlessly rewarding. The evidence is unequivocal that relationships are a vital protective force against toxic stress and trauma and that they are a foundational necessity for the emotional, social, and cognitive development of the child. Despite all the profound uncertainties NICU families face, it is certain that the prioritization of relationships—with the parent–infant relationship at the center—in the fetal care center, the NICU, and follow-up clinics needs to be ethical bedrock (Steinberg & Patterson, 2017).

REFERENCES

Benoit, D., Parker, K. C., & Zeanah, C. H. (1997). Mothers' representations of their infants assessed prenatally: Stability and association with infants' attachment classifications. *Journal of Child Psychology and Psychiatry, 38*(3), 307–313.

Boss, P. (1999). *Ambiguous loss.* Harvard University Press.

Boundy, E. O., Dastjerdi, R., Spiegelman, D., Fawzi, W. W., Missmer, S. A., Lieberman, E., Kajeepeta, S., Wall, S., & Chan, G. J. (2016). Kangaroo mother care and neonatal outcomes: A meta-analysis. *Pediatrics, 137*(1), e20152238.

Campbell-Jackson, L., & Horsch, A. (2014). The psychological impact of stillbirth on women: A systematic review. *Illness, Crisis, & Loss, 22*(3), 237–256.

Centers for Disease Control and Prevention, American Society for Reproductive Medicine, and Society for Assisted Reproductive Technology. (2015). *2013 Assisted reproductive technology fertility clinic success rates report.* U.S. Department of Health and Human Services.

Chambers, P. L., Mahabee-Gittens, E. M., & Leonard, A. C. (2011). Vulnerable child syndrome, parental perception of child vulnerability, and emergency department usage. *Pediatric Emergency Care, 27*(11), 1009–1013.

Clark, C. A., Woodward, L. J., Horwood, L. J., & Moor, S. (2008). Development of emotional and behavioral regulation in children born extremely preterm and very preterm: Biological and social influences. *Child Development, 79*(5), 1444–1462.

Crawford, A., & Benoit, D. (2009). Caregivers' disrupted representations of the unborn child predict later infant–caregiver disorganized attachment and disrupted interactions. *Infant Mental Health Journal, 30*(2), 124–144.

Cricco-Lizza, R. (2014). The need to nurse the nurse: Emotional labor in neonatal intensive care. *Qualitative Health Research, 24*(5), 615–628.

Davis, L., Edwards, H., Mohay, H., & Wollin, J. (2003). The impact of very premature birth on the psychological health of mothers. *Early Human Development, 73*(1–2), 61–70.

de Ocampo, A. C., Macias, M. M., Saylor, C. F., & Katikaneni, L. D. (2003). Caretaker perception of child vulnerability predicts behavior problems in NICU graduates. *Child Psychiatry and Human Development, 34*(2), 83–96.

Dumas, A. (1922). *The Count of Monteo Cristo.* Huntington Smith. (Original work published 1894)

Feldman, R., Rosenthal, Z., & Eidelman, A. I. (2014). Maternal–preterm skin-to-skin contact enhances child physiologic organization and cognitive control across the first 10 years of life. *Biological Psychiatry, 75*(1), 56–64.

Fenwick, J., Barclay, L., & Schmied, V. (2001). "Chatting": An important clinical tool in facilitating mothering in neonatal nurseries. *Journal of Advanced Nursing, 33*(5), 583–593.

Field, T. (2010). Postpartum depression effects in early interactions. *Infant Behavior and Development, 33*(1), 1–6.

Flacking, R., Lehtonen, L., Thomson, G., Axelin, A., Ahlqvist, S., Moran, V. H., Ewald, U., & Dykes, F. (2012). Closeness and separation in neonatal intensive care. *Acta Paediatrica, 101,* 1032–1037.

Forcada-Guex, M., Borghini, A., Pierrehumbert, B., Ansermet, F., & Muller-Nix, C. (2011). Prematurity, maternal posttraumatic stress and consequences on the mother–infant relationship. *Early Human Development, 87*(1), 21–26.

Gawande, A. (2002). *Complications: Notes from the life of a young surgeon.* Metropolitan.

Gerstein, E. D., Njoroge, W., Paul, R. A., Smyser, C. D., & Rogers, C. E. (2019). Maternal depression and stress in the neonatal intensive care unit: Associations with mother–child interactions at age 5 years. *Journal of the American Academy of Child and Adolescent Psychiatry, 58*(3), 350–358.e2.

Givrad, S., Dowtin, L. L., Scala, M., & Hall, S. L. (2021). Recognizing and mitigating infant distress in neonatal intensive care unit. *Journal of Neonatal Nursing, 27,* 14–20.

Golish, T. D., & Powell, K. A. (2003). "Ambiguous loss": Managing the dialectics of grief associated with premature birth. *Journal of Social and Personal Relationships, 20*(3), 309–334.

Greene, M. M., Rossman, B., Patra, K., Kratovil, A., Khan, S., & Meier, P. P. (2015). Maternal psychological distress and visitation to the neonatal intensive care unit. *Acta Paediatrica, 104*(7), e306–e313.

Hall, R. A. S., Hoffenkamp, H. N., Tooten, A., Braeken, J., Vingerhoets, A. J. J. M., & van Bakel, H. J. A. (2015). Longitudinal associations between maternal disrupted representations, maternal interactive behaviour and infant attachment: A comparison between full-term and preterm dyads. *Child Psychiatry & Human Development, 46,* 320–331.

Haward, M. F., Gaucher, N., Payot, A., Robson, K., & Janvier, A. (2017). Personalized decision making: Practical recommendations for antenatal counseling for fragile neonates. *Clinics in Perinatology, 44*(2), 429–445.

Karkowsky, C. E. (2020). *High risk: Stories of pregnancy, birth and the unexpected.* Norton.

Lasiuk, G. C., Comeau, T., & Newburn-Cook, C. (2013). Unexpected: An interpretive description of parental traumas associated with preterm birth. *BMC Pregnancy and Childbirth, 13*(Suppl. 1), S13.

Lefkowitz, D. S., Baxt, C., & Evans, J. R. (2010). Prevalence and correlates of posttraumatic stress and postpartum depression in parents of infants in the neonatal intensive care unit (NICU). *Journal of Clinical Psychology in Medical Settings, 17*(3), 230–237.

Mishel, M. H., & Braden, C. J. (1988). Finding meaning: Antecedents of uncertainty in illness. *Nursing Research, 37*(2), 98–103.

Morelius, E., & Anderson, G. C. (2015). Neonatal nurses' beliefs about almost continuous parent–infant skin-to-skin contact in neonatal intensive care. *Journal of Clinical Nursing, 24*(17–18), 2620–2627.

National Scientific Council on the Developing Child. (2004). *Young children develop in an environment of relationships* (Working Paper No. 1).

Penn, S. (2015). Overcoming the barriers to using kangaroo care in neonatal settings. *Nursing Child Young People, 27*(5), 22–27.

Peters, A., McEwen, B., & Friston, K. (2017). Uncertainty and stress: Why it causes diseases and how it is mastered by the brain. *Progress in Neurobiology, 156,* 164–188.

Reynolds, L. C., Duncan, M. M., Smith, G. C., Mathur, A., Neil, J., Inder, T., & Pineda, R. G. (2013). Parental presence and holding in the neonatal intensive care unit and associations with early neurobehavior. *Journal of Perinatology, 33*(8), 636–641.

Robertson Blackmore, E., Côté-Arsenault, D., Tang, W., Glover, V., Evans, J., Golding, J., & O'Connor, T. G. (2011). Previous prenatal loss as a predictor of perinatal depression and anxiety. *British Journal of Psychiatry, 198*(5), 373–378.

Sigurdson, K., Profit, J., Dhurjati, R., Morton, C., Scala, M., Vernon, L., Randolph, A., Phan, J., & Franck, L. (2020). Former NICU families describe gaps in family-centered care. *Qualitative Health Research, 30*(12), 1861–1875.

Staver, M., Moore, T., & Hanna, K. (2021). An integrative review of maternal distress during neonatal intensive care hospitalization. *Archives of Women's Mental Health, 24*(2), 217–229. doi:10.1007/s00737-020-01063-7

Steinberg, Z., & Kraemer, S. (2010). Cultivating a culture of awareness: Nurturing reflective practices in the NICU. *Zero to Three, 31*(2), 15–21.

Steinberg, Z., & Patterson, C. (2017). Giving voice to the psychological in the NICU: A relational model. *Journal of Infant, Child, and Adolescent Psychotherapy, 16*(1), 25–44.

White, Z., Gilstrap, C., & Hull, J. (2017). "Me against the world": Parental uncertainty management at home following neonatal intensive care unit discharge. *Journal of Family Communication, 17*(2), 105–116.

Wilson, C., & Cook, C. (2018). Ambiguous loss and post-traumatic growth: Experiences of mothers whose school-aged children were born extremely prematurely. *Journal of Clinical Nursing, 27*(7–8), e1627–e1639.

Winnicott, D. W. (1956). Primary maternal preoccupation. In *Through paediatrics to psychoanalysis: Collected papers* (pp. 300–305). Tavistock.

24

MENTAL HEALTH AND COPING CHALLENGES AMONG FAMILIES IN THE NICU

JENNIFER HARNED ADAMS, STACEY R. BROMBERG,
AND ANNA ZIMMERMANN ■

Perinatal mood and anxiety disorders (PMADs)—including depression, anxiety, obsessive–compulsive disorder, and post-traumatic stress disorder (PTSD)—are among the most common complications of pregnancy and childbirth for new parents. Factors related to high-risk pregnancy, premature delivery, and maternal and/or fetal health factors place parents of neonatal intensive care unit (NICU) infants at even greater risk for poor emotional adjustment after their infants' birth. The consequences of PMADs may extend beyond the parents, resulting in (a) a less optimal course in the NICU for the infant; (b) long-term challenges with cognitive, behavioral, and emotional development; (c) poor infant–parent relationship/dyad functioning; and (d) difficulties for older siblings and the family unit as a whole. Risk and protective factors for NICU parents, infants, and families are discussed in this chapter.

PREVALENCE AND COURSE OF PMADS AND TRAUMA IN THE NICU

When discussing concerns related to perinatal mental health, postpartum depression is often at the forefront, but current thinking encompasses both depression and anxiety-related disorders under the umbrella of PMADs.

Depression

As reviewed previously in this book and elsewhere (Wisner et al., 2013), PMADs affect approximately 10% of mothers during pregnancy and approximately 15% of mothers after delivery under "typical" circumstances. Risk factors for perinatal depression for mothers and fathers, such as financial concerns, separation from support networks, and maternal/fetal health complications, are often present within the context of a newborn hospitalization. Wyatt et al. (2019) found that although mothers may have similar rates of prenatal depression, mothers who experience a NICU stay are more likely to remain depressed (if depressed prenatally) or to report new or increased symptoms of depression over the course of 6 weeks compared to mothers of healthy term infants.

Several additional studies (Children's National, 2018; Johnson & Rubarth, 2020; Lefkowitz et al., 2010; Misund et al., 2014) have examined the course of depression in both mothers and fathers across the NICU stay. At 2–4 weeks after birth, studies show that 28–39% of parents meet criteria for depression (Alkozei et al., 2014; Children's National, 2018; Lefkowitz et al., 2010; Misund et al., 2014). Furthermore, an additional 16–18% of mothers endorsed subclinical levels of depression (Lefkowitz et al., 2010; Vasa et al., 2014). Although mothers are at greater risk of depression, research focused on NICU fathers shows they are at risk as well. Johnson and Rubarth (2020) found that 14% of NICU fathers were depressed; this finding is different than that of families who do not experience newborn hospitalization because paternal depression often starts later during the infant's first year. This suggests that the risk period for the development of perinatal depression in nongestational parents may start earlier in NICU families. Implementing screening protocols for all NICU parents and enhancing psychosocial support for parents experiencing symptoms of postpartum depression are critical.

Anxiety, "Stress," and PTSD/Trauma

Parents typically experience the NICU, in part or total, as a stressful or traumatic event. Parents may report feelings of fear, horror, and/or helplessness because of the birth or the events leading to the NICU hospitalization, even when they are anticipated. Parents often report symptoms consistent with acute stress disorder (symptoms <30 days) or (symptoms >30 days), including re-experiencing, avoidance, and physiological hyperarousal (Lefkowitz et al., 2010).

The course of PTSD in NICU parents during their hospital stay and after discharge has been a source of recent attention. Although there is some variability across studies as to the rates of trauma symptoms at the various time points, there is consensus that NICU families experience higher rates of trauma symptoms compared to both mothers and fathers of full-term healthy infants (Misund et al., 2014; Prouhet et al. 2018). Thus, it is important to provide care in a trauma-sensitive manner for all NICU families.

Lefkowitz et al. (2010) examined prevalence rates of trauma symptoms across the NICU stay in both mothers and fathers. They found that within the first 3– 5 days, 35% of mothers and 24% of fathers met criteria for acute stress disorder, and 16.3% of mother and 9.7% of fathers reported significant yet subclinical levels of trauma symptoms; almost all parents in the study reported at least one trauma-associated symptom. Depression during pregnancy, family history of depression, and fear of the death of their infant predicted the severity of the acute stress disorder diagnosis. These rates are similar to those reported by Shaw et al. (2013), who found that 18% of mothers of infants in the NICU met criteria for acute stress disorder at baseline assessment 7–10 days after birth.

It is less clear how trauma-related symptoms unfold as the NICU stay continues. These rates may increase from the start of the NICU stay, as Misund et al. (2014) found that at 2 weeks postpartum, up to 52% of mothers reported symptoms consistent with PTSD. Shaw et al. (2013) reported an increase from 18% to 35% of parents meeting criteria for PTSD at 1 month after birth, whereas Lefkowitz et al. (2010) reported a decrease in parents meeting criteria at 30 days after birth (15% of mothers and 8% of fathers). Risk factors such as prenatal and family history of anxiety and depression, life stressors (Lefkowitz et al., 2010), and higher levels of education may be associated with increased risk at this time interval.

The time of discharge can also be a difficult transition. Families are often relieved and excited to finally go home, but this may look quite different than the homecoming they imagined prior to their NICU stay, resulting in mixed feelings (Shaw et al., 2013). Leaving the protective and supportive environment of the NICU, with 24/7 access to medical professionals, may feel intimidating or even downright terrifying to parents. Shaw et al. (2013) found that up to 45% of parents reported significant symptoms of depression, anxiety, and stress upon discharge; furthermore, parents with higher levels of depression were also more likely to report higher levels of anxiety. Ensuring that parents have had an opportunity to receive emotional support while in the NICU and have a plan to access support after they go home is critical to the family's success.

Most research on parental well-being in the NICU is focused on mothers, but it is vital to also examine the NICU's impact on fathers and partners. Due to various factors, such as receiving less caretaking from the medical team than their birthing partner and juggling NICU life with a quicker return to work, NICU fathers are at increased risk for developing symptoms of depression and anxiety compared to fathers of healthy term infants. Prouhet et al. (2018) identified that fathers were less stressed overall than mothers of NICU infants, although they still experienced a great deal of distress associated with the NICU and were significantly more stressed than fathers of full-term infants. Fathers endorsed stress associated with juggling competing roles, concerns about infant appearance, worries about the NICU environment, and communication with staff.

Differences in psychological outcomes between NICU families and families of healthy infants continue to be evident even after the families go home, but these patterns appear to differ between NICU mothers and their partners. Garfield et al. (2018) measured parents' stress levels in the NICU and after discharge through cortisol testing. By measuring cortisol levels starting on the day of NICU discharge through the first 2 weeks at home, they observed that mothers displayed a more stable cortisol pattern, whereas fathers displayed a shift toward a less adaptive pattern. The authors hypothesized that mothers might be better prepared for the transition home, potentially due to having spent a greater amount of time learning about and caring for their infant in the NICU. The fathers' less adaptive cortisol patterns may reflect the impact of the stress of the care of their infant being shifted from the hospital to the home. Fathers often become the primary caregivers for both their partner and their infant while continuing to work and carry out other life tasks, whereas during the NICU stay, mother and infant receive additional support from the NICU team. Garfield et al. (2018) suggest that providing additional education and support to fathers and partners in anticipation of discharge may ease this transition.

KEY FACTORS IMPACTING NICU PARENTAL MENTAL HEALTH

Risk Factors

There are a myriad of mental health risk factors for families in the NICU, spanning physical and emotional health, logistical/environmental, and those related to relationships and role conflicts. Maternal health factors, such as difficulties during pregnancy or birth in the current or previous pregnancies, previous pregnancy loss, and history of chronic health problems, are known to be associated with greater risk for poorer mental health outcomes (Aftyka et al., 2017; Vasa et al., 2014). Health complications in infants, such as very low birth weight, younger gestational age, severity of associated illness, and/or fetal anomalies (Loewenstein, 2018; Prouhet et al., 2018), also put parents at greater risk for distress. Conversely, older gestational age is also associated with increased risk for parents (Misund, 2014), perhaps due to parents' beliefs that their infant was at lower risk for a NICU stay due to their status as a near-term or full-term infant.

Previous personal and family mental health histories also serve as risk factors for distress in NICU parents. Previous history of depression during pregnancy and family history of mental health concerns are both well-established risk factors for mothers, and these are exacerbated by the experience of the NICU (Loewnstein et al., 2018; Misund et al., 2014; Vasa et al., 2014). Symptoms of PTSD in mothers may be a risk factor for PTSD in fathers (Aftyka et al., 2017).

Having an infant in the NICU constitutes a major stress for any family system and can serve as an additional factor in the development of depression and anxiety. Factors such as distance between the home and hospital, financial stress, time lost from work, and juggling the care of older children represent significant stressors (Alkozei et al., 2014). These factors may be compounded by additional social risk factors, such as poor perceived social support, low family cohesion in the extended family, and conflicts in the parent relationship (Loewnstein et al., 2018; Misund et al., 2014).

Protective Factors

Due to the uncontrollable nature of many of the risk factors for poor parental adjustment (e.g., medical complications and previous mental health history), focusing on protective factors related to the NICU stay may be the most effective way to buffer the impact of the NICU on parental well-being. Williams et al. (2018) identified elements of the NICU experience that can be structured to provide greater support to families, thereby serving as a buffer to the development of parental depression and anxiety. Frequent and informative communication with the medical team, parental participation in rounds, and one-to-one teaching, when combined with professional, supportive, and nonjudgmental verbal communication and nonverbal behavior, were identified as having a positive impact on parental experience of the NICU and increasing parental sense of efficacy. Similarly, the findings of Hawes et al. (2016) identified the relationship between poor maternal mental health outcomes and low maternal perception of comfort with infant care. Mothers who feel more supported by NICU practices that enhance parental competence report better emotional outcome. Feeling excluded from their infant's care was cited as a primary stressor, whereas participation in bedside care, awareness of the importance of milestones such as first baths for parents, and flexible visiting and call-in policies eased parental distress. Receiving social support from other NICU families was also a protective factor, highlighting the importance of peer support in NICU settings (Williams et al., 2018).

CHALLENGES FOR THE DYAD, SIBLINGS, AND FAMILY SYSTEM

The birth of an infant, even under the most typical circumstances, can cause significant disruption and the need to reorganize the family system. However, the stress of the developmental shift around the birth of a new infant can feel especially salient for families for whom birth circumstances require NICU hospitalization and care. This stress can extend to parents, siblings, grandparents, and the extended support network.

Focus on the Dyad

Parent–infant attachment and bonding are natural processes that can be significantly interrupted and impaired in the NICU setting. The NICU stay often includes stressors such as technologically laden, bustling surroundings; emotional and physical distance from the infant and limited social support; and worries about the infant's health. The absence of more normative rituals around the introduction of the infant contributes to the traumatic experience of the NICU stay (Kim et al., 2020). The myriad of stressors noted previously place both parents and infants at great risk for long-term adverse outcomes related to toxic stress, including cycles of dysregulation and relationship disruption, re-traumatization, and poor long-term health conditions (Sanders & Hall, 2018).

As knowledge of the importance of parent–infant attachment for newborn growth and development has grown, NICU environments have worked to include deliberate, trauma-informed support and also methods to facilitate bonding between parents and their infants to help buffer the experiences of toxic stress (Kim et al., 2020). There is robust evidence highlighting the importance of facilitating dyadic interaction and support for caregiver–infant bonding in the NICU as protective, with findings supporting engagement of parents with hospitalized infants toward improved neurodevelopmental outcomes for infants and more positive experiences for their parents (Craig et al., 2015; Kim et al., 2020).

Recommendations around family-centered developmental care (FCDC) models of intervention center the integration of families as collaborators in care of the infant, with a focus on optimizing positive outcomes for the infant and scaffolding the building of long-term relationships between family members and their infant (Craig et al., 2015).

Successful interventions require a culture of shared vision and collaboration, a perspective of parents' roles both as essential caregivers and as part of the medical team, an integrated team approach among staff and the various disciplines interfacing with the family, and clear policies and procedures to formalize best practices that have FCDC at their core (Craig et al., 2015). In fact, due to the plasticity of the infant's brain, there is evidence that dyadic interactions with parents can influence physical brain architecture and maturation responsible for critical aspects of development (Smith et al., 2011). Parents who are supported in recognizing their infant's cues and provided guidance around ways to mitigate stressors of the NICU environment become integral to positive neurodevelopmental outcomes. Furthermore, parents' understanding of their potential positive and protective impact on their vulnerable infant can promote greater sense of confidence and efficacy around caregiving and positive attachment in relationship to their infant. Circumstances that honor the importance of close relationships between parent and infant become necessary components of translating the protective model of FCDC into applicable practice (Fleury et al., 2014).

Specific approaches to facilitate FCDC support include both environmental accommodations that support the natural progression around parent–child bonding and targeted interventions to support the dyad in the context of a healing environment centered on the infant's unique needs. For example, interventions that support physical closeness (e.g., kangaroo care, other forms of skin-to-skin contact, and breastfeeding) allow for the protective aspects of co-regulation and an experience of close connection between mother and infant that can minimize the potential adverse effects of stress (Baley et al., 2015; Fleury et al., 2014;

Head, 2014; Sanders & Hall, 2018). Core markers of FCDC include the presence of physical support, engagement of parents as experts in daily caregiving routines, understanding and promotion of strategies to facilitate infant regulation, pain management and protected sleep, and family-centered care (Coughlin et al., 2009).

There are multiple strategies that behavioral health clinicians and other NICU staff can implement to safeguard against otherwise adverse and lasting impacts of NICU stressors on the infant and family. These strategies include providing psychoeducation and hands-on practice in recognizing, interpreting, and responding to an infant's cues in a developmentally supportive manner; allowing for co-regulation in the context of trauma-informed care that honors the relationship between parent and infant; and scaffolding parents' understanding of the unique needs of their infant in the presence of supportive staff. The context in which such interventions are provided and supported requires a culture of understanding, training, and leadership support for the medical teams emotionally holding families' needs in mind and practice (Fleury et al., 2014), as families learn in turn to hold their infants' needs in mind and practice.

Focus on the Siblings

How parents experience support around their own needs and recognize family-centered ways to mitigate stressors of the NICU environment is integral to positive neurodevelopmental outcomes, positive experiences of parental efficacy, and positive attachment to their infant. The collaboration between professionals and families should be considered the optimal approach to support positive physical, cognitive, and psychosocial outcomes for both the infant and their family. However, despite acceptance of comprehensive models of FCDC as best practice to promote more positive outcomes, there remain obstacles to appropriate and consistent implementation of FCDC. The presence of a caregiver in the NICU contributes to more positive outcomes, and being "present" includes not only being physically present but also being psychologically open to engage emotionally and wholly in the caregiving routines and relationship-building required for the infant to develop healthy attachment to the parent and other family members. One facet of care that can inadvertently be underemphasized, yet is extremely meaningful, is the role of siblings, who are often overlooked because both parents and hospital providers can become focused on the hospitalized infant or the parent–infant dyad. Appropriate recognition of siblings is a powerful component to securing positive family outcomes. Infants in the NICU can be hospitalized for weeks to months, which can represent a significant loss for siblings, who often suffer a sudden and unexpected loss of parental presence and expectations around siblinghood (Beavis, 2007). Helping families discuss their concerns, find balance for the needs of all of their children, and build more robust interactions in the context of sibling relationships in the NICU is imperative in supporting families' developing narrative, shared experience, and reorganization in terms of roles and responsibilities.

Parents who experience a sense of feeling "split" or unsupported in managing multiple needs and roles are often riddled with a sense of failure, concern, distraction, and/or mood disturbance. The ongoing sense of loss of control, traumatization, anxiety, and grief in an attempt to manage the competing demands of supporting their infant in the NICU while also ensuring that their other children are appropriately cared for both physically and emotionally can become overwhelming and contribute to poor coping and negatively impact outcomes for parental mental health (Carvalho et al., 2019). Parental mental health concerns in turn can interfere with the ability to be effectively and consistently present in the context of the necessary dyadic support needed for neuroprotection and positive outcomes. Understanding the larger context of the family unit, with an emphasis on supporting parents' stress around securing care and support for other children, can be considered an essential piece of mitigating parental stress.

Siblings of infants hospitalized in the NICU can experience a tremendous sense of distress and confusion, guilt, fear, anger, and regression as their needs are often overlooked, ignored, or intentionally guarded from inclusion in the process of care (Beavis, 2007). This tendency to guard or protect is often borne out of a parental desire to shield siblings from difficult information or experience. However, the literature that exists considering sibling needs consistently underscores the importance of the opposite approach, positing the honest and intentional inclusion of siblings as part of family-centered developmental care as essential to better outcomes for the infant (Levick et al., 2010). Including siblings in the NICU experience allows for demystification of the process, whereas in the absence of accurate information, children may create their own narratives to make meaning of the experience and can wrongly or unnecessarily blame themselves or experience guilt or regret around negative feelings toward the infant (Beavis, 2007). For example, as parents grieve the hospitalization of their infant, their bereavement and preoccupation with the hospitalized infant can be perceived as a rejection by their other children. This in turn can lead to a cascade of difficulties for families, relationship functioning between parents and older children, as well as other children's role development as siblings to the hospitalized infant. More positive outcomes have been associated with sibling involvement with their new brother or sister, memory-making around cherished moments, and/or the opportunity to develop a narrative around their relationship as significant (Sombans et al., 2018).

The perspective of hospitalization of an infant in the NICU as a trauma experienced by the family as a whole allows for guidance around intervention and support that is inclusive and comprehensive (Davis et al., 2012). Adopting a family perspective supports families in creating a collective and shared understanding of their NICU journey and helps develop a cohesive narrative for meaning-making and adaptive coping. Maintaining as much normalcy around routine and communicating honestly and openly with siblings in age-appropriate ways can mitigate the experience of loss and allow a child to regain a sense of agency and make meaning of their experience (Davis et al., 2012). Providing opportunities for siblings to express their questions, concerns, and feelings is also of critical importance.

Teaching and training for professionals around how to best collaborate and support inclusion of siblings are imperative, with guidelines around age-appropriate ways to introduce difficult material, and best practices to support parents in supporting their children through the process. Such practices often include clear policies for families focused on inclusion of siblings as part of successful and quality care and open communication, including introductions and relationships with hospital staff and providers. Psychoeducation and structured visits work to guide siblings toward safe and appropriate interactions with the infant. Furthermore, providing physical space and/or on-site child care to accommodate opportunities to experience a sense of family unity, and special time with their parent to preserve pre-existing relationships, will facilitate the development of a positive new sibling relationship from the start. Positive sibling involvement can include making drawings, writing messages, and/or taking pictures of themselves at their sibling's bedside. Support includes developing a narrative explaining the situation, highlighting similarities or differences relative to that child's own birth and newborn stage. Siblings can engage in positive relationship-building with the hospitalized infant via talking, singing, and/or reading to the infant; assigning special "gifts" to the infant from the siblings and vice versa; marking milestones together (e.g., first sibling cuddle, birthdays, and holidays); and simple "jobs" to support physical care of the infant.

Because the duration of hospitalization varies, the medical staff and interdisciplinary providers often become an integral part of the families' NICU experience and often serve as avenues for guidance, reassurance, and social support. Attention to a supportive holding environment for families and the delicate interplay of relationships as they support meaning-making of the NICU experience is of critical importance beyond discharge.

The Interaction Between Parental Mental Health Symptoms and Parental Engagement

Parental well-being may impact participation within the NICU milieu, active partnership in their infant's care at bedside, as well as interactions with the medical team. Psychosocial challenges, including symptoms of depression, anxiety, trauma, substance abuse, and challenges in the partner relationship, can lead to a pattern of physical and/or emotional withdrawal from their infant and create barriers to effective parental engagement while in the NICU (e.g., parent–infant interactions and breastfeeding/pumping). Mothers who are more distressed also report feeling less confident, whereas more engaged mothers are more confident and feel less role disturbance (Harris et al., 2018). When the team implements family-centered care strategies, parents have the experience of feeling supported in their new role as they learn to care for their infant. As they begin to feel confident in this role, it has a reciprocal effect because this confidence is associated with a decrease in symptoms of anxiety and stress, leading to better outcomes for the infant (Lean et al., 2018).

Impact in the NICU Milieu

Samra et al. (2015) present the idea of "engagement," defined both by the amount of time parents spend in the NICU and how engaged the parents are while in the NICU. Due to the lack of opportunity for "typical" hands-on care with their infants, many parents gauge the quality of their parenting by the amount of time spent at the bedside. The findings of Samra et al. (2015) encourage parents to consider this time in terms of "optimal dosage," such that parents are available to support infant care and development while also preserving their own well-being and maintaining a balance between life in the NICU and other responsibilities.

The amount of time spent in the NICU and the level of engagement while at bedside can be balanced to create an optimal equation for each family (Samra et al., 2015). For example, a mother going to great lengths to stay at bedside 12–14 hours a day may be doing so at the cost of chaos in the home and tenuous child care arrangements for older siblings, potentially to the point that she constantly needs to be on the phone and is distracted from the infant's care. In this situation, it may be more optimal for her to dedicate a shorter time to the hospital each day to be fully present at bedside and attend to other tasks when away from the hospital.

Parental well-being has a significant impact on parental engagement, as problems with depression and anxiety can impede parents coming into the hospital or prevent them from engaging in care out of fear of harm to their infant or fear of incompetence. Additional factors that may impact engagement are cultural beliefs, education and health literacy, and emotional and logistical support (Samra et al., 2015). Programming that meets parents where they are (e.g., allowing parents to talk through their understanding and perceptions of circumstances before providing detailed medical information) and provides support and education will have a positive impact on engagement. Through optimal parental engagement, parents can better understand their infant's condition and needs, and staff can better understand the parents' needs for information and support. Through more frequent opportunities to discuss clinical progress, parents can better function as confident members of the medical team and be active participants in medical decision-making when appropriate. This can lead to lower levels of anxiety and stress in parents and better outcomes for infants (Lean et al., 2018).

Pumping and Breastfeeding

Boucher et al. (2011) highlighted that breastfeeding rates for mothers in the NICU are lower than those for mothers of healthy preterm infants, particularly when considering continuation after the first weeks post-birth. Newer research (Spatz et al., 2019) notes that close monitoring of milk supply and specialized support enabled NICU mothers to provide human milk to their infants throughout the first year. Although providing human milk through breast pumping and breastfeeding may be emotionally and physically optimal for both mother and infant, many barriers may still exist for NICU mothers, such as feeling stressed, worried, and overwhelmed by the NICU experience; a lack of privacy; and a sense of frustration with low supply and/or the need to supplement to encourage weight gain. The discomfort of pumping, the rigorous schedule, and the perceived impact of ability to simultaneously care for one's self and their infant are additional factors that may impact a mother's mental health and/or decision to cease pumping despite initiation after birth (Lewis et al., 2019). Even with those challenges, mothers may view their ability to provide milk for their infants and breastfeed as a mechanism for continuing their in utero attachment, particularly in light of premature birth (Boucher et al., 2011). Mothers report that education and encouragement from their nurses helped them better understand the importance and benefits of providing human milk to their infants and provided them with the support to continue to do so even in light of frustration and challenges (Lewis et al., 2019). While in the NICU, mothers tend to perceive that breastfeeding will be less stressful at home, and although this may be true for some dyads, this may not be the case for most (Lewis et al., 2019). Without the additional support of the NICU nurse and lactation teams when at home, breastfeeding may become difficult or discouraging. We stress the importance of ongoing lactation education and support for mothers after discharge from the NICU.

Holding and Kangaroo Care

Physical touch with the infant through holding and kangaroo care is well established as having a positive impact on NICU infants' growth and development, milk production and breastfeeding success, parent–infant bonding, and parental perceptions of competence. However, these practices can be costly in terms of time and emotional investment for both parents and the NICU team (Lewis et al., 2019). Parents' (particularly mothers') stress levels, recovery from childbirth, perceived burden (i.e., financial or logistical difficulty getting to the hospital), and communication challenges with the NICU team may be barriers to successful engagement in holding and kangaroo care. Lewis et al. (2019) identified several factors that enhanced mothers' ability to engage in care, including access to the hospital (including transportation); sufficient time to be present at the hospital whether due to child care, transportation, or maternity leave; and logistical support from hospital staff for transportation, financial, or child care concerns. Outside the hospital, both the family's and friends' instrumental and social support will enable the mother to meet her own needs for physical and emotional recovery while caring for her infant and other children.

Communication to Support Family Engagement

A number of supports and strategies appear to be beneficial to all NICU families. Utilizing a proactive approach when interacting with parents, through offering choice whenever possible, while being clear about situations in which medical expertise is required for decision-making will allow parents to feel a sense of agency and control in their infant's care and create trust that the team is still relying on medical expertise when needed. The use of language that reflects partnership status will reinforce the norm that parents are crucial team participants in their infant's care. Providing families with frequent and consistent updates through practices such as family-centered rounds creates a sense of trust and security for parents because they are not having to actively seek out information about their infant's status. Furthermore, encouraging parents to reach out to the medical team at any time and ensuring accessibility and prompt provision of information will create a trusting relationship based on clear two-way communication. To whatever degree possible, ensuring that the medical team is on the same page prior to giving important updates, news, and/or discussing critical changes to the care plan may also lessen confusion and anxiety for parents. These strategies will create a foundation for a strong partnership between the medical team and the family, serving the best interests of the infant.

IDEAS WORTH SHARING

- Perinatal mood and anxiety disorders are common among NICU parents, even in the most "typical" pregnancy, labor and delivery, and postpartum situations. Due to complications during this vulnerable time, NICU parents are at even higher risk of mental health complications.
- Mothers are more likely to experience symptoms of depression, anxiety, and PTSD than are fathers, but it is still crucial to be aware that fathers and partners may also be struggling and to provide support for them. Finding effective ways of connecting with fathers and partners may require additional flexibility and creativity from staff, especially if they are less present on the unit due to location, work, or family demands.
- In addition to risk factors inherent with a NICU stay, additional support for parents who have a personal or family history of depression and anxiety, who are experiencing low social support, or who are experiencing a high number of concurrent stressors may be indicated.
- PMADs may impact parental behavior in many ways, from the amount of time spent on the unit to the level of engagement in care for their infant and their interactions with staff members. Often, this behavior may be impacted by trauma and anxiety, and it may appear to be avoidant or controlling. Approaching parents from a trauma-sensitive

perspective may allow them to connect with their infant and their NICU experience more effectively.

- Dyadic support in the context of the parent–infant relationship leads to reliable and measurable outcomes in terms of neurodevelopment.
- Supporting parents in effectively caring for siblings' needs allows for more psychological availability of parents to engage appropriately with the needs of their infant. Honest communication and inclusion of siblings in the process of care for the hospitalized infant are protective for family adjustment and improved long-term outcomes for all.

CONCLUSION

Parents of NICU infants are under a great deal of stress and are at greater risk for PMADs, including PTSD. Poor emotional adjustment in parents may impact parental health and well-being, engagement in the NICU, outcomes for infants, as well as the larger family unit, including older siblings. Although a number of factors increase the likelihood of emotional distress in NICU families, implementing best practice for communication with families and providing comprehensive education and support can provide a buffering effect.

REFERENCES

Aftyka, A., Rybojad, B., Rosa, W., Wróbel, A., & Karakuła-Juchnowicz, H. (2017). Risk factors for the development of post-traumatic stress disorder and coping strategies in mothers and fathers following infant hospitalisation in the neonatal intensive care unit. *Journal of Clinical Nursing, 26*(23–24), 4436–4445.

Alkozei, A., McMahon, E., & Lahav, A. (2014). Stress levels and depressive symptoms in NICU mothers in the early postpartum period. *Journal of Maternal–Fetal & Neonatal Medicine, 27*(17), 1738–1743. https://doi.org/10.3109/14767058.2014.942626

Baley, J., Watterberg, K., Cummings, J., Eichenwald, E., Poindexter, B., Stewart, D. L., ... & Goldsmith, J. P. (2015). Skin-to-skin care for term and preterm infants in the neonatal ICU. *Pediatrics, 136*(3), 596–599.

Beavis, A. G. (2007). What about brothers and sisters? Helping siblings cope with a new baby brother or sister in the NICU. *Infant, 3*(6), 239–242.

Boucher, C. A., Brazal, P. M., Graham-Certosini, C., Carnaghan-Sherrard, K., & Feeley, N. (2011). Mothers' breastfeeding experiences in the NICU. *Neonatal Network, 30*(1), 21–28. https://doi.org/10.1891/0730-0832.30.1.21

Carvalho, S. C., Facio, B. C., Souza, B. F., Abreu-D'Agostini, F., Leite, A. M., & Wernet, M. (2019). Maternal care in the preterm child's family context: A comprehensive look towards the sibling. *Revista Brasileira de Enfermagem, 72*(Suppl. 3), 50–57. https://doi.org/10.1590/0034-7167-2017-0780

Children's National. (2018, November 5). *Resiliency in NICU parents may be linked to lower depression and anxiety.* Retrieved September 27, 2020, from https://childrensn

ational.org/news-and-events/childrens-newsroom/2018/resiliency-in-nicu-pare
nts-may-be-linked-to-lower-depression-and-anxiety

Coughlin, M., Gibbins, S., & Hoath, S. (2009). Core measures for developmentally supportive care in neonatal intensive care units: Theory, precedence and practice. *Journal of Advanced Nursing*, *65*(10), 2239–2248. https://doi.org/10.1111/j.1365-2648.2009.05052.x

Craig, J. W., Glick, C., Phillips, R., Hall, S. L., Smith, J., & Browne, J. (2015). Recommendations for involving the family in developmental care of the NICU baby. *Journal of Perinatology*, *35* (Suppl. 1), S5–S8. https://doi.org/10.1038/jp.2015.142

Davis, C. G., Harasymchuk, C., & Wohl, M. J. (2012). Finding meaning in a traumatic loss: A families approach. *Journal of Traumatic Stress*, *25*(2), 142–149. https://doi.org/10.1002/jts.21675

Fleury, C., Parpinelli, M. A., & Makuch, M. Y. (2014). Perceptions and actions of healthcare professionals regarding the mother–child relationship with premature babies in an intermediate neonatal intensive care unit: A qualitative study. *BMC Pregnancy and Childbirth*, *14*, 313. https://doi.org/10.1186/1471-2393-14-313

Garfield, C. F., Simon, C. D., Rutsohn, J., & Lee, Y. S. (2018). Stress from the neonatal intensive care unit to home: Paternal and maternal cortisol rhythms in parents of premature infants. *Journal of Perinatal & Neonatal Nursing*, *32*(3), 257–265. https://doi.org/10.1097/JPN.0000000000000296

Harris, R., Gibbs, D., Mangin-Heimos, K., & Pineda, R. (2018). Maternal mental health during the neonatal period: Relationships to the occupation of parenting. *Early Human Development*, *120*, 31–39. https://doi.org/10.1016/j.earlhumdev.2018.03.009

Hawes, K., McGowan, E., O'Donnell, M., Tucker, R., & Vohr, B. (2016). Social emotional factors increase risk of postpartum depression in mothers of preterm infants. *Journal of Pediatrics*, *179*, 61–67. https://doi.org/10.1016/j.jpeds.2016.07.008

Head, L. M. (2014). The effect of kangaroo care on neurodevelopmental outcomes in preterm infants. *Journal of Perinatal & Neonatal Nursing*, *28*(4), 290–299. https://doi.org/10.1097/JPN.0000000000000062

Johnson, E., & Rubarth, L. (2020). *Implementation of postnatal depression screening for NICU fathers*. Doctor of Nursing Practice scholarly project, Creighton University.

Kim, A. R., Kim, S. Y., & Yun, J. E. (2020). Attachment and relationship-based interventions for families during neonatal intensive care hospitalization: A study protocol for a systematic review and meta-analysis. *Systematic Reviews*, *9*(1), 61. https://doi.org/10.1186/s13643-020-01331-8

Lean, R. E., Rogers, C. E., Paul, R. A., & Gerstein, E. D. (2018). NICU hospitalization: Long-term implications on parenting and child behaviors. *Current Treatment Options in Pediatrics*, *4*(1), 49–69.

Lefkowitz, D. S., Baxt, C., & Evans, J. R. (2010). Prevalence and correlates of posttraumatic stress and postpartum depression in parents of infants in the neonatal intensive care unit (NICU). *Journal of Clinical Psychology in Medical Settings*, *17*(3), 230–237. https://doi.org/10.1007/s10880-010-9202-7

Levick, J., Quinn, M., Holder, A., Nyberg, A., Beaumont, E., & Munch, S. (2010). Support for siblings of NICU patients: An interdisciplinary approach. *Social Work in Health Care*, *49*(10), 919–933. https://doi.org/10.1080/00981389.2010.511054

Lewis, T. P., Andrews, K. G., Shenberger, E., Betancourt, T. S., Fink, G., Pereira, S., & McConnell, M. (2019). Caregiving can be costly: A qualitative study of barriers and facilitators to conducting kangaroo mother care in a US tertiary hospital neonatal intensive care unit. *BMC Pregnancy and Childbirth, 19*(1), Article 227. https://doi.org/10.1186/s12884-019-2363-y

Loewenstein, K. (2018). Parent psychological distress in the neonatal intensive care unit within the context of the social ecological model: A scoping review. *Journal of the American Psychiatric Nurses Association, 24*(6), 495–509.

Misund, A. R., Nerdrum, P., & Diseth, T. H. (2014). Mental health in women experiencing preterm birth. *BMC Pregnancy and Childbirth, 14*(1), 263. https://doi.org/10.1186/1471-2393-14-263

Prouhet, P., Gregory, M., Russell, C., & Yaeger, L. (2018). Fathers' stress in the neonatal intensive care unit—A systematic review. *Advances in Neonatal Care, 18*(2), 105–120. https://doi.org/10.1097/ANC.0000000000000472

Samra, H. A., McGrath, J. M., Fischer, S., Schumacher, B., Dutcher, J., & Hansen, J. (2015). The NICU Parent Risk Evaluation and Engagement Model and Instrument (PREEMI) for neonates in intensive care units. *Journal of Obstetric, Gynecologic, and Neonatal Nursing, 44*(1), 114–126. https://doi.org/10.1111/1552-6909.12535

Sanders, M. R., & Hall, S. L. (2018). Trauma-informed care in the newborn intensive care unit: Promoting safety, security and connectedness. *Journal of Perinatology, 38*(1), 3–10. https://doi.org/10.1038/jp.2017.124

Shaw, R. J., Bernard, R. S., Storfer-Isser, A., Rhine, W., & Horwitz, S. M. (2013). Parental coping in the neonatal intensive care unit. *Journal of Clinical Psychology in Medical Settings, 20*(2), 135–142. https://doi.org/10.1007/s10880-012-9328-x

Smith, G. C., Gutovich, J., Smyser, C., Pineda, R., Newnham, C., Tjoeng, T. H., Vavasseur, C., Wallendorf, M., Neil, J., & Inder, T. (2011). Neonatal intensive care unit stress is associated with brain development in preterm infants. *Annals of Neurology, 70*(4), 541–549. https://doi.org/10.1002/ana.22545

Sombans, S., Ramphul, K., & Sonaye, R. (2018). The impact of a sibling's death in intensive care unit: Are we doing enough to help them? *Cureus, 10*(4), e2518. https://doi.org/10.7759/cureus.2518

Spatz, D. L., Froh, E. B., Bartholomew, D., Edwards, T., Wild, K. T., Hedrick, H., & Nawab, U. (2019). Lactation experience of mothers and feeding outcomes of infants with congenital diaphragmatic hernia. *Breastfeeding Medicine, 14*(5), 320–324.

Vasa, R., Eldeirawi, K., Kuriakose, V. G., Nair, G. J., Newsom, C., & Bates, J. (2014). Postpartum depression in mothers of infants in neonatal intensive care unit: Risk factors and management strategies. *American Journal of Perinatology, 31*(5), 425–434. https://doi.org/10.1055/s-0033-1352482

Williams, K. G., Patel, K. T., Stausmire, J. M., Bridges, C., Mathis, M. W., & Barkin, J. L. (2018). The neonatal intensive care unit: Environmental stressors and supports. *International Journal of Environmental Research and Public Health, 15*(1), 60. https://doi.org/10.3390/ijerph15010060

Wisner, K. L., Sit, D. K. Y., McShea, M. C., Rizzo, D. M., Zoretich, R. A., Hughes, C. L., Eng, H. F., Luther, J. F., Wisniewski, S. R., Constantino, M. L., Confer, A. L., Mose-Kolko, E. L., Famy, C. S., & Hanusa, B. H. (2013). Onset timing, thoughts of self-harm, and diagnoses in postpartum women with screen-positive depression

findings. *JAMA*, *70*(5), 490–498. https://jamanetwork.com/journals/jamapsychia
try/fullarticle/1666651

Wyatt, T., Shreffler, K. M., & Ciciolla, L. (2019). Neonatal intensive care unit admission
and maternal postpartum depression. *Journal of Reproductive and Infant Psychology*,
37(3), 267–276. https://doi.org/10.1080/02646838.2018.1548756

Neonatal Follow-Up Settings

25

A BRIEF HISTORY OF NEONATAL FOLLOW-UP AND WHY IT IS DONE

HOWARD NEEDELMAN, BEATRICE EGBOH, WHITNEY STRONG-BAK, AND GRACE WINNINGHAM ■

HISTORY OF NEONATAL FOLLOW-UP

In 1880, the French obstetrician Tarnier first introduced the warm air incubator for premature infants in Paris (Dunn, 2002). Convinced of the value of the incubator, Budin and Couney exhibited the incubators at the 1896 World Expo in Berlin (Columbia Surgery, 2015). Eventually, the incubators and their incubator babies were displayed in Coney Island's amusement park and could be seen for 25 cents. The understanding of the importance of the neutral thermal environment was perhaps the groundwork upon which the newborn intensive care unit (NICU) was built.

The formation of neonatal follow-up programs came much later. At Michael Reese Hospital in Chicago, Illinois, in 1953 Hess reported on the long-term outcomes of preterm survivors of the Michael Reese nursery. Among infants weighing less than 1,251 g, less than 25% had poor developmental outcomes. In Edinburgh, United Kingdom, Drillien (1958) reported approximately 50% of low-birth-weight infants to have normal development. These reports—whether viewed as positive or negative—can help put the importance and ethics of neonatal intensive care in some perspective.

As neonatal intensive care underwent what Robertson (2003) describes as "therapeutic exuberance," it also made some significant stumbles. Silverman (Gartner, 1997) describes some 10,0000 infants with retrolental fibroplasia, presumably the result of overenthusiastic oxygen use. Years later, chloramphenicol, commonly used as the "rule out sepsis" therapy, was found associated with the gray baby syndrome (St. Geme, 1960). And more recently, dexamethasone, used to help ameliorate some of the respiratory complications of bronchopulmonary dysplasia (BPD), was found to lead to an increased likelihood of microcephaly and cerebral palsy (Watterberg et al., 2010). These admitted misadventures have been countered with many significant victories. The use of artificial surfactant has significantly aided in the therapy for respiratory distress syndrome (Mandile, 2020). Cooling as a treatment for a hypoxic–ischemic encephalopathy has by almost all studies reduced the morbidity in many of these cases.

As the care for the high-risk infant in the NICU was advancing, the understanding of the needs of all children, including those with disabilities, was also growing. The exposure of children to a nurturing environment, even to such apparently simple things as the number of words to which a young child is exposed, is now understood and taken as fact to benefit the child's development. Head Start was established in the 1960s to help children believed to need further support as they approach school age. Furthermore, the 1975 Education for All Handicapped Act and its subsequent modifications through the Individuals with Disabilities Education Improvement Act of 2004 (IDEA 2004) have guaranteed a free and appropriate public education to all, and early intervention to those aged 0–3 years with defined needs is now also guaranteed with an Individualized Family Service Plan. An appreciation of the value of these interventions can be seen in the Infant Health and Development Program (1990), which documents prolonged positive effects of early intervention on heavier low-birth-weight infants and notes the importance of considering environmental factors, including maternal characteristics. Part C of IDEA 2004 requires states to have a "child find" system to identify those believed to need intervention.

FORMATION OF NICU FOLLOW-UP CLINICS

As both the need to assess the long-term neurodevelopmental effect of interventions in the NICU and the need to provide a program to identify at-risk infants believed to be most likely to benefit from early intervention services grew, many institutions developed NICU follow-up clinics. The structure of these clinics has generally been established by the individual institution, and little agreement on programmatic synchrony exists. Thus, there is no consensus as to whom these clinics should serve, how they should be structured, and even how to appropriately evaluate the individual child. The timing of the evaluations, the age at which the children are evaluated, and the duration of follow-up vary from clinic to clinic. Confusing matters even more, assuming the clinics are to serve a child find function, the guidelines and eligibility for early intervention programs in the United States differ between and even within states (Dempsey et al., 2020).

Despite the lack of consistency as to how they are structured, according to an American Academy of Pediatrics (AAP)/American College of Obstetrics and Gynecology (2002) policy statement, infants who are deemed high risk should be enrolled in a follow-up clinic that specializes in the neurodevelopmental assessment of graduates at risk for delays. These clinics can also provide educational resources and information to the family about developmental delays and provide experienced support around such diagnoses, offer guidance for feeding and growth problems, provide parents with information on parenting, and acknowledge and support the mental health needs of the family. Infants discharged with significant medical issues can be co-managed by a neonatologist or other medical subspecialist in conjunction with the primary care physician. The role of the clinic in managing medical issues such as pulmonary support for chronic lung disease or nutritional support for a short bowel syndrome varies.

Regardless of the program's structure, to both assist the individual graduate in getting services and evaluate NICU interventions, neonatal follow-up programs are designed to monitor growth and development of infants who have been identified with various risk factors for disability after discharge from the NICU. Once identified, these medical and developmental needs ideally should be addressed as early as possible and families provided with services and resources to address these needs.

ELIGIBILITY AND GRADUATION CRITERIA FOR FOLLOW-UP CLINICS

At the inception of follow-up clinics, most children served were those deemed at greatest risk for significant neurodevelopmental sequelae such as cerebral palsy, intellectual disability, blindness, and deafness. These less common outcomes were more likely in the smaller, more premature infants and therefore many clinics primarily followed these very low-birth-weight (VLBW) infants (i.e., those with birth weight <1,500 g). However, more recent literature has documented the increased risk for both major and especially minor sequelae, such as specific learning disorders, speech and language delays, and behavior problems, in both VLBW infants and heavier premature infants with birth weights of 1,500–2,500 g (You et al., 2019). For example, cerebral palsy afflicts the smallest premature infants at the greatest prevalence and also affects children born with late preterm birth at a rate approximately 10 times greater than that of the term population (Hirvonen et al., 2014). Thus, although historically NICU follow-up clinics have seen primarily VLBW infants and focused on the outcome of these premature infants in the first 2 years of life, questions now arise as to the appropriate need for follow-up in the early years of life of the late preterm given a heightened risk for even major sequelae.

In addition to calls for systematic follow-up of children born with later degrees of prematurity, there are also calls for longer follow-up until school entry, given the clear risk of minor sequelae in NICU graduates. An increased likelihood of autism in NICU graduates has also added to the question of the appropriate timing and length of follow-up required for these infants, given the data on the increased effectiveness of early diagnosis and treatment of autism in children (Agrawal et al., 2018). Use of the General Movement Assessment has caused the issue of timing of the first visit to follow-up clinic to be revisited because advocates of this exam believe it aids in diagnosing cerebral palsy at 3 months corrected age (Morgan et al., 2015).

PRACTICES OF FOLLOW-UP CLINICS

Adverse Childhood Experiences

Whereas earlier follow-up clinics generally focused on sequelae of medical diagnoses associated with the newborn's admission to the NICU, more recent concern has been raised regarding a broader definition of disability (World Health Organization [WHO], 2020) and potential risk for problems associated with the environmental factors children at risk for delays are likely to face (Vanderbilt et al., 2018). The NICU graduate population is more likely to experience several adverse childhood experiences (ACEs), such as maternal mental health problems and instability in the home environment associated with parental separation or even parental substance abuse. In a life course model, the toxic stress caused by these ACEs can lead to a myriad of subsequent long-term problems. As such, many pediatric clinics and some follow-up clinics have begun to screen for maternal post-traumatic stress disorder and postpartum depression in an attempt to not only guide the guardian to mental health help for themself but also help ameliorate the negative developmental and health effects on the graduate.

Developmental and Behavioral Functioning

Because the earlier follow-up programs generally dealt with major developmental sequelae, they were usually established under the auspices of a neonatologist. Several issues have led to restructuring some of these follow-up programs. The diagnostic evaluation and treatment of major sequelae have changed over time based on statements such as the WHO's definition of disability and the goals of treatment. As noted previously, there has also been increasing concern for minor and behavioral sequelae seen in graduates. With these changes, programs have morphed, each in their own ways. Recommendations to standardize the programs have not been heeded. There are no standards established for the appropriate follow-up assessment, testing timetable, or follow-up staff in clinics.

Variations in Practices and Barriers to Care

Needelman and colleagues (2015) surveyed members of the AAP Section on Perinatal Pediatrics regarding the follow-up clinic with which they were associated. Although the response rate was less than ideal (27.5%), the responses represented a range of academic and private institutions over a geographic range throughout the United States and Canada. A common constraint for these programs is funding; for at least 50% of these clinics, costs were greater than income. Furthermore, because one of the purposes of NICU follow-up clinics is to evaluate the success of neonatal interventions, it is concerning that only approximately 50% of clinics in academic institutions participated in research networks such as the Vermont Oxford Network, the National Institute of Child Health and Human Development's Neonatal Research Network, or the Canadian Neonatal Network.

Composition of the teams varied considerably, per survey respondents. Whereas the neonatologist and clinic nurse were the most common members of the clinic team, representation from occupational and physical therapy was more limited. Even less frequently present in clinics were speech and language pathologists and psychologists. Other pediatric subspecialists, such as a pediatric neurologist or developmental/behavioral pediatrician, sometimes participated. Although not present at every visit, a social worker and dietitian were sometimes available. The composition of the clinics is also indicative of variations in practices and domains of care.

Developmental Monitoring and Assessment in Neonatal Follow-Up Programs

Assuming that a primary role for the clinic is that of child find (i.e., to connect young children with appropriate services), it seemed appropriate that in the survey by Needelman and colleagues (2015) described in the previous section, approximately 75% of clinics referred children to early intervention programs. Some clinics worked directly with early intervention programs and performed eligibility evaluations. Most clinics used varying schedules of follow-up, seeing graduates until approximately age 2 years, although some saw graduates for much longer. Developmental evaluations were performed in the majority of clinics, typically with the Bayley Scales of Infant and Toddler Development or its related screening tool (Bayley, 2006). However, there was also significant variation in the developmental assessment instruments used across clinics, with at least nine different assessment tools being reported.

High-quality assessment measures are crucial to the mission of NICU follow-up clinics because they are instrumental in the clinics' goals of early identification and referral for early intervention services. Instruments used for the assessment of infant and toddler development must have demonstrated validity in detecting deficits of early milestones across several domains, including language, cognition, social interaction, and motor development. Clinicians in follow-up programs must have a working knowledge of quality assessments and screeners of early childhood development to ensure proper identification and provision of services for their patients.

COMMON MEDICAL CONCERNS IN NEONATAL FOLLOW-UP CLINICS

Cerebral Palsy

Cerebral palsy (CP) has been known since ancient times, and Shakespeare's Gloucester describes his affliction as having him "deform'd, unfinish'd, sent before my time Into this breathing world, scarce half made up" (Rhodes, 1977, p. 1650). William Little, an English orthopedist with an equinus deformity as the result of polio, had an interest in spasticity and in 1861 described "Little's disease," which is now called CP (Little, 1966). At a meeting devoted to the state of the art in CP in Brioni, Yugoslavia, in 1990, CP was described as "an umbrella term covering a group of non-progressive, but often changing, motor impairment syndromes secondary to lesions or anomalies of the brain arising in the early stages of its development" (Mutch et al., 1992, p. 549).

The term CP describes a motor problem associated with delayed acquisition of motor skills in conjunction with abnormalities of muscle tone, persistent primitive reflexes, and delayed postural responses. Because of the plasticity seen in early development, there has been some hesitancy in the past to make the diagnosis before approximately age 2 years. However, correlation of motor development with imaging abnormalities, such as periventricular leukomalacia (PVL), and with examination findings, such as Prechtl's GMA (Einspieler & Prechtl, 2005), has led to an earlier diagnosis in many cases (as early as 3 months chronological age).

The prevalence of CP is generally reported to be in the range of 1.5–2.5 per 1,000 live births (Pellegrino, 2002). The condition is usually separated into two general types—spastic (or pyramidal) and extrapyramidal. In spastic CP, increased tone generally can be appreciated in the first year of life, whereas those with extrapyramidal CP usually have a longer period of hypotonia with abnormal movements beginning later, often around age 2 years. Among those with spastic CP, there is further subclassification based on limbs involved, with spastic diplegia being most commonly seen in the VLBW infant. Extrapyramidal CP is most often seen in term infants and is often seen in conjunction with spastic CP, giving it a "mixed" picture. With approximately 40–50% of all cases of CP being associated with prematurity, it is clear why this symptom complex is of interest to those working in NICU follow-up clinics.

Whereas CP is by definition a motor problem, its associated comorbidities (Nickel, 2000) result in significant added stress to the child and family. Especially for those with spastic quadriplegia and mixed-type CP, intellectual disability is common. Seizures are also not unusual, nor are sensory conditions such as visual and hearing impairment. Feeding issues eventually requiring gastrostomy feedings are not uncommon, nor is the sequela of failure to thrive. Abnormalities in tone can lead to hip dislocation and kyphoscoliosis, which may lead to later cardiopulmonary disease.

Therapy decisions can often be made with the guidance of tools such as the WHO or National Center for Medical Rehabilitation Research (NCMRR) disability terminology (Butler et al., 1999). The NCMRR describes five dimensions of function: pathophysiology, impairment, functional limitation, disability, and societal limitation. For CP, Butler et al. equate these with, respectively, PVL; spasticity and contractures; awkward walking; participation in a restricted environment; and exclusion from school sports, for example. Therapy will not eliminate PVL, but it may help the toddler navigate the living room. Appropriate intervention probably should be directed toward realistic objectives and goals and those of most importance to the family.

Bronchopulmonary Dysplasia

Bronchopulmonary dysplasia is a chronic respiratory illness that is primarily seen in preterm infants who have required mechanical ventilation and supplemental oxygen for the treatment of respiratory distress syndrome. The condition is known to result in significant morbidity and mortality. In the NICU and even after discharge, these patients may present with tachypnea, retractions, and cyanosis without oxygen.

Despite significant advances in perinatal care, BPD remains one of the most common, complex, and intriguing diseases in perinatal medicine (Jensen & Schmidt, 2014). Although the requirement to meet criteria for the diagnosis differs among various groups, the Vermont Oxford Network, an organization whose recommendations are followed by many in neonatal/perinatal medicine and that has several quality improvement initiatives, defines BPD based on a fraction of inspired oxygen requirement at 36 weeks PMA (Gomez Pomar et al., 2018).

It is unclear whether the incidence of BPD is changing. The majority of studies suggest that rates have remained stable or even increased during the past two or three decades, possibly due to increased survival of the highest risk infants. Prematurity is the primary risk factor for BPD, with the incidence increasing with decreasing gestational age. Whereas BPD is seen as frequently as in one-third of newborns with birth weights of less than 1,000 g (Walsh et al., 2006), it is infrequent in infants weighing more than 1,500 g.

As they grow older, infants with BPD are more likely to have asthma in later childhood and, in fact, many develop adult chronic obstructive pulmonary disease (Cheong & Doyle, 2018). They are more likely to have chronic cough, wheezing, episodes of pneumonia, hospitalizations, limitation of exercise capacity, and long-term medication use.

In addition, infants with BPD may have feeding issues eventually requiring gastrostomy and also delayed growth with failure to thrive. This may be due to increased caloric expenditure in the work of breathing, intermittent hypoxia, restricted fluids, diuretic and postnatal steroid therapy, and comorbidities such as sepsis and pneumonia (Theile et al., 2012).

BPD is a risk factor for significant major neurodevelopmental sequelae, including CP, cognitive delays, and poor academic outcome. Children with BPD are also at risk for hearing and vision impairment, receptive and expressive language delays, and impairment in visuospatial perception.

Feeding Difficulties/Failure to Thrive

Feeding is an interplay of medical factors, infant developmental level and behaviors, infant temperament, caregiver sensitivity, nutritional requirements, psychosocial factors and environment, cultural variations, and caregiver–child interaction. Physiologically, feeding is a complex process requiring sufficient neurodevelopmental maturation; control of tone; and coordinated sucking, swallowing, and breathing (McGrath & Braescu, 2004).

The evaluation of the infant's growth starts with review of maternal health factors that may impact the neonate's growth. Despite several varying criterion used to diagnose failure to thrive, the overarching theme is a state of undernutrition that occurs when caloric intake is insufficient to maintain growth. Assessing for any feeding difficulties includes an evaluation of an array of signs and symptoms: choking, gagging, difficulty latching/sucking, swallowing difficulties, excessive drooling, respiratory distress while feeding, and regurgitation. Obtaining a feeding history includes the frequency and amount of feeding and, if formula fed, how the bottle was prepared. A comprehensive physical exam should include examining the infant's tone, particularly low muscle tone, which may disrupt the development of oral–motor skills; hard and soft palate, examining for cleft; breathing, with perhaps residual distress due to BPD; and reviewing the infant's length, weight, and head circumference measurements—both current measurements and the growth trajectories. The assessment in the clinic should also include the child's developmental skills, including social interaction, attachment with caregiver, infant temperament, and caregiver response (Phalen, 2013).

For some concerns about feeding difficulties and failure to thrive, clinicians may need to refer to an individual or team for a feeding evaluation that includes an oral sensorimotor and feeding evaluation and video fluoroscopic swallow study. This feeding evaluation should be performed by a specialized feeding therapist with experience in this area, generally a speech–language pathologist or occupational therapist. Other integral team members may include a dietician reviewing the nutritional needs of the infant, a lactation specialist for breastfeeding mothers, a developmental pediatrician to evaluate any global developmental delays and attachment difficulties, a social worker and psychologist facilitating parent–child conflict and maladaptive mealtime behaviors, and a pediatric gastroenterologist assessing any higher acuity needs for nutrition.

Feeding difficulties and suboptimal growth impact development, behaviors, and family functioning. The feeding event, as a whole, influences the infant's social and emotional development. Impaired motor and cognitive performance is often seen in very preterm infants with poor postnatal growth (Cooke & Foulder-Hughes,

2003; Corbett & Drewett, 2004). Feeding difficulties may also cause distress in families. Delays in the attainment of full oral feeds can result in psychological distress among mothers, altering the mother–infant relationship (Silberstein et al., 2009). Optimizing nutrition and feeding behaviors and also implementing early management and intervention can provide long–term developmental benefits for the NICU graduate (Black et al., 2007).

Neurosensory Impairments

The NICU graduate is at risk for a spectrum of neurosensory impairments, including hearing impairment, blindness and visual impairments, and other sensory deviations. In general, as gestational age decreases, these neurosensory impairment risks increase.

HEARING AND VISION

Hearing impairment covers the range from mild to profound hearing loss. Hearing impairment is multifactorial and can be due to conductive hearing loss, sensorineural hearing loss, mixed conductive–sensorineural hearing loss, or auditory neuropathy. In the NICU population, a number of risk factors for hearing impairment are related to prematurity and other conditions, including side effects of various treatments and environmental factors. Evaluation, identification, and intervention should start as early possible, while the infant is in the NICU, and continue throughout follow-up.

The most common vision difficulty in NICU graduates is retinopathy of prematurity (ROP), but several other ophthalmologic conditions also need to be assessed, including cataracts, optic nerve hypoplasia, and cortical visual impairment. ROP is a disease in which retinal blood vessels of premature infants fail to grow and develop normally. The earlier the gestational age and lower the birth weight, the greater the risk of ROP. ROP is one of the most common causes of visual impairment in the United States. All infants born at less than 30 weeks of gestation or weighing less than 1,500 g should be screened, as should any infants with a birth weight between 1,500 and 2,000 g or a gestational age of greater than 30 weeks (Fierson, 2018). Early identification of visual impairment is crucial. The follow-up clinic team should be aware that infants who have had ROP, even if the ROP resolves, are at increased risk for other visual disorders, such as strabismus, amblyopia, high refractive errors, cataracts, glaucoma, and later retinal detachments (Early Treatment for Retinopathy of Prematurity Cooperative Group, 2005; Fierson, 2018).

SENSORY PROCESSING DIFFICULTIES

Sensory processing disorders are included as a neurosensory impairment in this section because NICU infants, particularly preterm infants, are at risk for sensory sensitivities (Ryckman et al., 2017). These sensory processing difficulties include a hyper- or hyporesponsiveness to tactile, auditory, or visual stimuli and self-stimulatory behaviors. If a child presents with these symptoms, additional diagnoses should also be investigated (i.e., autism spectrum disorder, attention-deficit/hyperactivity disorder, and developmental delays). In addition to providing support for these diagnoses, occupational therapists may be part of the therapeutic team to provide sensory integration therapy (Schaaf et al., 2017).

Complex Medical Conditions

Whereas complex medical conditions may be the most difficult to deal with in the NICU and generally involve the participation of multiple subspecialists, they can often be rather straightforward during graduate follow-up. For example, although predicting the needs of VLBW infants with some degree of neurological impairment is uncertain, it is clear that the child with trisomy 21 and congenital heart disease will need follow-up by cardiology and other subspecialists providing care as documented in the AAP policy statement on health supervision of children with Down syndrome (Bull et al., 2011). These children will also almost certainly qualify for early intervention services in all states based on the genetic diagnosis and not need to go through an evaluation for verification of needs for these services. In these complex cases, the goals of long-term management can often be determined by the diagnosis, and the difficulty is in navigating a path to those goals. This navigation often rests in the hands of the NICU discharge team, often led by an experienced nurse or social worker.

Unfortunately, there are also conditions diagnosed for which further medical care aimed at "cure" may be considered futile, and care in follow-up may instead focus on supporting the family in providing comfortable care to the infant/young child, such as for children/families with specific genetic conditions (e.g., trisomy 18 and spinal muscular atrophy type 1) or congenital anomalies (e.g., anencephaly). Although hospital pastoral care is seldom included in follow-up program planning, community support from local clergy should not be refused if desired by the family.

CONCLUSION

Since the beginning of the 20th century, both the field of medicine and society at large have been fascinated with the outcome for infants born at risk for death and neurodevelopmental disabilities. Physicians skilled in these infants' diseases have made great progress in treating them, but these diseases still persist and iatrogenic ones have arisen. Psychologists and other professionals debate the best way to evaluate the survivors. The medical system works in various ways with the educational system to provide the best care possible.

REFERENCES

Agrawal, S., Rao, S. C., Bulsara, M. K., & Patole, S. K. (2018). Prevalence of autism spectrum disorder in preterm infants: A meta-analysis. *Pediatrics, 142*(3), e20180134. https://doi.org/10.1542/peds.2018-0134

American Academy of Pediatrics and American College of Obstetrics and Gynecology. (2002). Neonatal complications. In *Guidelines for perinatal care* (5th ed., pp. 237–283).

Bayley, N. (2006). *Bayley Scales of Infant and Toddler Development—Third edition: Administration manual.* Harcourt.

Black, M. M., Dubowitz, H., Krishnakumar, A., & Starr, R. H. (2007). Early intervention and recovery among children with failure to thrive: Follow-up at age 8. *Pediatrics, 120*(1), 59–69. doi:10.1542/peds.2006-1657

Bull, M. J.; Committee on Genetics. (2011). Health supervision for children with Down syndrome. *Pediatrics, 128*(2), 393–406. https://doi.org/10.1542/peds.2011-1605

Butler, C., Chambers, H., Goldstein, M., Harris, S., Leach, J., Campbell, S., Adams, R., & Darrah, J. (1999). Evaluating research in developmental disabilities: A conceptual framework for reviewing treatment outcomes. *Developmental Medicine and Child Neurology, 41*(1), 55–59.

Cheong, J., & Doyle, L. W. (2018). An update on pulmonary and neurodevelopmental outcomes of bronchopulmonary dysplasia. *Seminars in Perinatology, 42*(7), 478–484.

Columbia University Irving Medical Center. (2015, August 6). *History of Medicine: The Incubator Babies of Coney Island.* https://columbiasurgery.org/news/2015/08/06/history-medicine-incubator-babies-coney

Cooke, R. W., & Foulder-Hughes, L. (2003). Growth impairment in the very preterm and cognitive and motor performance at 7 years. *Archives of Disease in Childhood, 88*(6), 482–487. doi:10.1136/adc.88.6.482

Corbett, S., & Drewett, R. (2004). To what extent is failure to thrive in infancy associated with poorer cognitive development? A review and meta-analysis. *Journal of Child Psychology and Psychiatry, 45*(3), 641–654. doi:10.1111/j.1469-7610.2004.00253.x

Dempsey, A. G., Goode, R. H., Colon, M. T., Holubeck, P., Nsier, H., Zopatti, K., & Needelman, H. (2020). Variations in criteria for eligibility determination for early intervention services with a focus on eligibility for children with neonatal complications. *Journal of Developmental & Behavioral Pediatrics, 41*(8), 646–655.

Drillien, C. M. (1958). Growth and development in a group of children of very low birth weight. *Archives of Disease in Childhood, 33*(167), 10–18. https://doi.org/10.1136/adc.33.167.10

Dunn, P. M. (2002). Stéphane Tarnier (1828–1897), the architect of perinatology in France. *Archives of Disease in Childhood: Fetal and Neonatal Edition, 86*(2), F137–F139. https://doi.org/10.1136/fn.86.2.f137

Early Treatment for Retinopathy of Prematurity Cooperative Group. (2005). The incidence and course of retinopathy of prematurity: Findings from the Early Treatment for Retinopathy of Prematurity Study. *Pediatrics, 116*(1), 15–23.

Einspieler, C., & Prechtl, H. F. (2005). Prechtl's assessment of general movements: A diagnostic tool for the functional assessment of the young nervous system. *Mental Retardation and Developmental Disabilities Research Reviews, 11*(1), 61–67. https://doi.org/10.1002/mrdd.20051

Fierson, W. M. (2018). Screening examination of premature infants for retinopathy of prematurity. *Pediatrics, 142*(6), e20183061. doi:10.1542/peds.2018-3061

Gartner, L. (1997, June 10). *Interview with William A. Silverman* [Interview]. American Academy of Pediatrics Pediatric History Center. https://www.aap.org/pediatrichistorycenter

Gomez Pomar, E., Concina, V. A., Samide, A., Westgate, P. M., & Bada, H. S. (2018). Bronchopulmonary dysplasia: Comparison between the two most used diagnostic criteria. *Frontiers in Pediatrics, 6*, 397.

Hess, J. H. (1953). Experiences gained in a thirty-year study of prematurely born infants. *Pediatrics, 11*(5), 425–434.

Hirvonen, M., Ojala, R., Korhonen, P., Haataja, P., Eriksson, K., Gissler, M., Luukkaala, T., & Tammela, O. (2014). Cerebral palsy among children born moderately and late preterm. *Pediatrics*, 134(6), e1584–e1593. doi:10.1542/peds.2014-0945

Infant Health and Development Program. (1990). Enhancing the outcomes of low-birth-weight, premature infants. *JAMA, 263*(22), 3035–3042. https://doi.org/10.1001/jama.1990.03440220059030

Jensen, E. A., & Schmidt, B. (2014). Epidemiology of bronchopulmonary dysplasia. *Birth Defects Research. Part A: Clinical and Molecular Teratology, 100*(3), 145–157.

Little, W. J. (1966). On the influence of abnormal parturition, difficult labors, premature birth, and asphyxia neonatorum, on the mental and physical condition of the child, especially in relation to deformities. *Clinical Orthopedics and Related Research, 46*, 7–22.

Mandile, O. (2020). Neonatal respiratory distress syndrome and its treatment with artificial surfactant. In *The Embryo Project Encyclopedia*. http://embryo.asu.edu/handle/10776/12981.

McGrath, J. M., & Braescu, A. V. (2004). State of the science: Feeding readiness in the preterm infant. *Journal of Perinatal & Neonatal Nursing, 18*(4), 353–368. doi:10.1097/00005237-200410000-00006

Morgan, C., Crowle, C., Goyen, T., Hardman, C., Jackman, M., Novak, I., & Badawi, N. (2015). Sensitivity and specificity of General Movements Assessment for diagnostic accuracy of detecting cerebral palsy early in an Australian context. *Journal of Pediatrics and Child Health, 52*(1), 54–59. doi:10.1111/jpc.12995

Mutch, L., Alberman, E., Hagberg, B., Kodama, K., & Perat, M. V. (1992). Cerebral palsy epidemiology: Where are we now and where are we going? *Developmental Medicine and Child Neurology, 34*(6), 547–551. https://doi.org/10.1111/j.1469-8749.1992.tb11479.x

Needelman, H., Contompasis, S., Steingass, K., Boyd, L., & Tang, B. (2015). *Creating systems of developmental follow up for NICU graduates: Lessons from the past, current challenges, and collaborations for the future* [Conference presentation]. Society of Developmental Pediatrics annual meeting, October 2–5, Las Vegas, NV.

Nickel, R. E. (2000). Cerebral palsy. In R. E. Nickel & L. W. Desch (Eds.), *The physician's guide to caring for children with disabilities and chronic conditions* (pp. 141–185). Brookes.

Pellegrino, L. (2002). Cerebral Palsy. In M. Batshaw, N. J. Roizen, & L. Pellegrino (Eds.), *Children with disabilities* (5th ed., pp. 443–466). Brooks.

Phalen, J. A. (2013). Managing feeding problems and feeding disorders. *Pediatrics in Review, 34*(12), 549–557. doi:10.1542/pir.34-12-549

Rhodes, P. (1977). Physical deformity of Richard III. *British Medical Journal, 2*(6103), 1650–1652.

Robertson, A. F. (2003). Reflections on errors in neonatology: II. The "heroic" years, 1950 to 1970. *Journal of Perinatology, 23*(2), 154–161.

Ryckman, J., Hilton, C., Rogers, C., & Pineda, R. (2017). Sensory processing disorder in preterm infants during early childhood and relationships to early neurobehavior. *Early Human Development, 113*, 18–22. doi:10.1016/j.earlhumdev.2017.07.012

Schaaf, R. C., Dumont, R. L., Arbesman, M., & May-Benson, T. A. (2017). Efficacy of occupational therapy using Ayres Sensory Integration: A systematic review. *American Journal of Occupational Therapy, 72*(1), 7201190010p1–7201190010p10. doi:10.5014/ajot.2018.02

Silberstein, D., Geva, R., Feldman, R., Gardner, J. M., Karmel, B. Z., Rozen, H., & Kuint, J. (2009). The transition to oral feeding in low-risk premature infants: Relation to infant neurobehavioral functioning and mother–infant feeding interaction. *Early Human Development, 85*(3), 157–162. doi:10.1016/j.earlhumdev.2008.07.006

St. Geme, J. (1960). On the "Gray Syndrome" and Chloramphenicol Toxicity. *Pediatrics, 25*(6), 1088–1090.

Theile, A. R., Radmacher, P. G., Anschutz, T. W., Davis, D. W., & Adamkin, D. H. (2012). Nutritional strategies and growth in extremely low birth weight infants with bronchopulmonary dysplasia over the past 10 years. *Journal of Perinatology, 32*(2), 117–122.

Vanderbilt, D., Mirzaian, C., & Schifsky, K. (2018). Environmental risks to NICU outcomes. In H. Needelman & B. Jackson (Eds.), *Follow-up for NICU graduates* (pp. 199–203). Springer. https://doi.org/10.1007/978-3-319-73275-6_10

Walsh, M. C., Szefler, S., Davis, J., Allen, M., Van Marter, L., Abman, S., Blackmon, L., & Jobe, A. (2006). Summary proceedings from the Bronchopulmonary Dysplasia Group. *Pediatrics, 117*(3 Pt. 2), S52–S56.

Watterberg, K. L.; American Academy of Pediatrics, Committee on Fetus and Newborn. (2010). Policy statement—Postnatal corticosteroids to prevent or treat bronchopulmonary dysplasia. *Pediatrics, 126*(4), 800–808. https://doi.org/10.1542/peds.2010-1534

World Health Organization. (2020). *Disability*. https://www.who.int/health-topics/disability

You, J., Shamsi, B., Hao, M., Cao, C., & Yang, W. (2019). A study on the neurodevelopment outcomes of late preterm infants. *BMC Neurology, 19*(1), 108. doi:10.1186/s12883-019-1336-0

COMMON NEURODEVELOPMENTAL AND BEHAVIORAL HEALTH CHALLENGES IN NEONATAL FOLLOW-UP

KATHRYN E. GUSTAFSON AND MOLLIE G. WARREN ■

High-risk infants are those who receive prolonged care in a neonatal intensive care unit (NICU), such as infants born prematurely, or infants with congenital anomalies including heart disease or congenital diaphragmatic hernia, prenatal insults such as intrauterine stroke or in utero drug exposure, or perinatal complications such as birth asphyxia or hypoxic ischemic encephalopathy (HIE). Outpatient developmental follow-up of high-risk infants is an essential component of ongoing medical care because these children are at risk for numerous neurodevelopmental morbidities. A vast body of research during the past several decades has shown that these infants are at risk for ongoing developmental and behavioral challenges that continue well into adulthood. Neurodevelopmental outcomes research on children born extremely premature is abundant. This chapter reviews the common neurodevelopmental and behavioral health challenges exhibited by children who were high-risk infants and who are typically referred to NICU follow-up clinics (NFUs). The focus of this chapter is on infancy through early school age, given that children of these ages are those most typically seen in NFUs.

CASE EXAMPLE

Isaiah was born at 24 weeks of gestation to a 19-year-old mother following a pregnancy complicated by placental abruption and no prenatal care. Isaiah's 4-month course was complicated by bronchopulmonary dysplasia (BPD), necrotizing enterocolitis, retinopathy of prematurity (ROP) requiring laser surgery, grade IV intraventricular hemorrhage (IVH) requiring shunt placement, and poor oral feeding requiring gastrostomy tube placement. His parents both had histories of learning and mental health disorders, had not completed high school, and were unemployed. They had difficulties managing his home care needs and reliably attending his medical appointments. At age 3 years, he was placed in foster care. Developmental follow-up in the high-risk infant clinic at 18 months and again at age 3 years resulted in diagnoses of spastic diplegic cerebral palsy (CP) and developmental delay. Behavioral problems were evident, including distractibility and inattention. Isaiah learned to ambulate independently by age 3 years, although he required orthotics and had a slow and clumsy gait. He received occupational, physical, and speech therapy (OT, PT, and ST, respectively) through his county early intervention program and attended developmental preschool starting at age 3 years. A neuropsychological assessment at age 6 years revealed mild intellectual disability, with particular challenges with visual spatial processing, working memory, and processing speed, and relatively stronger verbal reasoning abilities. He also exhibited very low reading and math achievement scores relative to age and grade expectations. Isaiah received a diagnosis of attention-deficit/hyperactivity disorder (ADHD), combined type, and was prescribed methylphenidate. He was placed in a self-contained special education classroom with some mainstreaming, and he continued to receive OT, PT, and ST at school. His biological parents maintained regular visitation with him but have thus far been unable to meet the requirements for family reunification. Isaiah remains with the same foster family, who are very devoted to his care and development.

DEVELOPMENTAL DELAY

Developmental delay is common in children followed in high-risk infant follow-up clinics, as seen with Isaiah (described above). Although mortality has decreased for extremely preterm infants due to advances in medical care, rates of developmental problems remain high. However, the rates of developmental delay in extremely preterm children vary across studies, in part due to varying methods of defining or classifying developmental delay, use of different developmental assessment tools, and differing child ages at the time of follow-up assessment.

In a review of large developmental outcomes studies of extremely premature infants (<28 weeks of gestation) conducted in several countries, rates of mild developmental delay during early childhood ranged from 16% to 37%, moderate developmental delay ranged from 19% to 32%, and severe developmental delay ranged from 9% to 19%. There was a shift toward the lower end of the developmental distribution. The mean score was lower than average, more children fell in the lower developmental ranges, and fewer children fell in the higher developmental ranges (Rogers & Hintz, 2016).

As with Isaiah, neurodevelopmental impairment is particularly evident in children born near the limits of viability, although rates of neurodevelopmental impairment may be decreasing over time with improved neonatal care, at least in some infants. Younge and colleagues (2016) examined neurodevelopmental outcomes during the toddler age in infants born at less than 25 weeks gestational age (GA). Infants born between 1998 and 2004 (Epoch 1) were compared with infants born between 2005 and 2011 (Epoch 2). Despite similar birth weight and GA, infants born during Epoch 2 had significantly lower rates of mortality and medical morbidities, but they also had significantly lower neurodevelopmental impairment defined by moderate or severe CP, significant cognitive or motor impairment on the Bayley Scales of Infant and Toddler Development, or bilateral blindness. Neurodevelopmental impairment declined from 68% in Epoch 1 to 47% in Epoch 2, indicating improvement over time but high rates of impairment, nonetheless. Moreover, when further divided by birth GA, risk of death or neurodevelopmental impairment was lower in Epoch 2 in infants born at 24 weeks of gestation but not in infants born at 23 weeks or less, indicating that high rates of mortality and morbidity are still evident in the most extremely premature infants.

Problems in development persist into early school age and are associated with neurologic findings in infancy. As described in the case example, Isaiah experienced a brain hemorrhage during infancy, exhibited brain abnormality on magnetic resonance imaging (MRI), and continued to show developmental delay at early school age—a pattern that has been supported by research. The National Institute of Child Health and Human Development's Neonatal Research Network (NRN) assessed neurodevelopmental outcomes at ages 6 and 7 years as part of the Neuroimaging and Neurodevelopmental Outcomes study, a prospective study of early and near-term cranial ultrasound (CUS) and near-term brain MRI among extremely preterm infants born from 24 through 27 weeks GA (Hintz et al., 2018). Follow-up data were available for 386 children. Forty-five percent of children had a full-scale intelligence quotient (FSIQ) <85 and 13% had FSIQ <70. Adverse late CUS findings and significant cerebellar lesions on MRI were associated with significant disability, as defined by FSIQ <70; moderate to severe CP; and/or severe vision or hearing impairment. Adverse late CUS findings were associated with FSIQ <70 at early school age.

Neurodevelopmental impairment or developmental delay is also evident in early childhood in children with other neonatal insults that occur in the first 28 days of life. A recent meta-analysis and systematic review of 52 studies from throughout the world that evaluated long-term outcomes in 94,978 children aged 6 years or older found that the neurodevelopmental domain was commonly affected by neonatal insults (Magai et al., 2020). This meta-analysis found a median rate of 22% neurodevelopmental impairment across studies and diagnosis, although rates varied by disease: bacterial meningitis, 36.9%; HIE, 34.1%; congenital rubella, 32.7%; congenital cytomegalovirus, 27.5%; fetal growth restriction, 26.1%; preterm birth, 25.1%; birth asphyxia, 24.1%; and neonatal jaundice, 11.6%.

Developmental follow-up clinics are increasingly providing care for infants with in utero opioid exposure. The number of children exposed to opioids in utero has increased drastically, with an increase of greater than 300% from 1999 to 2014. The majority of these neonates experience opioid withdrawal or neonatal opioid withdrawal syndrome (NOWS), which includes neuroirritability, sleep disturbance, tremors, feeding difficulty, hypertonia, temperature instability, and gastrointestinal and respiratory issues. Despite this dramatic increase in the number of children exposed to opioids in utero, there has been relatively little research on short- and long-term neurodevelopmental outcomes, and most studies have lacked methodological rigor. A review article identified relatively few studies of neurodevelopmental outcomes in exposed infant- and toddler-aged children, and these studies were limited by small sample sizes, confounded by social environmental risk factors, or based on retrospective chart review (Conradt et al., 2019). Few differences emerged and effect sizes tended to be small, with most children developing within normal expectations. However, there were more studies of neurodevelopmental outcomes in school-age children. Although findings were again variable and complicated by methodological limitations, there does seem to be emerging evidence of poorer neurocognitive, academic, and behavioral outcome in opioid-exposed children relative to controls. However, to adequately understand the short- and long-term neurocognitive outcomes in these children, large-scale, multicenter, prospective, longitudinal studies are needed that evaluate diverse populations and that control for confounding pre- and postnatal biological, social, and environmental factors.

CEREBRAL PALSY AND DEVELOPMENTAL COORDINATION DISORDER

Care for children with motor problems is also important in high-risk infant follow-up clinics because high-risk infants are at increased risk for CP and other motor problems. CP encompasses a wide range of movement disorders and is clinically diagnosed based on neurological signs and motor impairments. The diagnosis often includes standardized motor assessments and brain imaging such as an MRI. As seen with Isaiah, there is an increased rate of CP in children born preterm, associated with increased rates of IVH and periventricular leukomalacia (PVL). Other neonatal complications, such as HIE, are also associated with CP and other motor impairments due to damage to the motor cortex. However, as noted by McGowan and Vohr (2019), with improvements in NICU care, rates of CP have declined over time. A NRN study of extremely preterm infants born from 2011 to 2014 found that the rate of CP declined from 16% to 12% during the study period. Although the rate of severe CP declined by 43%, the rate of mild

CP increased by 13%, suggesting that motor problems persist but may be milder (McGowan & Vohr, 2019). In children with HIE, treatment with whole body hypothermia has resulted in lower rates of CP. In a large randomized controlled trial, rates of CP were 19% in the hypothermia group and 30% in the control group (Natarajan et al., 2016).

In addition to CP, high-risk infants are at risk for other forms of motor impairment, such as balance abnormalities, poor manual dexterity, and general coordination problems that interfere with everyday life. These problems may result in a diagnosis of developmental coordination disorder (DCD). A prospective population-based investigation examined rates of DCD at age 61/ 2 years in otherwise healthy children born at 22–26 weeks GA compared with full-term controls (Bolk et al., 2018). The researchers intentionally excluded extremely preterm children with known medical problems such as CP, significant cognitive delay, and/or vision or hearing impairment. They found that 37% of preterm children compared with just 5.5% of full-term controls demonstrated DCD. Moreover, DCD at school age is associated with lower performance on cognitive and academic assessments and increased behavior problems (Bolk et al., 2018).

LEARNING AND ACADEMIC DIFFICULTIES

Children spend significant amounts of time in school, and academic performance is a major contributor to short- and long-term social–emotional functioning as well as economic outcomes in adulthood. As is evident with Isaiah, children who were high-risk infants demonstrate higher rates of learning difficulties and problems in school compared to their full-term peers. A meta-analysis of 17 studies that assessed academic achievement in children who were born premature found that the premature children scored below full-term peers by 0.71 standard deviations (SD) in arithmetic, 0.44 SD in reading, and 0.52 SD in writing (Twilhaar et al., 2018). In addition, premature children were almost three times more likely to receive special education services at school. Children with a history of BPD had the poorest academic outcomes. When limited to studies of children with GA <32 weeks, 78% of children with BPD had special education needs.

Learning problems in children who were high-risk infants may be associated with other neuropsychological deficits, such as poor working memory, impaired attention, and deficits in mental processing speed (Mulder et al., 2009). Therefore, developmental follow-up programs that continue to support children into early school age should monitor the academic outcomes of their patients and provide support for diagnostic assessment, school consultation, and referral for academic support and intervention. Indeed, school failure can have a profound and lifelong effect on an individual's economic success and mental and physical health outcomes.

EXECUTIVE FUNCTIONING

Executive functioning (EF) involves higher order cognitive processes necessary for self-regulation and organized goal-directed behavior and includes skills such as inhibitory control, working memory, planning and organization, cognitive flexibility, fluency, and selective and sustained attention. These skills are important to academic and social functioning. However, children who were former high-risk infants show an increased risk of impairment in EF and dysregulation. Our patient, Isaiah, demonstrated difficulties in several EF skills that contributed to his academic and learning challenges.

In a meta-analysis that included 29 studies, EF and attention emerged as areas of weakness for preterm children, although effect sizes ranged from small to moderate, and many of the findings on specific EF skills varied as a function of GA, assessment measure used, or age at assessment (Mulder et al., 2009). Impairments in EF may decrease with increasing GA, meaning that children who were the most premature are likely at greatest risk, although there is evidence of some difficulties with EF even in moderate or late preterm children (Taylor & Clark, 2016). Risk for EF impairment increases in children with neonatal complications such as BPD, ROP, sepsis, and neurosensory impairment and also in children, like Isaiah, with early brain abnormalities, such as PVL or IVH.

Moreover, social environmental factors, such as socioeconomic status (SES), parent mental health, and parenting styles, have been associated with EF difficulties (Taylor & Clark, 2016). Impairments in EF are also highly associated with academic achievement and behavioral functioning across childhood. Therefore, it is crucial that efficacious interventions are identified for EF problems in former preterm or other high-risk infants. NICU interventions (e.g., kangaroo care [skin-to-skin contact] and parent training programs), school programs that focus on development of self-regulation skills, and computerized cognitive training programs have shown mixed success with improving EF in preterm children (Taylor & Clark, 2016).

AUTISM SPECTRUM DISORDER

Autism spectrum disorder (ASD) is among the most common developmental disabilities affecting children, with the Centers for Disease Control and Prevention reporting a prevalence of 1 in 44 children (Maenner et al., 2021). Children who were high-risk infants, particularly those born prematurely, are at increased risk for ASD. A large population-based retrospective study of almost 200,000 children born across the gestational age range from 24 to 42+ weeks found that children born at less than 27 weeks GA were three times more likely to have ASD compared to term infants and that risk increased with each week of lower GA (Kuzniewicz et al., 2014). Moreover, increased risk for ASD was associated with being small for gestational age independent of GA. Relative to matched full-term peers, extremely premature children may demonstrate higher rates of impaired social and communication development, even when they do not meet diagnostic threshold for ASD (Johnson et al., 2010).

A systematic review and meta-analysis of 3,366 premature infants from 18 studies that used autism diagnostic methodologies, rather than ASD screening measures, found a rate of 7% in children born prematurely (GA: 25–31 weeks; body weight: 719–1,565 g), with a slightly, although not significantly, higher rate (9%) when children with disabilities were excluded (Agrawal et al., 2018).

Additional research is necessary to provide a better understanding of the biomedical and environmental factors that increase this risk. However, most researchers believe there is a multifactorial pathogenesis, with children who develop ASD having underlying biologic vulnerability combined with exogenous stressors affecting brain development during the intrauterine or early postnatal periods.

OTHER BEHAVIORAL HEALTH DIFFICULTIES

Behavioral and mental health issues are common in children who were high-risk infants, particularly those born premature. These challenges may emerge early. An NRN study of 2,505 children born at less than 27 weeks of gestation evaluated on a parent report measure of behavior problems and social competence at 18–22 months corrected age found that 35% of children had behavior problems and 26% showed deficits in social competence. At 30–33 months of age, the rate of parent-reported behavior problems was almost 47% and the rate of deficits in social competence was 20% (Peralta-Carcelen et al., 2017).

Given these high rates of behavioral problems, understanding the specific behavioral diagnoses can potentially target empirically validated treatment approaches. A prospective longitudinal study evaluated psychiatric diagnoses at age 7 years in children born very preterm (<30 weeks of gestation) compared with their full-term peers and found that very preterm children had a three times higher rate of psychiatric diagnosis than their peers, with 24% of the very preterm children having a psychiatric diagnosis at age 7 years (Treyvaud et al., 2013). Anxiety disorders (11%), ADHD (10%), and ASD (4.5%) were the most common diagnoses in the very preterm group, whereas the greatest rate difference between the very preterm group and the term controls was that for ASD (4.5% vs. 0%, respectively). Specific phobia and separation anxiety disorder were the most common anxiety disorders in the very preterm group. Factors associated with psychiatric diagnosis at age 7 years in the preterm group were global brain abnormalities on MRI at term equivalent, parent-reported significant social–emotional problems at age 5 years, and high family social risk.

Symptoms of inattention or diagnoses of ADHD have frequently emerged as among the most common behavioral challenges presented by children born prematurely. As described in the case example, Isaiah began exhibiting significant problems of distractibility and inattention by age 3 years and received a diagnosis of ADHD requiring treatment with stimulant medication by age 6 years.

A recent meta-analysis that included 12 studies and 1,787 children found that both very premature (VP; <32 weeks of gestation) and very low-birth-weight (VLBW; <1,500 g) and extremely preterm (EP; <28 weeks of gestation) and extremely low-birth-weight (ELBW; <1,000 g) children have a significantly higher risk of ADHD diagnosis than term controls, with an odds ratio of 3.04 (Franz et al., 2018). Findings were even stronger for EP/ELBW children than for VP/VLBW children, suggesting greater risk for ADHD in situations of more extreme prematurity. Moreover, when assessing ADHD symptomatology rather than diagnoses in 29 of the studies with 3,504 children, there were higher rates of inattention, impulsivity, hyperactivity, and combined symptoms in children born preterm relative to controls (Franz et al, 2018). Therefore, it is crucial that follow-up programs consider this increased risk for ADHD and related symptoms and provide intervention or referrals, particularly given the association of poorer academic achievement, lower self-esteem, higher rates of social problems, and greater conduct and antisocial behavior and substance use later in life in individuals with ADHD.

SLEEP

Good-quality sleep is crucial to child development and quality of life, yet sleep problems are common across childhood. Moreover, infant and child sleep can affect parental mental health and quality of life. Therefore, developmental follow-up clinic staff are frequently asked by parents to address child sleep problems. Evidence indicates a higher rate of sleep problems throughout childhood in children born prematurely; however, studies vary in terms of GA of participants, age at sleep assessment, and comorbidities such as neurological pathology (Romeo et al., 2019). Romeo and colleagues examined sleep problems in preschool-age children. They found that elevations on a sleep problems scale were only slightly higher in preterm children without neurological disorders (7%) compared to a matched sample of full-term peers (3%), although specific types of sleep problems were evident in almost 21% of these children and in only 4% of their matched peers. Higher rates of sleep-disordered breathing, sleep hyperhidrosis, and difficulty initiating and maintaining sleep were all evident in the preterm group (Romeo et al., 2019). Assessment of specific sleep problems in children who were high-risk or premature infants should therefore be included as a standard component of developmental follow-up care. Parents may benefit from psychoeducation about the benefits of and strategies for sleep training. Moreover, these children may need a referral to a pediatric specialty sleep clinic, particularly in more medically fragile children or in situations of parental anxiety about sleep training. Sleep training, which typically involves extinction or modified extinction approaches, can be very difficult for some parents, particularly parents who already worry about their children's medical and developmental status.

PARENTAL STRESS AND COPING

Parental stress and distress in the presence of childhood chronic illness have been documented for decades, although parent resilience is also common (Thompson & Gustafson, 1996). Parents of children who were high-risk infants are no exception, and parent support programs, such as Hand to Hold for parents of premature infants, Hope for HIE for parents of children with HIE, or Little Hearts for parents of children with congenital heart disease, can provide important coping resources for these families. When providing family-centered care in developmental follow-up clinics, it is important that members of developmental follow-up teams be aware of risk and resiliency factors for individual families. Availability of high-quality emotional and social support for parents is crucial. The significance of social support to child and parent outcomes in the presence of childhood chronic illnesses has long been a robust finding in the literature. More recently, a study of ELBW children participating in NRN studies assessed family resources and social support using the Family Resource Scale, which assesses family access to physical and health necessities, financial resources, personal resources, and social support (Fuller et al., 2019). Families who had higher levels of resources and social support had children who showed greater gains in cognitive outcomes between ages 18 and 30 months. Social support was a significant predictor of improvement in cognitive development, independent of income and demographic variability. Addressing parental social support is a potentially modifiable social ecological factor for NFU teams.

SOCIAL ENVIRONMENTAL CHALLENGES

Neurodevelopmental and behavioral health outcomes in children with chronic illness are determined by complex transactions between biomedical and social environmental factors (Thompson & Gustafson, 1996). In much of the research reviewed above, the role of social environmental factors in developmental outcome is evident. Our patient, Isaiah, was affected by social environmental factors such as having parents with poor economic stability, low education, and mental health problems. Indeed, social environmental factors such as lower SES, poverty, parental mental health problems, lower parental education, and poorer quality neighborhoods and schools are associated with poorer developmental outcomes in high-risk infants (Fuller, 2019). In our society, these factors are associated with economic adversity, and economic adversity is in turn associated with worse medical, developmental, and behavioral outcomes. Recognition of these factors points to the crucial importance of advocating for social policy reform as necessary to improve outcomes for families and children.

In addition, some former high-risk infants with complicated social histories may end up in foster care or kinship care, as happened with our patient, Isaiah. Although foster care or kinship care can result in improved social environments for many children, family reunification is often the goal, and efficacious family support programs are needed to help birth parents manage their own challenges with mental health, addiction, child neglect, or maltreatment. The effects of social and environmental factors on outcomes in high-risk infants provide a challenge for NFU staff. Clinic staff must recognize the contributions of these factors to patients' medical and neurodevelopmental functioning, appropriately and sensitively evaluate these factors in individual patients, access effective family support programs in their communities, and become vocal advocates for increased resources and more effective social policies.

IDEAS WORTH SHARING

- Routine assessment for cognitive, language, motor, and learning problems is crucial at least into early school age given high rates of developmental, motor, and learning problems in children who were former high-risk infants.
- Routine screening for behavioral health challenges is crucial at least into early school age, especially given higher rates of behavioral difficulties as well as disorders such as ADHD, ASD, and anxiety in this population.
- Children with prenatal drug exposure or NOWS need close follow-up, particularly given the comorbid social risks often confronted by these children.
- Children with brain abnormalities may be particularly at risk for cognitive, language, motor, learning, and behavioral health problems.
- Children who were high-risk infants may require behavioral health services, and NFU teams should develop consulting relationships with local child support agencies, including counseling centers and behavioral health clinics, to facilitate referrals.
- Children who were high-risk infants may require social and academic support at school, and follow-up clinic staff should develop consulting relationships with schools.
- All children seen in developmental follow-up clinics should be screened for sleep problems, and staff should provide/refer for behavioral sleep training or medical treatment, as needed.
- Parents of high-risk infants are also at risk for stress and distress, although resiliency is also possible. Parents may benefit from support from other parents or members of the follow-up team, such as social workers or psychologists, or require referral for behavioral health services in their home communities.
- Children's developmental needs should be considered within the context of their sociocultural and socioeconomic environment, including consideration of both risk and resiliency factors.

CONCLUSION

As reviewed in this chapter, high-risk infants are at increased risk for problems in neurodevelopment, including developmental delay; neuromotor problems such as CP and DCD; academic difficulties in reading, math, and spelling; and neuropsychological deficits such as impaired EF or other skills that are important to learning and effective daily functioning. Many of these children may need developmental intervention and therapies, as well as academic support and special educational services, throughout their development. In addition, these children are at increased risk for behavioral health challenges such as increased rates of behavioral dysregulation, ASD, ADHD, and anxiety disorders, and they may need high-quality, empirically validated behavioral health services. Disordered sleep is also evident in many children who were high-risk infants, with associated implications for quality of life for both children and parents. Social and environmental factors have a significant effect on developmental outcomes independent of biomedical risk factors, and poorer outcomes are evident in children who also confront the challenges of poverty, parental mental health problems, and other adverse childhood experiences. Research is just beginning to elucidate the potential role of prenatal, perinatal, and postnatal environmental stress on the developmental trajectories of high-risk infants through epigenetic changes in stress-related genes. Finally, parents and caregivers of these children are at increased risk for stress and distress but can also exhibit resiliency, particularly when provided with social support as well as appropriate resources to address their children's needs.

Given the myriad of neurodevelopmental and behavioral health challenges in children who were high-risk infants and the associated challenges for families, comprehensive, multidisciplinary developmental follow-up of these infants is crucial. Ideally, the NFUs continue to follow children at least until early school age. Ongoing developmental follow-up, with associated monitoring, screening, assessment, and intervention services, either as part of clinic services or through well-developed relationships with community referral resources, can affect the short- and long-term outcomes for these children. Health care providers who work with these children can also make a significant difference in the lives of these children through remaining aware of and advocating for effective social programs, policies, and resources that effectively and efficiently support high-risk infants and their families.

REFERENCES

Agrawal, S., Rao, S. C., Bulsara, M. K., & Patole, S. K. (2018). Prevalence of autism spectrum disorder in preterm infants: A meta-analysis. *Pediatrics, 142*(3), e20180134.

Bolk, J., Farooqi, A., Hafström, M., Åden, U., & Serenius, F. (2018). Developmental coordination disorder and its association with developmental comorbidities at 6.5 years in apparently healthy children born extremely preterm. *JAMA Pediatrics, 172*(8), 765–774.

Conradt, E., Flannery, T., Aschner, J. L., Annett, R. D., Croen, L. A., Duarte, C. S., Friedman, A. M., Guille, C., Hedderson, M. M., Hofheimer, J. A., Jones, M. R., Ladd-Acosta, C., McGrath, M., Moreland, A., Neiderhiser, J. M., Nguyen, R. H. N., Posner, J., Ross, J. L., Savitz, D. A., . . . Lester, B. M. (2019). Prenatal opioid exposure: Neurodevelopmental consequences and future research priorities. *Pediatrics*, *144*(3), e20190128.

Franz, A. P., Bolat, G. U., Bolat, H., Matijasevich, A., Santos, I. S., Silveira, R. C., Procianoy, R. S., Rohde, L. A., & Moreira-Maia, C. R. (2018). Attention-deficit/hyperactivity disorder and very preterm/very low birth weight: A meta-analysis. *Pediatrics*, *141*(1), e20171645.

Fuller, M. G., Vaucher, Y. E., Bann, C. M., Das, A., & Vohr, B. R. (2019). Lack of social support as measured by the Family Resource Scale screening tool is associated with early adverse cognitive outcome in extremely low birth weight children. *Journal of Perinatology*, *39*, 1546–1554.

Hintz, S., Vohr, B., Bann, C., Taylor, H. G., Das, A., Gustafson, K. E., Yolton, K., Watson, V., Lowe, J., DeAnda, M. E., Ball, M. B., Finer, N., Van Meurs, K., Shankaran, S., Pappas, A., Barnes, P., Bulas, D., Newman, J., Wilson-Costello, D., . . . Higgins, R. (2018). Preterm neuroimaging and school-age cognitive outcomes. *Pediatrics*, *42*(1), e20174058.

Johnson, S., Hollis, C., Kochhar, P., Hennessy, E., Wolke, D., & Marlow, N. (2010). Autism spectrum disorders in extremely preterm children. *Journal of Pediatrics*, *156*(4), 525–531.

Kuzniewicz, M. W., Wi, S., Qian, Y., Walsh, E. M., Armstrong, M. A., & Croen, L. A. (2014). Prevalence and neonatal factors associated with autism spectrum disorders in preterm infants. *Journal of Pediatrics*, *164*(1), 20–25.

Maenner, M. J., Shaw, K. A., Bakian, A. V., Bilder, D. A., Durkin, M. S., Esler, A., Furnier, S. M., Hallas, L., Hall-Lande, J., Hudson, A., Hughes, M. M., Patrick, M., Pierce, K., Poynter, J. N., Salinas, A., Shenouda, J., Vehorn, A., Warren, Z., Constantino, J. N., . . . & Cogswell, M. E. (2021). Prevalence and characteristics of autism spectrum disorder among children aged 8 years—autism and developmental disabilities monitoring network, 11 sites, United States, 2018. *MMWR Surveillance Summaries*, *70*(11), 1–16. doi:http://dx.doi.org/10.15585/mmwr.ss7011a1

Magai, D. N., Karyotaki, E., Mutua, A. M., Chongwo, E., Nasambu, C., Ssewanyana, D., Newton, C. R., Koot, C. M., & Abubakar, A. (2020). Long-term outcomes of survivors of neonatal insults: A systematic review and meta-analysis. *PLoS One*, *15*(4), e0231947.

McGowan, E. C., & Vohr, B. R. (2019). Neurodevelopmental follow-up of preterm infants. *Pediatric Clinics of North America*, *66*(2), 509–523.

Mulder, H., Pitchford, N. J., Hagger, M. S., & Marlow, N. (2009). Development of executive function and attention in preterm children: A systematic review. *Developmental Neuropsychology*, *34*(4), 393–421.

Natarajan, G., Pappas, A., & Shankaran, S. (2016). Outcomes in childhood following therapeutic hypothermia for neonatal hypoxic-ischemic encephalopathy (HIE). *Seminars in Perinatology*, *40*(8), 549–555.

Peralta-Carcelen, M., Carlo, W. A., Pappas, A., Vaucher, Y. E., Yeates, K. O., Phillips, V. A., Gustafson, K. E., Payne, A. F., Duncan, D. H., Newman, J. E., & Bann, C. (2017).

Behavioral problems and socioemotional competence at 18–22 months of extremely premature children. *Pediatrics, 139*(6), e20161043.

Rogers, E. E., & Hintz, S. R. (2016). Early neurodevelopmental outcomes of extremely preterm infants. *Seminars in Perinatology, 40*(8), 497–509.

Romeo, D. M., Leo, G., Lapenta, L., Leone, D., Turrini, I., Brogna, C., Gallini, F., Cota, F., Vento, G., & Mercuri, E. (2019). Sleep disorders in low-risk preschool very preterm children. *Sleep Medicine, 63*, 137–141.

Taylor, H. G., & Clark, C. A. C. (2016). Executive function in children born preterm: Risk factors and implications for outcome. *Seminars in Perinatology, 40*(8), 520–529.

Thompson, R. J., Jr., & Gustafson, K. E. (1996). *Adaptation to chronic childhood illness.* American Psychological Association.

Treyvaud, K., Ure, A., Doyle, L. W., Lee, K. J., Rogers, C. E., Kidokoro, H., Inder, T. A., & Anderson, P. J. (2013). Psychiatric outcomes at age seven for very preterm children: Rates and predictors. *Journal of Child Psychology and Psychiatry, 54*(7), 772–779.

Twilhaar, E. S., de Kieviet, J. F., Aarnoudse-Moens, C. S. H., van Elburg, R. M., & Oosterlaan, J. (2018). Academic performance of children born preterm: A meta-analysis and meta-regression. *Archives of Disease in Childhood: Fetal and Neonatal Edition, 103*, F322–F330.

Younge, N., Smith, P. B., Gustafson, K. E., Malcolm, W., Ashley, P., Cotten, C. M., Goldberg, R. N., & Goldstein, R. F. (2016). Improved survival and neurodevelopmental outcomes among extremely premature infants born near the limit of viability. *Early Human Development, 95*, 5–8.

27

ROLE OF BEHAVIORAL HEALTH CLINICIANS IN NEONATAL FOLLOW-UP SETTINGS

CASEY HOFFMAN AND ANNIE MARKOVITS ■

Medically complex infants often receive ongoing assessment after hospital discharge in neonatal follow-up clinics (NFUs) to best meet their multiple needs (American Academy of Pediatrics Committee on Fetus and Newborn, 2008). These clinics are often multidisciplinary and may include providers from diverse backgrounds, such as physicians from various pediatric specialties (e.g., neonatology, neurology, rehabilitation medicine, and developmental/general pediatrics), nurse practitioners, nurses, social workers, psychologists/neuropsychologists, developmental specialists, physical therapists, occupational therapists, and/or speech–language pathologists (Orton et al., 2018). Behavioral health clinicians (BHCs) are not yet ubiquitous, but when present they are significant assets to these teams and serve a variety of roles for both the infant and growing child and their families: screening, assessment, diagnosis, support, psychoeducation, referral, liaison, brief intervention, and multidisciplinary collaboration. When part of an academic medical center, BHCs may also contribute to the supervision of trainees as well as outcomes research.

TRANSITION TO HOME

I know how to be a parent in the NICU, but once she is discharged I will have no idea how to be parent at home!

—*Anonymous NICU parent*

Before families arrive at NFUs, there is a significant transition that occurs after neonatal intensive care unit (NICU) discharge. A BHC such as a social worker can play a key role in bridging this transition. In institutions in which inpatient and outpatient social workers comprise different teams, a handoff between the two groups of providers is essential for continuity of care. When possible, the outpatient social worker should meet families prior to discharge because this can help build rapport and continuity. Social workers can help caregivers understand the scope of the NFU and how the clinic can be helpful to them and their infant. Despite careful discharge planning, families may need support after discharge with the logistics of home nursing, medical daycare, medical equipment, referral to early intervention, and help knowing which specialists to contact for specific needs. Social workers can also help families with challenges in managing home life, employment, and finances with an infant who has complex medical needs. Social disparities can negatively impact some families' attendance in follow-up. Social workers are well positioned to identify and assist with some of the barriers that may exist, such as limited transportation or lack of child care for siblings (Swearingen et al., 2020). Social workers also guide parental expectations about their role in their infant's care after NICU discharge—specifically that parents will play a central role in advocating for their infant's needs and coordinating their care moving forward. The transition home is often not linear. Medically complex infants are at high risk for hospital readmission, and social workers help families cope with the multiple transitions that may occur.

CAREGIVER SCREENING IN FOLLOW-UP

Elevations in parental mood and anxiety symptoms often persist beyond infant NICU discharge, and some studies have indicated that post-traumatic stress can be persistent after an infant with complex medical history transitions home (Schecter et al., 2020). In addition to processing a traumatic pregnancy, labor, and delivery, as well as the loss of a typical infancy and trauma incurred during the NICU stay, parents may be faced with new stressors, including management of their infant's chronic medical conditions, ongoing feeding challenges, difficulties with equipment and home nursing, developmental concerns, and financial stressors related to loss of income. After NICU discharge, parents are often more likely to present to pediatric appointments than see their own adult providers, and even at their own appointments, thorough mental health screening for both parents is not likely to occur. Screening for depression and anxiety at a mother's postpartum obstetrics visit is only at one time point and often does not include screening of a second caregiver (American College of Obstetricians and Gynecologists, 2018).

Behavioral health clinicians can be instrumental in establishing a screening program in the NFU setting. Selecting the most appropriate screening tools to detect parental symptoms should be based on the time since birth and type of symptoms. In the initial follow-up period, screening should be performed for postpartum mood and anxiety, as well as trauma. As time passes from the postpartum period, more general symptoms of depression, anxiety, and family stress may also present. Screening for additional concerns, including interpersonal violence, substance use, and family stress, is often part of social workers' verbal screening with families and can provide important contextual information when interpreting the results of mental health screeners. Due to the potential adverse impact of parental mental health concerns on the developing infant, screening should attempt to capture all primary caregivers of the infant, including parents, foster parents, and grandparents who may serve in a primary caretaking role. Other important considerations include building a screening process for caregivers with limited English proficiency as well as for caregivers with low literacy. Screening can be accomplished on paper or electronically, and BHCs can help establish a process that provides adequate protection for caregivers' screening information that may be stored within an infant's chart.

Administration is only the first step in screening, and a clear process for scoring, follow-up safety assessment for positive scores, and a referral process for further evaluation and/or treatment is needed. BHCs can be helpful in identifying when these steps will occur and which providers will complete them. A brief safety assessment following positive screening results should occur the day of screening, prior to the family leaving the clinic. Although serious safety concerns such as a caregiver with active suicidal intent are rare, a process for triaging caregivers with these types of concerns needs to be identified ahead of time. For clinics with embedded social workers or psychologists, these providers may perform some of these steps, although medical and nursing providers can also play a role. All providers will benefit from a decision tree to guide clinical decision-making following screening results.

BEHAVIORAL HEALTH TREATMENT RECOMMENDATIONS FOR CAREGIVERS

There may be a clear path for caregiver referral within the organization when treatment is indicated and/or a list of local providers may be provided. BHCs can be helpful in creating parental education documents that explain what positive results on the screeners indicate (including their limitations), how to obtain a follow-up evaluation, empirically supported treatments for the condition(s) being screened, as well as considerations in locating a BHC. When infants are followed longitudinally in the clinic, changes or consistency in screening results over time can be used as an educational tool to validate caregivers' impressions that symptoms are decreasing or highlight that ongoing concerns remain and build motivation for further evaluation. Caregivers often defer their own health needs, both physical and emotional, in favor of attending to their infant's needs. Attending a multitude of follow-up appointments for a high-risk infant often means caregivers have little time for their own appointments. BHCs can provide education about the impact of parental mental health on child development and counsel parents that attending to their own needs will lead to improvements for both them and their infant.

Several different approaches may be effective in the treatment of caregivers' symptoms of depression, anxiety, trauma, and/or stress within the family system. Treatment may include a range of modalities, such as individual therapy, family therapy, group therapy, peer support, and/or medication evaluation and management. For the treatment of postpartum mood and anxiety disorders, cognitive–behavioral therapies, interpersonal therapy, and psychotropic medications have been found to be effective (Fitelson et al., 2011). Depressive symptoms that cause disruption in caregiver–infant interactions, and evolving attachment may also benefit from dyadic approaches such as parent–infant psychotherapy. For post-traumatic stress disorder, trauma-focused cognitive–behavioral therapies such as cognitive processing therapy or prolonged exposure have been shown to be the most effective, with positive effects also found for eye movement desensitization and reprocessing and with the addition of certain antidepressant medications (Merz et al., 2019).

Support groups and peer-to-peer support can also help caregivers experiencing grief related to the loss of a typical parenting experience and feelings of isolation from their existing support network due to their infant's chronic health needs (Levick et al., 2014). These groups may be facilitated by BHCs and may meet in person or virtually. Given the expectation that medically vulnerable infants should be kept away from others due to infection risk, in addition to the logistical challenges of traveling with an infant with medical equipment and/or the need to find child care for the infant during the group meeting, virtual options may offer the best opportunity for caregivers to attend. These support groups may be administered locally, or caregivers can participate in a group hosted by a national organization (Box 27.1). Other caregivers may prefer one-on-one support from a trained parent mentor who can provide individual guidance. Finally, when an infant's condition causes strain within the family system, including siblings, family therapy can be a useful modality to explore ways to promote adaptive family dynamics.

COMPREHENSIVE PSYCHOLOGICAL ASSESSMENT OF HIGH-RISK INFANTS AND CHILDREN

Infants with complex medical histories are known to be at high risk for developing a range of neurodevelopmental, behavioral, and social–emotional comorbidities. Longitudinal assessment of infants and children is necessary to detect the full range of these concerns, as they emerge at different points along a child's developmental trajectory. For example, whereas delays in developmental milestones such as motor skills and cognitive exploration may be visible from infancy, social–emotional, behavioral, and persistent communication concerns appear more prominently in toddlerhood, and difficulties with attention, learning, and more complex cognitive processing may emerge in the preschool years and beyond. Identification of each

---

Box 27.1

RESOURCES FOR NEONATAL FOLLOW-UP FAMILIES

American Academy of Pediatrics for Parents: https://www.healthychildren.org
Attachment & Biobehavioral Catch-up: http://www.abcintervention.org
Autism Speaks: https://www.autismspeaks.org/tool-kit
Baby Sign Language: https://www.babysignlanguage.com
Center for Parent Information & Resources: https://www.parentcenterhub.org
Cerebral Palsy Foundation: https://www.yourcpf.org
CHADD (attention-deficit/hyperactivity disorder resources): https://chadd.org
Feeding Tube Awareness Foundation: https://www.feedingtubeawareness.org
Hand to Hold (parent support): https://handtohold.org
Hearing Loss Association of America: https://www.hearingloss.org
Individual with Disabilities Education Act: https://sites.ed.gov/idea
Lighthouse Guild, Cortical Visual Impairment (CVI):
    https://www.lighthouseguild.org/vision-health/cortical-visual-
    impairment-cvi
Make-A-Wish Foundation: https://wish.org
National Center for PTSD: https://www.ptsd.va.gov
National Disability Rights Network: https://www.ndrn.org
National Domestic Violence Hotline: https://www.thehotline.org
National Federation of the Blind: https://www.nfb.org
National Lekotek Center (assistive technology and toys for children with
    disabilities): https://www.facebook.com/NationalLekotek
National Organization for Rare Disorders: https://rarediseases.org
Parent–Child Interaction Therapy International: http://www.pcit.org
Parent to Parent Network: https://parent-parent.org
Pediatric Sleep Council: http://www.babysleep.com
Postpartum Support International: https://www.postpartum.net
The Arc (intellectual and developmental disabilities): https://thearc.org
WarmLine Family Resource Center: http://www.warmlinefrc.org
Zero to Three: https://www.zerotothree.org

---

concern at the earliest possible time point allows for intervention to optimize a child's functioning and facilitates family adjustment. Psychologists are well positioned to conduct these assessments due to their expertise in (a) selection of appropriate assessment instruments for each developmental domain; (b) standardized administration of testing instruments, including making needed testing accommodations and understanding their impact; (c) interpretation of assessment findings in the context of clinical observations, child medical and sensory conditions, knowledge of limitations of testing measures, parent report, and family factors; (d) diagnosis of neurodevelopmental disabilities and mental health disorders; (e) provision of family feedback with recommendations tailored to the unique needs of the child and family; and (f) knowledge of empirically supported interventions.

Standardized Testing

Testing in the NFU setting should include assessment of multiple domains, including cognition and learning, play, language, motor skills, social–emotional functioning, behavior, adaptive skills, and relationships. Attention to both age-based protocols and individual needs is important when selecting specific measures. At each stage, the goal of assessment is not only to identify where a child's skills fall in relation to same-aged peers but also to better understand the child's strengths as well as identify areas for improvement and the child's relative gains over time along their own developmental trajectory. For preterm infants born at less than 37 weeks of gestation, corrected age should be used for developmental expectations and when selecting and scoring tests (D'Agostino et al., 2013). Switching to chronological age typically occurs at age 2 years, although for extremely preterm infants, corrected age scores may provide a more accurate assessment of their progress until preschool age.

The BHC also needs to consider the impact of any sensory or motor impairments on the child's ability to engage with testing tasks. For example, significant vision impairment may impact the acquisition of developmental milestones across a range of domains and may interfere with demonstration of skills such as object permanence, imitation, and fine motor coordination. Children with significant muscle tone abnormality may have difficulty engaging in cognitive tasks that are play-based or language tasks that require pointing or turning to find sounds. The BHC must consider if traditional assessment measures provide meaningful information about the child's skills or if other alternative approaches would better capture their strengths and weaknesses, such as a skills checklist for children with visual impairment that also takes adaptation to visual impairment into consideration. During testing, children should use any adaptive equipment they have, such as eyeglasses, hearing aids, or adaptive seating, to elicit their best performance. Children with orthotics, splints, or gait trainers could be assessed with or without these devices depending on the skill being assessed. For example, adaptive equipment may be beneficial if the child's reaching is important to demonstrate object exploration, whereas assessment without the equipment may be helpful to reveal baseline grasp patterns. The BHC should decide if the goal is to obtain baseline information without supports or to obtain information about the child's highest level of functioning with current supports; a combination of approaches is often most helpful.

Ongoing medical conditions can also impact children's performance on standardized testing. For children with severe chronic lung disease and pulmonary hypertension, their stamina for activity may be reduced and they may require a slower pace of assessment. Children with reflux and feeding tubes may have differing tolerance for certain positions, depending on whether a feed is running or has recently finished. Children with tracheotomy and ventilator support also may need breaks for suctioning, and tubing and other medical equipment may limit mobility. Children with tracheotomy will benefit from assessment of communication skills such as gestures and sign language separate from a language scale that combines verbal and nonverbal skills.

Finally, cultural and family language preferences need to be considered during assessment, from the perspective of both testing the child and communicating with the family. Particularly for young children who may be primarily exposed to languages spoken at home, an accurate assessment depends on test administration in a familiar language(s). Use of an interpreter is crucial when the BHC does not speak the language at the level of professional proficiency. If multiple languages are spoken to the child, the clinician should determine which languages are spoken and in what proportions to determine interpreter needs (International Test Commission, 2019). Even with interpretation, the test measures may not be validated for administration in other languages, and cultural bias can impact findings (Goh et al., 2017). Providers should be aware of implicit cultural bias in assessment measures and the potential impact on the categorization of children and subsequent educational opportunities (Worrell & Roberson, 2016).

Interpretation

The results of testing in early childhood need to be interpreted with caution and attention to several factors. Young children's rate of acquisition of developmental skills does not occur at a consistent pace but, rather, amid spurts and plateaus. Skills in different domains show some degree of interdependence, particularly early on, but also may develop at quite different rates. Skills may be emerging at the time of assessment but not yet consistently demonstrated, which the assessment measure may not recognize but the clinician should consider when interpreting the results. Conversely, some skills may be readily demonstrated by young children at home but not in the testing environment. Several contextual and individual factors may influence a child's skill demonstration, including comfort in the assessment environment versus anxiety in medical settings, temperament in willingness to explore new materials, fatigue, hunger, behavior such as oppositionality, ability to sustain attention, and developmental phase (e.g., "stranger anxiety"). In addition to the initial underlying medical conditions, developmental skill acquisition may be impacted by proximity from hospital discharge, surgeries, hospital readmissions, feeding difficulties, or the need for continued respiratory support. Stressors or transitions in the home environment, especially out-of-home placements such as foster care or care in a skilled nursing facility, can have a significant impact on development. Therefore, test scores should not be considered in isolation but, rather, combined with caregivers' report, clinical judgment of the BHC, and information from medical providers in interpreting their meaning.

Testing results can certainly be meaningful indicators of how a child is progressing in relation to age expectations, but perhaps equally if not more meaningful to a useful interpretation of testing results in early childhood is how a child is progressing over time. This rate of gain can be thought of like a physical growth chart as a depiction of how a child is moving along a developmental trajectory. The child may not be performing within age expectations but may be demonstrating a steady rate of gain over time versus slowing in development or regressing in their progress. A child may also not yet be at age level but may be showing an accelerated rate of gain, referred to as "catching up." Early developmental test scores are not intended to predict later functioning but, rather, provide a snapshot at a particular time point. These longitudinal patterns are likely to provide the most helpful information to aid caregivers in understanding their child's development and guide treatment planning.

Diagnosis

Developmental and psychological evaluations in NFUs serve not only to provide information about a child's current functioning across important domains but also to provide a context for observing early signs of neurodevelopmental disorders. For example, medically complex infants are at especially high risk for autism spectrum disorder (ASD), attention-deficit/hyperactivity disorder (ADHD), intellectual disability, and learning disorders, and psychologists are trained to recognize and diagnose these. Children may present with signs of ASD particularly early, at times in toddlerhood. Given that early intervention with symptoms of ASD is crucial to improve long-term outcome, a protocol should be in place for routine screening for ASD in NFUs. A diagnosis of ASD may be complicated by co-occurring developmental delay as well as sensory impairments. In some cases, other providers may suspect the presence of ASD but attribute the symptoms to these comorbidities. In other cases, sensory issues can be mistaken for signs of ASD. For example, Kuban et al. (2009) examined the Modified Checklist for Autism in Toddlers (MCHAT), a commonly used screener for ASD, and found that several items were strongly related to the use of vision, hearing, and motor skills. Therefore, careful follow-up for a concerning score is needed to understand if symptoms of ASD exist above and beyond sensory impairment and developmental delay. The revised screening tool (MCHAT-R) has a follow-up questionnaire, which significantly improves the specificity of the measure. If concerns about ASD persist, psychologists are well positioned to provide a thorough assessment and provide the diagnosis when indicated, allowing for the initiation of ASD-specific interventions.

In early childhood, it is common for children to exhibit symptoms that may significantly impact their functioning in daily life yet not meet full diagnostic criteria for a neurodevelopmental or other psychological disorder as defined by the fifth edition of the *Diagnostic and Statistical Manual of Mental Disorders* (American Psychiatric Association, 2013) or the *International Statistical Classification of Diseases and Related Health Problems* (World Health Organization, 2019). For example, signs of ADHD may be present in older toddlers or preschool-aged children, yet because several symptoms are less relevant for young children, they may not meet full criteria. Likewise, young children may present with early challenges in emotion and behavior regulation or sensory processing that do not clearly link to specific diagnoses. However, when these symptoms interfere with important developmental and adaptive goals, a path to intervention is needed. Therefore, psychologists should be familiar with the *Diagnostic Classification of Mental Health and Developmental Disorders of Infancy and Early Childhood* (Zero to Three, 2016), which seeks to address this gap in describing clinically significant challenges of early childhood. Its multi-axial format includes not only clinical disorders but also the relational context, physical health conditions, psychosocial stressors, and developmental competence.

Family Feedback

By the time they present to NFUs, caregivers may have been anxiously awaiting information about their infant's or child's neurodevelopmental outcomes for months. Some caregivers describe their child's visit to the clinic as the most stressful of all specialty visits due to their fears about what they might hear. Effective, supportive, and helpful feedback begins with a clear understanding of caregivers' concerns at the start of the visit. Questions could include "What are you most worried about?" "How do you think your child is doing?" and "What would you like help with?" Providers should understand caregivers' goals for the visit, which should shape both the information that is delivered and how it is delivered. Providing caregivers an opportunity to have a conversation about their child rather than delivering a list of strengths and weaknesses allows them to engage as a partner in understanding their child's needs and problem-solving the solutions. The active role of caregivers in the assessment of young children in providing support and reinforcement to elicit best performance creates a natural context to engage them in a dialogue throughout the assessment rather than just at the end. This enables the BHC to point out examples of the child's approach, strategies, and reactions in real time. The goal of feedback from the assessment is to enhance caregivers' knowledge of their child's competencies and areas for growth, facilitate appropriate developmental expectations, and build motivation to pursue recommendations. Caregivers should leave the visit believing that their child's strengths as a unique individual were recognized and celebrated and that their efforts with their child were acknowledged. It is critical that BHCs make recommendations while being mindful of families' diversity with respect to culture, socioeconomic status, and other important life experiences. For example, beliefs about ideal parent–child interactions vary widely, and these should be understood before changes in parenting behaviors are recommended. Recommendations should always reflect a reasonable level of caregiver follow-through and be sensitive to the families' resources. Some caregivers have many competing demands and so a long list of activities may only serve to further overwhelm them; more targeted areas to focus on may be more helpful.

Interdisciplinary Team Collaboration

Behavioral health clinicians work closely with other members of the multidisciplinary team. Social workers can act as liaisons between the family and other providers, ensuring that caregivers have understood the feedback and plan of care and helping them cope with the emotional impact of that information. They are ideally positioned to support the treatment plan and help the family overcome any barriers to moving forward with the plan. Social workers can also help other members of the team understand a family's needs and frame of reference. This can be essential in helping the team provide individualized care. They also validate caregivers' role as their child's advocate and can help them effectively communicate with the team.

Psychologists also work closely with other team members and exchange assessment results so that all providers can interpret their findings in the context of the whole child and family. They help guide other team members' expectations about the child by providing an understanding of the child's developmental level. Psychologists help other providers conceptualize the child's behavioral presentation in a relational context. This interpretation helps differentiate behaviors that occur as the result of parenting style and family dynamics from a biologically driven developmental regression that would indicate additional medical follow-up is needed, such as referral to neurology or genetics. Psychologists are also well positioned to detect concerns about vision, hearing, or motor functioning that would benefit from further evaluation.

CROSS-SYSTEMS LIAISON

Behavioral health clinicians in NFUs should connect children and families to community resources and act as a liaison between the family and community agencies. Social workers play a key role in linking families to financial resources and must be knowledgeable about funding sources available to families of children with disabilities and chronic medical needs. Social workers also help families with obtaining insurance, social security, nutrition programs, home nursing, transportation, legal services, immigration services, housing programs, and other resources that are important social determinants of young children's well-being and should be addressed in the NFU setting (Horbar et al., 2020). Social workers facilitate letters from providers that families may need to qualify for these services. They also help create a linkage back to the child's primary medical home and to other specialty medical care. Social workers collaborate with child protective services and can assist the team in making a new report if there is a suspicion of child abuse or neglect. Social workers also communicate with staff at skilled nursing facilities when children are in residential care.

Early intervention services, Part C of the Individuals with Disabilities Act, is a federally funded program administered in each state to provide young children with developmental intervention during the first 3 years of life. Each state administers the program and may have slightly different eligibility requirements. The intent across states is for a child to receive a multidisciplinary evaluation with a resulting individualized family service plan if the child is found eligible for services. These services are delivered in a naturalistic environment, such as home or daycare. Although child referral programs are part of each state's early intervention system, BHCs in clinic often play important roles in helping families understand the scope and possible benefits of early intervention (Spittle & Treyvaud, 2016), connect to early intervention, advocate for additional services through early intervention, and provide recommendations for specific goals that could be addressed through early intervention. At times it is advised to supplement early intervention services with outpatient developmental therapies. Psychologists can help caregivers decide the best fit for the family and their child, and social workers can help families overcome any barriers to receiving appropriate developmental intervention.

Social workers can also assist caregivers in navigating the challenges that often come with recommendations to pursue behavioral health services for young children. For example, if a diagnosis of ASD is made, diagnosis-specific therapies such as applied behavioral analysis may be recommended (Makrygianni et al., 2018). Other behavioral health services may be recommended for challenging behaviors, anxiety, or relationship difficulties. These services can be difficult to find due to the comparatively small number of BHCs who treat young children, particularly those who will take insurance. Although some states have mandated that insurance companies must provide coverage for autism-related services, there can be a lengthy intake process and long wait for these services.

Both psychologists and social workers are critical advocates for children's medical, behavioral, emotional, and educational needs in the school setting. They communicate with teachers, school counselors, principals, preschool directors, and the child study team to ensure that children receive the support, accommodations, and opportunities to maximize their potential to learn and thrive at school. Sharing information with schools, with caregiver permission, can accelerate the processes of evaluation and the creation of an Individualized Education Program (IEP) or a plan of accommodations (504 plan). The information that teachers and other school staff provide about children's functioning at school is also invaluable for the psychologist's evaluation of the child. BHCs can help caregivers understand their rights with respect to special education, suggest items that should be included in the IEP or 504 plan, identify challenges in communication between the family and school, and/or participate in meetings. Caregivers may also benefit from connection to a parent mentor or advocate, or educational law assistance, found through local agencies. Due to the wide variability that exists among preschool programs, psychologists can relay important considerations to maximize the fit for the caregivers' child. They also guide caregivers in considerations for the transition to kindergarten. Some caregivers may erroneously assume that a child who was born prematurely should delay kindergarten entry; this is not always advantageous.

RECOMMENDATIONS FOR PARENT–CHILD INTERVENTIONS

Challenges in the parent–infant relationship can be revealed in the NFU visit. Parents of infants with high-risk medical histories may continue to view their infants as vulnerable even as their medical challenges subside. Perception of vulnerability can lead in parental overprotection, resulting in increased anxiety, behavioral difficulties, and school challenges for children and a reluctance of parents to set limits and provide consequences for negative behaviors (Horwitz et al., 2015). Starting in infancy, parents may feel heightened distress when their infant cries, and they may have difficulty with sleep training or allowing their infant to self-soothe. In toddlerhood, parents may inadvertently reward tantrums by giving into their child's demands and be reluctant to set limits for misbehavior. At times, these patterns are readily apparent during the assessment and interfere with the child's engagement in psychologist-directed tasks. The psychologist can use these opportunities during the assessment to model use of positive reinforcement, selective ignoring, effective time-out sequences, and loss of privilege. Psychologists can also help parents think through how they might apply these strategies to common challenges at home and what supports they need to tolerate normative distress in their child. Sometimes parents can carry over these strategies at home and create more adaptive patterns, whereas other times parents benefit from more in-depth intervention.

In cases in which more support is needed, the psychologist can refer the family for behavioral health intervention such as Parent–Child Interaction Therapy (PCIT) or other parent training programs. PCIT is an evidenced-based treatment for noncompliance that focuses both on relationship building and effective strategies for providing discipline for misbehavior, ideally suited for children aged 2–7 years. However, the treatment has also been shown to be effective for difficulties beyond noncompliant behavior, including behaviors associated with ADHD, and, more recently, with adaptations in the treatment of internalizing disorders and other populations (Lieneman et al., 2017). Sometimes difficulties in parent–child interactions are related to pervasive negative attributions of the child by the parent, a lack of sensitivity in parental responses, and an inability of the child to effectively use the parent as a source of support. Medically high-risk infants are particularly prone to conditions that can result in agitation and difficulty soothing, which may be a particularly challenging fit for a parent who has a history of mood lability or attachment disruption in their family of origin. In these cases of insecure parent–child attachment relationships, particularly in cases of maltreatment, other approaches, such as Attachment and Biobehavioral Catch-up, have been shown to produce lasting gains (Zajac et al., 2019). Parents may also benefit from seeking individual therapy to address challenges contributing to a dysfunctional pattern of interactions with their child. Although parents may be reluctant to pursue therapy, they may be motivated by a discussion of the parenting stress they are experiencing and also by the BHC conveying a sense of hope that more positive interactions are possible.

IDEAS WORTH SHARING

Behavioral health clinicians should be aware of both local and national organizations that may assist caregivers as they continue their journey after NICU discharge (Box 27.1). When implementing psychological assessments in the NFU setting, several decisions must be made with respect to visit timing, domains assessed, and age-/developmental stage-specific considerations. Areas of focus will depend on other assessments being conducted within the NFU and how the psychological assessment fits within this structure. Key considerations in designing a timeline for assessment are the transitions for children at different ages. For example, the transition to early intervention programs is important, as is the transition that occurs out of these services at age 3 years. Assessment just prior to age 3 years can be helpful in providing recommendations for continued developmental intervention in other systems when indicated. Likewise, preschool and kindergarten entry are key transition periods, and assessment results can help guide decision-making about the types of settings and supports that would be most appropriate for each child. Finally, not every child in the NFU program may need the same schedule. Depending on the specific population, providers may wish to have separate timelines for higher and lower risk subpopulations or may wish to alter the schedule based on a child's progress over time. A sample schedule with age-specific considerations is provided in Table 27.1.

CONCLUSION

Behavioral health clinicians play many key roles in the follow-up of NICU graduates. When both psychologists and social workers are part of the NFU team, the program can more holistically meet the needs of children with complex medical conditions. This includes contributions to caregiver screening and support, connection to needed resources, thorough evaluation of the child, liaison with community entities, and recommendations to optimize outcomes. The NICU journey can have a lasting impact on both children and their families, and BHCs provide essential support to promote adjustment for children, their parents, and the entire family and help these children achieve their potential.

Table 27.1 SAMPLE SCHEDULE FOR PSYCHOLOGICAL EVALUATIONS IN
NEONATAL FOLLOW-UP

Child Age	Testing Domains	Additional Areas of Focus
6 months[a]	Cognition/play Language Motor skills	Temperament Social interest Parent–infant interactions/bonding Play/floor-time opportunities Daily routines/sleep Connection with early intervention Family adjustment post discharge Caregiver mental health screening
12 months[a]	Cognition/play Language Motor skills Social–emotional and behavioral functioning	Parent–child attachment Early discipline strategies Daily routines/sleep Caregiver mental health screening
18 months[a]	Cognition/play Language Motor skills Social–emotional and Behavioral functioning Autism screening[b]	Parent–child interactions Early discipline strategies Daily routines/sleep Caregiver mental health screening
24 months[a]	Cognition/play Language Motor skills Social–emotional and behavioral functioning Autism screening[b]	Parent–child interactions Early semistructured social experiences Evolving discipline strategies Toilet training readiness Daily routines/sleep Caregiver mental health screening

30 months
(2½ years)
	Cognition/play
	Language
	Motor skills
	Social–emotional and
	  behavioral functioning
	Autism screening[b]
		Parent–child interactions
		Early semistructured social experiences
		Transition from early intervention
		Consider evaluation for preschool
		  individualized education
		Preschool placement suggestions
		Evolving discipline strategies
		Toilet training readiness
		Daily routines/sleep
		Caregiver mental health screening

3 years
(scheduled
if concerns
present at
2½ years)
	Cognition/play
	Language
	Motor skills
	Social–emotional and
	  behavioral functioning
	Adaptive functioning
	Autism screening[b]
		Parent–child interactions
		Discipline strategies
		Social opportunities
		Adjustment and functioning in
		  the preschool setting, including
		  teacher report
		Daily routines/sleep
		Caregiver mental health screening

Table 27.1 CONTINUED

Child Age	Testing Domains	Additional Areas of Focus
4½–5 years (winter/ early spring prior to kindergarten eligibility)	Cognition School readiness/early achievement Visual–motor integration[c] Adaptive functioning Social–emotional and behavioral functioning Attention/early executive functioning Autism screening[b]	Parent–child interactions Discipline strategies Kindergarten entry decisions Consider an Individualized Education Program or 504 plan Early friendship development Participation in community activities (e.g., soccer and dance) Child's beginning understanding of medical course and conditions Daily routines/sleep Referral for continued specialty follow-up as needed Caregiver mental health screening

[a]Ages should be corrected for prematurity.

[b]Follow-up assessment for autism spectrum disorder when indicated.

[c]Add visual perception and motor coordination when indicated.

REFERENCES

American Academy of Pediatrics Committee on Fetus and Newborn. (2008). Hospital discharge of the high-risk neonate. *Pediatrics, 122*(5), 1119–1126.

American College of Obstetricians and Gynecologists. (2018). ACOG committee opinion: Screening for perinatal depression. *Obstetrics and Gynecology, 132*(5), e208–e212.

American Psychiatric Association. (2013). *Diagnostic and statistical manual of mental disorders* (5th ed.).

D'Agostino, J., Gerdes, M., Hoffman, C., Manning, M., & Phalen, A. (2013). Provider use of corrected age during health supervision visits for premature infants. *Journal of Pediatric Health Care, 27*(3), 172–179.

Fitelson, E., Kim, S., Scott, A., & Leight, K. (2011). Treatment of postpartum depression: Clinical, psychological, and pharmacological options. *International Journal of Women's Health, 3*, 1–14.

Goh, S. K. Y., Tham, E. K. H., Magiati, I., Sim, L., & Sanmugam, S. (2017). Analysis of item-level bias in the Bayley-III language subscales: The validity and utility of standardized language assessment in a multilingual setting. *Journal of Speech Language and Hearing Research, 60*(9), 2663–2671.

Horbar, J. D., Edwards, E. M., & Ogbolu, Y. (2020). Our responsibility to follow through for NICU infants and their families. *Pediatrics, 146*(6), e20200360.

Horwitz, S. M., Stofer-Isser, A., Kerker, B. D., Lilo, E., Leibovitz, A., St. John, N., & Shaw, R. J. (2015). A model for the development of mothers' perceived vulnerability of preterm infants. *Journal of Developmental & Behavioral Pediatrics, 36*(5), 371–380.

International Test Commission. (2019). ITC guidelines for the large-scale assessment of linguistically and culturally diverse populations. *International Journal of Testing, 19*(4), 301–336.

Kuban, K. C. K., O'Shea, T. M., Allred, E. N., Tager-Flusberg, H., & Goldstein, D. J. (2009). Positive screening on the Modified Checklist for Autism in Toddlers (M-CHAT) in extremely low gestational age newborns. *Journal of Pediatrics, 154*(4), 535–540.

Levick, J., Quinn, M., & Vennema, C. (2014). NICU parent to parent partnerships: A comprehensive approach. *Neonatal Network, 33*(2), 66–73.

Lieneman, C. C., Brabson, L. A., Highlander, A., Wallace, N. M., & McNeil, C. B. (2017). Parent–child interaction therapy: Current perspectives. *Psychology Research and Behavior Management, 10*, 239–256.

Makrygianni, M. K., Gena, A., Katoudi, S., & Galanis, P. (2018). The effectiveness of applied analytic behavior interventions for children with autism spectrum disorder: A meta-analytic study. *Research in Autism Spectrum Disorders, 51*, 18–31.

Merz, J., Schwarzer, G., & Gerger, H. (2019). Comparative efficacy and acceptability of pharmacological, psychotherapeutic, and combination treatments in adults with posttraumatic stress disorder: A network meta-analysis. *JAMA Psychiatry, 76*(9), 904–913.

Orton, J. L, Olsen, J. E., Ong, K., Lester, R., & Spittle, A. J. (2018). NICU graduates: The role of the allied health team in follow-up. *Pediatric Annals, 47*(4), e165–e171.

Schecter, R., Pham, T., Hua, A., Spinazzola, R., Sonnenklar, J., Li, D., Papaioannou, H., & Milanaik, R. (2020). Prevalence and longevity of PTSD symptoms among parents of NICU infants analyzed across gestational age categories. *Clinical Pediatrics, 59*(2), 163–169.

Spittle, A., & Treyvaud, K. (2016). The role of early developmental intervention to influence neurobehavioral outcomes of children born preterm. *Seminars in Perinatology, 40*, 542–548.

Swearingen, C., Simpson, P., Cabacungan, E., & Cohen, S. (2020). Social disparities negatively impact neonatal follow-up clinic attendance of premature infants discharged from the neonatal intensive care unit. *Journal of Perinatology, 40*, 790–797.

World Health Organization. (2019). *International statistical classification of diseases and related health problems* (11th ed.).

Worrell, F. C., & Roberson, C. C. B. (2016). 2014 standards for educational and psychological testing: Implications for ethnic minority youth. In S. L. Graves & J. J. Blake (Eds.), *Psychoeducational assessment and intervention for ethnic minority children: Evidenced-based approaches* (pp. 41–57). American Psychological Association.

Zajac, L., Raby, K. L, & Dozier, M. (2019). Sustained effects on attachment security in middle childhood: Results from a randomized clinical trial of the Attachment and Biobehavioral Catch-up (ABC) intervention. *Journal of Child Psychology and Psychiatry, 61*(4), 417–424.

Zero to Three. (2016). *Diagnostic classification of mental health and developmental disorders of infancy and early childhood: DC:0–5*.

28

AFTER THE NICU

PRIMARY CARE BEHAVIORAL HEALTH SERVICES

VERENEA J. SERRANO, JONNA H. VON SCHULZ,
MELISSA BUCHHOLZ, KRISTINA MALIK,
AMY WRENN, AND AYELET TALMI ■

Pediatric primary care provides a universal, accessible, nonstigmatizing setting for children to receive comprehensive and preventative health care focused on supporting the whole child in the context of their environment (Stille et al., 2010). Children are seen early and often at routine well-child visits, where their development, growth, and wellness are carefully monitored and interventions are put in place to address concerns. A medical home model of primary care (referred to as a medical home) includes comprehensive care, care team collaboration to address all patient care needs, care coordination across settings, and support for an ongoing patient–provider relationship (Stille et al., 2010). Pediatric primary care settings can also screen for and address caregiver mental health and social determinants of health, which impact child well-being (Garg & Dworkin, 2011).

Primary care providers are charged with covering a broad range of topics and tasks within a relatively limited amount of time. The brief duration of well-child visits in the United States leaves insufficient time to comprehensively meet the needs of the whole child and family. A medical home is optimal for integrating behavioral health clinicians (BHCs) who can assist with addressing developmental, behavioral, and mental health concerns that arise in the context of well-child care. Behavioral health needs often present in primary care settings first due to the trusting relationships families frequently have with their child's medical provider. BHCs embedded into the medical home can increase accessibility for behavioral health services. Furthermore, integrated behavioral health (IBH) services in primary care are associated with improved behavioral health outcomes relative to usual care (Asarnow et al., 2015).

Primary care is particularly important for neonatal intensive care unit (NICU) graduates who are children and youth with special health care needs (CYSHCN). For NICU graduates, the medical home can support the transition home after NICU discharge; provide support to caregivers as they develop and adapt their parenting style to their child over time; provide care coordination with other specialties or community resources as needed; and provide ongoing surveillance and standardized screening for physical, developmental, cognitive, behavioral, and emotional needs. Furthermore, caregivers of CYSCHN are at risk for increased stress, which can impact caregiver and family well-being. Due to NICU graduates' risk for developmental delays and their caregivers' risk for mood symptoms and impaired well-being, the medical home provides an opportunity for ongoing discussion and monitoring of symptoms.

INTEGRATED BEHAVIORAL HEALTH SERVICES IN PRIMARY CARE

Although IBH service delivery in pediatric primary care settings can vary widely, benefits include early identification; addressing concerns before they impair functioning; providing intervention in a nonstigmatized environment; and engaging in care coordination, triage, and referral to expand access to necessary services (Talmi et al., 2016). IBH services can include health promotion and prevention, behavioral health screening, consultation and intervention, and care coordination. Universal child and family screening and care coordination are important approaches to identify those who may benefit from IBH services.

Given the relatively small number of specialty NICU follow-up clinics, many NICU graduates receive primary care in a general clinic. This chapter considers the wide range of presentations of NICU graduates across childhood and focuses on the role integrated BHCs play with screening, consultation and intervention, care coordination, and collaboration.

SCREENING

Following hospital discharge, NICU graduates often transition to primary care services. It is not uncommon for NICU graduates to have complex needs at the time of discharge and over the course of childhood, including, but not limited to, ongoing care of chronic medical conditions, neurodevelopmental delays, and utilization of complex medical technology. In primary care, universal screening for the child, caregiver, and family provides routine opportunities for monitoring child development and behavioral health, caregiver behavioral health, and family psychosocial stressors. A BHC can inform the development of the screening process; respond to elevated screening scores; and provide intervention, referrals, and recommendations when needed.

Child-Level Screening

DEVELOPMENT

The American Academy of Pediatrics (AAP, 2019) recommends developmental screening with a validated instrument at ages 9, 18, and 30 months and autism screening at ages 18 and 24 months, in addition to developmental surveillance at all visits. NICU graduates are at risk for developmental delays and neurodevelopmental disorders, and the risk increases for children who have prolonged stays in the NICU (Subedi et al., 2017). Therefore, ongoing monitoring of a child's development over time through routine screening is warranted and can facilitate early identification of developmental concerns, discussion of developmental strategies to support concerns, and referrals for additional evaluation and/or therapy (Lipkin & Macias, 2020). Although NICU graduates are often already referred to early intervention services at the time of discharge, ongoing developmental screening is advantageous to monitor a child's progress and routinely assess for concerns that may emerge over time (for details regarding developmental screening measures and processes, see Lipkin & Macias, 2020).

When discussing the results of developmental screening with families, it is important to consider the score in the context of the child's medical conditions, in addition to cultural and environmental factors. For example, if a child receives all nutrition via feeding tube, screener items related to adaptive or fine motor skills may be affected due to lack of opportunity for the child to self-feed. In addition, it is important to consider the child's current developmental services to determine what additional follow-up is needed. If a child is receiving early intervention speech therapy services and concerns related to a child's problem-solving and social–emotional development are identified, the BHC could contact the speech therapist to discuss screening results and the focus of speech therapy prior to recommending additional developmental services. Furthermore, for some children with medical complexity and severe developmental delays, who are already receiving appropriate developmental therapies and specialty care, a BHC may choose not to administer standardized screening measures due to the limited incremental utility of the measures and possible negative emotional impact for the family. For some families, completing an age-appropriate, but not developmentally appropriate, screener is a difficult reminder of the ways their child is not meeting expected developmental milestones and differs from same-aged children. The BHC could instead assess progress in developmental therapies and discuss the child's developmental trajectory with the caregiver.

When conducting developmental screening for children who are born prematurely, adjusting the child's age based on their gestational age at time of birth (i.e., corrected age) is recommended, but there are differing recommendations regarding for which domains to correct and for how long. The AAP recommends using corrected age for the first 3 years of life (Engle et al., 2004; guidelines reaffirmed in 2014). However, the extent of prematurity, domains assessed, reason for developmental screening or assessment, and impact on access to services are all relevant factors when determining whether and for how long to correct for prematurity. In clinical practice, the BHC or pediatrician may choose to provide developmental screeners that best match the child's current developmental level.

Autism Spectrum Disorder

Children who experience perinatal complications (e.g., preterm birth and low birth weight) are at higher risk for autism spectrum disorder (ASD; Schieve et al., 2014). ASD is also associated with certain fetal abnormalities (e.g., macrocephaly and brain overgrowth; Sacco et al., 2015). The Modified Checklist for Autism in Toddlers (M-CHAT; ages 16–30 months) and Social Communication Questionnaire (ages 4 years or older with mental age of at least 2 years) are two ASD screeners used in primary care. Screening at well-child visits allows for early discussion of symptoms, psychoeducation around early signs of ASD, and early referrals for a comprehensive diagnostic evaluation when appropriate. When screening for ASD, it is important to consider the screener results in the context of how a child's medical needs may impact scores (e.g., visual impairment, hearing impairment, and motor delay). Furthermore, it is important to consider limitations in screeners for this population. For example, the M-CHAT can result in increased false positives and negatives for children with hearing and vision impairments and increased false positives for children with motor and/or cognitive delays in addition to emotional and/or behavior regulation difficulties (Kim et al., 2016).

Attention-Deficit/Hyperactivity Disorder

When NICU graduates transition to school age, they are at risk for attention-deficit/hyperactivity disorder (ADHD; Franz et al., 2018). AAP guidelines recommend screening for ADHD in children aged 4–18 years when academic or behavioral concerns and ADHD symptoms are present (Wolraich et al., 2019), and there are several standardized screeners to consider (AAP, 2010). For children younger than age 4 years, behavioral parenting interventions can be recommended, but there is not sufficient evidence to recommend a diagnosis of ADHD. Behavioral parenting interventions may also be recommended for other types of disruptive behavior concerns (e.g., oppositional behavior and noncompliance). When reviewing ADHD screening results, it is important to consider to what extent difficulties in learning, cognitive ability, behavior, or physical health may be contributing to inattention and hyperactivity/impulsivity concerns. This can help avoid misinterpretation of ADHD screeners and inappropriate treatment or referrals. For example, if a child with a history of medical-related trauma presents as inattentive during daily medical care at home and school but does not exhibit these symptoms outside of medical care interactions, then the symptoms may be more related to anxiety or trauma than ADHD. The BHC may refer for a comprehensive learning or neuropsychological evaluation for further diagnostic clarification if needed.

Caregiver- and Family-Level Screening

Postpartum Depression

Postpartum depression (PPD) is not uncommon following childbirth and can negatively impact child–caregiver relationships, early infant brain development, and child and family well-being (Earls et al., 2019). Mothers of infants who are born prematurely or have low birth weight are at increased risk for PPD due to increased stressors that impact caregiver and family well-being (Vigod et al., 2010). Early and routine screening for PPD allows for early identification of symptoms, ongoing discussion about strategies to manage PDD symptoms, and referral to behavioral health services. The Edinburgh Postnatal Depression Scale is used to screen for PPD, and the Patient Health Questionnaire 2 or 9 are options for caregiver mood screening (AAP, 2010). PPD screening is recommended at each child's well-child visits until age 6 months (Earls et al., 2019). However, PPD screening for caregivers of NICU graduates can be advantageous until age 12 months to account for prolonged hospital stays, complex medical needs, and changes in medical status that impact caregiver well-being. Fathers can also experience depression in the postpartum period (Earls et al., 2019) and should be screened for depression when possible.

Medical-Related Trauma

Caregivers of NICU graduates experience increased risk for post-traumatic stress disorder (PTSD) as a result of their child's medical experiences (e.g., delivery, medical procedures, or life-threatening events) and the NICU stay (Lefkowitz et al., 2010). For these caregivers, PPD screening items may not capture the mental health difficulties associated with NICU-related PTSD symptoms. Thus, screening for caregiver medical-related trauma symptoms is valuable in understanding the impact of a NICU admission on family well-being and providing support for a topic that may otherwise not be discussed at well-child visits.

The Impact of Events Scale–Revised (IES-R) and the Perinatal PTSD Questionnaire have been used to screen for medical-related trauma among caregivers of CYSHCN and NICU graduates. The IES-R can be applied to any type of traumatic event. When administering the IES-R in our practice, we ask caregivers to consider significant child medical events from pregnancy, birth, the NICU, or surgeries as a collective. This may result in caregivers considering events that do not meet the definition of a traumatic event; however, given that the population is NICU graduates, there is a high likelihood that the family experienced a traumatic event. This administration process has led to clearer and more clinically relevant administration than asking families to consider one specific event. We administer the measure once within the first year of life (ideally within the first month of meeting the family), once in the second year of life, and once in the third year of life. Clinical judgment is used to decide the most appropriate administration time within each year of life.

Psychosocial Stressors

Caregivers of NICU graduates are at risk for increased psychosocial stressors related to caring for CYSHCN (e.g., change in caregiver roles and identity, managing their child's complex medical care, and coordinating therapy and medical appointments). Accordingly, routine screening of psychosocial factors that may impact child and family well-being is recommended (Garg & Dworkin, 2011). Psychosocial screening that assesses for intimate partner violence, financial stressors, and difficulties navigating health care waivers or benefits allows for early identification of stressors and discussion about barriers to accessing care. Once these psychosocial stressors have been identified, they can be further discussed to understand the family's unique needs and next steps in supporting each family member. In addition, nonbiological caregivers (e.g., foster, adoptive, and kinship) can experience stress in caring for CYSHCN; thus, they should be included in caregiver and family screening.

Once a NICU graduate transitions to the primary care setting, routine screening for child development and behavior, caregiver well-being, and psychosocial stressors provides routine opportunities to discuss concerns, offer support and psychoeducation to the family, and discuss additional referrals when necessary. Routine screening also allows for additional follow-up with a BHC and other support staff so that concerns can be discussed further.

CONSULTATION AND INTERVENTION

In addition to responding to concerns noted on screening measures, BHCs can provide consultation and intervention, including health and behavior assessment and intervention, for patients, families, and providers in the medical home. In contrast to behavioral health services provided during an inpatient hospital admission, IBH services can be provided throughout childhood as part of overall care in the medical home.

Child and Family

The scope of IBH services in primary care is wide (Talmi et al., 2016), and given the range of developmental, behavioral, and mental health outcomes among NICU graduates, a broad range of topics can be addressed in consultation and intervention. However, there are common consultation themes for NICU graduates across childhood. These include (a) adjustment to the child's medical diagnosis and implications of the diagnosis for child and family in the short and long term; (b) adapting parenting strategies and expectations to the child's specific developmental level and health needs; (c) supporting children and their families as they navigate various systems (e.g., health care, education, community, and medical needs–specific networks); and (d) monitoring for and addressing developmental, behavioral health, and academic concerns. Support for siblings who have witnessed frightening medical events (e.g., significant seizure and resuscitation attempts) and for caregivers as they navigate complexities in family planning after their NICU graduate may also be relevant. The consultation and intervention approach and recommendations will depend on the BHC's training and theoretical orientation, as well as the level of integration and IBH services available (e.g., consultation only or brief therapy). In addition to general consultation themes across childhood, common themes emerge during specific age periods (Table 28.1).

RESPONDING TO SCREENERS

Behavioral health clinicians can respond to concerns identified via any of the screening domains previously discussed or via other providers in the medical home. For concerns related to child development, behavior, or mental health, the BHC can support the family in understanding the concerns in the context of the child's medical history; provide psychoeducation intervention strategies; and facilitate referrals for further therapy, evaluation (e.g., comprehensive developmental assessment), or other services. When there is an elevated caregiver PPD or PTSD screener, the BHC can support the caregiver in recognizing mental health symptoms, understanding the connection between the symptoms and child and family well-being, identifying wellness activities, and accessing community supports (e.g., parent support groups and individual mental health therapy). When intimate partner violence concerns are identified, a BHC can address safety concerns and provide referrals to community services.

INTERVENTION

After behavioral health needs are identified, a BHC may provide behavioral health intervention during a consultation as part of the medical visit or via individual or group therapy scheduled separately from the medical visit. Short-term therapy services provided in the medical home are a strategy to help address acute, mild behavioral or mental health concerns that arise in the context of medical visits (e.g., management of behavioral concerns, adherence to medical recommendations, and caregiver adjustment difficulties). Based on the behavioral health need, the BHC may refer the family for long-term therapy services in the community or refer for further developmental, learning, or neuropsychological testing. In addition, health and behavior assessment and intervention services are well-suited to the NICU graduate population. Examples of health and behavior services include supporting medical adherence, adjustment to illness for child or caregiver, child or adolescent involvement in their medical care, and adapting caregiving strategies for a child's specific needs. Intervention services may be provided once as part of a brief consultation, ongoing in therapy or health prevention efforts, or as needed as the child grows. The flexibility of service provision allows the BHC to meet the child and family needs as they arise and to develop relationships over time that can enhance the quality and child and family experience of behavioral health care.

Regardless of the consultation or intervention approach used, the BHC must balance the initial presenting concern with additional concerns that arise during

Table 28.1 COMMON INTEGRATED BEHAVIORAL HEALTH CONSULTATION THEMES

Age Period	Common Consultation Themes for Children and Families
Infancy	Adjustment Adjustment to life at home after NICU discharge and significant life changes as a result of the infant's medical needs (e.g., caregiver not returning to work or relocate closer to medical center) Caregiver, siblings, and other family member adjustment to the infant's diagnoses and needs Navigating differences in adjustment process among caregivers Developing responses for strangers, acquaintances, and close family or friends who ask about the infant's health and well-being Coping with hospital readmissions or additional medical procedures that occur after initial NICU discharge Parenting Developing relationships with their infant when caregivers may feel like their child's "nurse" Uncertainty of the infant's prognosis and/or future developmental level Caregiver behavioral health Grief related to loss of expected perinatal experience, infant developmental milestones, and parenting experiences Managing caregiver behavioral health symptoms that are impacting caregiver well-being or relationships, or caregiver's ability to engage with medical team or adhere to recommendations Balancing high rate of service needs with other aspects of family life
Early childhood	Child and caregiver behavioral health Child or caregiver behavioral health concerns in response to medical traumatic stress Child behavior or emotional issues that affect adherence to medical care or recommendations Promoting developmentally appropriate strategies to encourage child compliance with required medical care Helping child develop their own medical narrative as is developmentally appropriate Supporting caregivers in developing and adapting their parenting strategies to manage behavioral and emotional concerns Development and school Learning further about patient's developmental level or about additional neurodevelopmental diagnoses that are identified Transitioning from early intervention developmental services to special education services in preschool and transition to school overall

Table 28.1 CONTINUED

Age Period	Common Consultation Themes for Children and Families
School age	Child behavioral health Child adjustment to own medical diagnoses and needs Child development of responses to others who ask about their health or medical technology Addressing bullying or peer/social difficulties related to developmental, behavioral, mental health, or medical needs Development and school Monitoring for developmental, learning, executive functioning, or mental health difficulties Caregiver and provider collaboration with school to provide necessary academic supports
Adolescence	Development and behavior Development of sexual identity and behavior, with consideration to developmental level and medical diagnoses Puberty-related concerns, including menstruation and hygiene Continued support related to developmental, behavioral, or academic concerns that arise Adolescent adjustment to medical diagnoses and needs and further development of medical narrative as part of overall identity Adolescent and caregiver safety for adolescents with developmental delays and unsafe behavior (e.g., self-injurious behavior, aggression, and elopement) Transition preparation Planning for transition to adulthood and changes that occur after the adolescent turns age 18 years (e.g., medical decision-making, service eligibility, and care team)

the consult and triage concerns that arise across domains (e.g., child, family, health status, and various systems). The BHC and primary care team should work with the family to determine not only what type and level of support maximizes child health and well-being but also what is feasible for the family. For example, applied behavioral analysis (ABA) therapy may be indicated to address behavior concerns in a child with developmental delays, but if the child is already receiving multiple developmental therapies, the family may not feasibly have time for another therapy. Thus, ABA therapy may be deferred to a future time. Furthermore, it is important to consider that for caregivers of NICU graduates and medical professionals, there are similarities and notable differences between what they believe constitutes higher and lower quality of life for a child (Adams et al., 2020). The differences can lead to caregiver and medical team disagreement in medical care and treatment planning (e.g., the level of medical technology that is required and the necessity of certain evaluations, appointments, or therapies). BHCs can provide support for caregivers in communicating care preferences and discussing factors that may contribute to care preferences.

The level of communication with the medical provider and the degree to which the BHC is integrated into the clinic can affect the content of the consultation. The medical needs of NICU graduates can be complex, and communication with the medical provider about the child's medical diagnoses, care, and prognosis should inform BHC recommendations. For example, the medical provider can describe to the BHC the expected course of a child's diagnosis and how development may be affected. This, in turn, allows the BHC to support caregiver and child adjustment to illness and provide recommendations that align with current and predicted developmental level. In addition, information learned by the BHC may also inform the child's medical care. If the caregiver and BHC are discussing toilet training and the caregiver notes constipation is resulting in the child avoiding using the toilet, the BHC could coordinate with the medical provider for follow-up for the constipation.

Provider Consultation

Medical provider and BHC collaborations can vary depending on the needs of the patient. The foremost importance is to develop a relationship with all care team members that recognizes the unique contributions each member brings to patient care depending on their training and experience. Medical providers may have varying degrees of comfort addressing behavioral health needs, depending on their training. Recognizing strengths, areas for support, and scope of practice of each care team member will help prevent misunderstandings that can lead to poor patient care. In addition, stressing the importance of team member communication can help facilitate care and development of a relationship between the provider and the BHC, which can lead to peer support for emotionally difficult situations when both are involved.

For providers, BHCs can provide consultation to inform care of complex patients and make plans for possible support, recommendations, follow-up, and/or referral. This can include assessing the acuity of a patient's needs and coordinating further direct patient care through a primary or specialty care visit. Other options can include providing guidance to the medical provider without direct BHC–patient interaction. Discussions with BHCs can aid the provider in differentiating which psychological screening and testing and subsequent support(s) may be most useful for the patient. BHCs can also recommend and facilitate referrals to other mental and behavioral health resources, including community programs and admissions to intensive mental and behavioral health service programs such as day treatment or inpatient programs.

CARE COORDINATION AND COLLABORATION

For caregivers, the work of caring for CYSHCN can require substantial time for care coordination outside of typical parenting responsibilities. Enhanced care coordination among professionals can help reduce caregiver work of care as they aim to integrate recommendations from multiple sources and manage their child's needs. A primary care BHC may collaborate with any of the professionals who comprise the child's extensive network of care or supports. Some key areas for care coordination are within the primary care clinic, school or early childhood care, community developmental agencies, and specialty medical clinics.

Within the medical home, the BHC can communicate with medical providers, nursing staff, administrative staff, and other professionals as available (e.g., social work and care coordinator) to enhance patient care. Based on information from the consultation, BHCs can relay to others on the care team caregiver questions or concerns about the medical plan or communicate when caregivers may need re-teaching for a care task that elicits anxiety or distress (e.g., feeding tube changes, tracheostomy care, and medication administration). For example, in a consultation related to nighttime fussiness and sleep difficulties following NICU discharge, a caregiver may discuss that the infant's nighttime feeding schedule impacts when the infant wakes and that they feel anxious completing gastronomy tube feeds because the feeding tube is newly placed. The BHC can then ask the medical provider if any adjustments to feeding schedule are possible and ask the clinic nurse to conduct re-teaching for gastronomy tube feeds.

Behavioral health consultation may also include supporting medical trauma-informed care during medical procedures in clinic, such as asking the child if they want to watch vaccine administration or close their eyes or by providing them with distracting and/or relaxing activities during anxiety-provoking medical procedures. Ideally, BHC recommendations are integrated with medical recommendations to the maximal extent possible. For example, for children with Prader–Willi syndrome, the medical provider and BHC can provide integrated recommendations for diet and addressing behavior difficulties when limits are set related to food.

Regarding collaboration with school professionals, the BHC can collaborate to learn if the needs identified during consultation can be addressed at school (e.g., school-based therapy and revision for formal or informal school supports) and, with caregiver permission, share diagnostic or medical history information that can inform school supports. Furthermore, information regarding the type of supports that have been effective at school can help the BHC work with caregivers to generalize these strategies to home to the extent possible. For children, school and primary care are two important sources of monitoring and support for health and well-being. Thus, collaboration between the two systems can decrease the care coordination burden on caregivers.

Opportunities for care coordination with BHCs in other medical clinics (e.g., inpatient, outpatient, and specialty clinics) include information sharing and identification of who will take the lead on addressing a need to avoid redundancy or confusion. The primary care BHC can communicate areas of support related to the BHC's specialty clinic (e.g., solid organ transplant readiness and medical adherence for chronic conditions) or provide a warm handoff between primary care and inpatient units if the child is admitted to the hospital. For infants newly discharged from the NICU, the warm handoff could address stress and possible trauma triggers associated with return to the NICU if readmission is necessary. It is also important to identify which BHC will provide assessment, intervention, resources, and/or follow-up monitoring for an identified issue. Specialty clinic BHCs may refer to primary care BHCs for ongoing monitoring that the specialty clinic BHCs cannot perform closely due to less frequent visits in their setting.

In addition, an estimated 5–10% of the U.S. foster care population are children in foster care specifically because of their medical complexity (Seltzer et al., 2016), and CYSHCN are at risk for maltreatment (Van Horne et al., 2018). Thus, care coordination with child protective services caseworkers or with multiple caregivers may be required. For BHCs, possible areas of collaboration with child protective services include monitoring and reporting for medical neglect or abuse, providing relevant medical information to caseworkers and guardian ad litems, and supporting continuity in care and recommendations as a child may change caregiving settings.

CASE EXAMPLE

Bisa is a 4-year-old African American female who was born at 31 weeks gestational age, spent 3 months in the NICU after birth, and had two inpatient admissions for feeding concerns by the age of 2 years. Bisa has a history of feeding difficulties, malnutrition, intolerance of nasogastric tube, constipation, and feeding therapy. Bisa's caregivers are her mother and father, Mr. and Mrs. Kamara, who were born in Africa and immigrated to the United States a few years before Bisa's birth. Bisa is their only child, and psychosocial screening did not identify concerns. At age 4 years, overall, Bisa is physically healthy, developmentally typical, and her oral motor feeding issues have resolved. However, Bisa requires her mother to spoon-feed her at each meal. Bisa is physically and developmentally able to feed herself and eats a typical diet. Bisa previously received feeding therapy for the concern, but her mother did not find it helpful.

At a primary care visit, Mrs. Kamara discussed that mealtime is stressful due to the feeding concern. The pediatrician discussed that it is medically acceptable for Bisa to miss a meal now that she is healthy and noted that Bisa would eventually become hungry and eat if her mother did not spoon-feed her. Mrs. Kamara did not feel comfortable with this plan. The pediatrician requested that the BHC speak with Mrs. Kamara about the feeding concern. The BHC asked Mrs. Kamara what her goal was related to feeding and her thoughts on recommendations provided thus far. Mrs. Kamara would like Bisa to feed herself but given Bisa's history of feeding difficulties, it felt too emotionally difficult to allow Bisa to miss a meal.

Mrs. Kamara also discussed the cultural importance of food and growth for her family.

The BHC provided psychoeducation related to behavior and parent–child relationships and reflected upon the connections between Bisa's medical history and the current feeding pattern. Together, the BHC and Mrs. Kamara developed a plan to meet Bisa at her current motivation level of taking one bite herself, develop a reward system to encourage gradual increases in independent feeding, and increase parent–child intentional time together outside of mealtime. They planned for follow-up in 1 month with the pediatrician and BHC. At the follow-up visit, Mrs. Kamara reported that Bisa was taking up to five bites herself for most meals and enjoyed earning special time with her mother. The BHC highlighted parenting efforts that led to this improvement and recommended behavior system revisions to continue encouraging self-feeding. They planned for a follow-up visit in 3 months with primary care pediatrician and the BHC or as needed.

IDEAS WORTH SHARING

Over the course of providing IBH services in a complex care clinic, we have developed the following questions that are effective in eliciting rich information that shapes services and recommendations provided:

- How has it been caring for [your child]?
- What are the best parts about parenting [child]?
- What are the most difficult or stressful parts about parenting [child] at this time?
- What is going well for [child]?
- How did you choose [child's] name?
- Is there anything that [child] is not doing that you think he/she should be doing? Is there anything that [child] is doing that you think is unusual or just want to ask about?
- Who can you count on for emotional support? Does that feel like enough support?
- How have you and your family coped with stressful times in the past?
- How are your other children coping with [child's] special health care needs?

CONCLUSION

A BHC integrated into the medical home of NICU graduates can provide a range of services that flexibly address concerns and bring valuable contributions to the care of children and families at risk for behavioral health difficulties. Furthermore, integration into the medical home allows for coordinated physical and behavioral health care, which enhances the overall quality of care provided and reduces care coordination burden on families.

ADDITIONAL RESOURCES

The following are resources for caregivers of CYSHCN to connect with other caregivers, obtain information, and/or identify support networks:

- Medical Home Portal—an extensive resource for kids with complex medical conditions: https://www.medicalhomeportal.org/liv ing-with-child
- Courageous Parents Network—website on education and empowerment for families of children with chronic illness: https://www.courageouspar entsnetwork.org
- Hand to Hold—website on information and peer support options for families of children currently or previously in the NICU: https://www. handtohold.org
- Complex Child—a monthly online magazine by parents: https://www. complexchild.org
- Parent to Parent—a support network for families: https://www.p2p usa.org
- Family Voices—local and national advocacy: https://www.familyvoices.org

REFERENCES

Adams, S. Y., Tucker, R., Clark, M. A., & Lechner, B. E. (2020). "Quality of life": Parent and neonatologist perspectives. *Journal of Perinatology*, *40*(12), 1809–1820. doi:10.1038/ s41372-020-0654-9

American Academy of Pediatrics. (2010). Mental health screening and assessment tools for primary care. In *Addressing Mental Health Concerns in Primary Care: A Clinician's Toolkit*. https://www.aap.org/en-us/advocacy-and-policy/aap-health-init iatives/Mental-Health/Documents/MH_ScreeningChart.pdf

American Academy of Pediatrics. (2019). 2019 Recommendations for preventive pedi- atric health care. *Pediatrics*, *143*(3), e20183971. doi:10.1542/peds.2018-3971

Asarnow, J. R., Rozenman, M., Wiblin, J., & Zeltzer, L. (2015). Integrated medical– behavioral care compared with usual primary care for child and adolescent be- havioral health: A meta-analysis. *JAMA Pediatrics*, *169*(10), 929–937. doi:10.1001/ jamapediatrics.2015.1141

Earls, M., Yogman, M., Mattson, G., & Rafferty, J. (2019). Incorporating recognition and management of perinatal depression into pediatric practice. *Pediatrics*, *143*(1), e20183259. doi:10.1542/peds.2018-3259

Engle, W. A.; American Academy of Pediatrics Committee on Fetus and Newborn. (2004). Age terminology during the perinatal period. *Pediatrics*, *114*(5), 1362–1364. doi:10.1542/peds.2004-1915

Franz, A. P., Bolat, G. U., Bolat, H., Matijasevich, A., Santos, I. S., Silveira, R. C., Procianoy, R. S., Rohde, L. A., & Moreira-Maia, C. R. (2018). Attention-deficit/hyperactivity disorder and very preterm/very low birth weight: A meta-analysis. *Pediatrics, 141*(1), e20171645. doi:10.1542/peds.2017-1645

Garg, A., & Dworkin, P. H. (2011). Applying surveillance and screening to family psychosocial issues: Implications for the medical home. *Journal of Developmental and Behavioral Pediatrics, 32*(5), 418–426. doi:10.1097/DBP.0b013e3182196726

Kim, S. H., Joseph, R. M., Frazier, J. A., O'Shea, T. M., Chawarska, K., Allred, E. N., Leviton, A., Kuban, K. K.; Extremely Low Gestational Age Newborn (ELGAN) Study Investigators. (2016). Predictive validity of the Modified Checklist for Autism in Toddlers (M-CHAT) born very preterm. *Journal of Pediatrics, 178*, 101–107 e102. doi:10.1016/j.jpeds.2016.07.052

Lefkowitz, D. S., Baxt, C., & Evans, J. R. (2010). Prevalence and correlates of posttraumatic stress and postpartum depression in parents of infants in the neonatal intensive care unit (NICU). *Journal of Clinical Psychology in Medical Settings, 17*(3), 230–237. doi:10.1007/s10880-010-9202-7

Lipkin, P. H., & Macias, M. M. (2020). Promoting optimal development: Identifying infants and young children with developmental disorders through developmental surveillance and screening. *Pediatrics, 145*(1), e20193449. doi:10.1542/peds.2019-3449

Sacco, R., Gabriele, S., & Persico, A. M. (2015). Head circumference and brain size in autism spectrum disorder: A systematic review and meta-analysis. *Psychiatry Research: Neuroimaging, 234*(2), 239–251. doi:10.1016/j.pscychresns.2015.08.016

Schieve, L. A., Tian, L. H., Baio, J., Rankin, K., Rosenberg, D., Wiggins, L., Maenner, M. J., Yeargin-Allsopp, M., Durkin, M., Rice, C., King, L., Kirby, R. S., Wingate, M. S., & Devine, O. (2014). Population attributable fractions for three perinatal risk factors for autism spectrum disorders, 2002 and 2008 Autism and Developmental Disabilities Monitoring Network. *Annals of Epidemiology, 24*(4), 260–266. doi:10.1016/j.annepidem.2013.12.014

Seltzer, R. R., Henderson, C. M., & Boss, R. D. (2016). Medical foster care: What happens when children with medical complexity cannot be cared for by their families? *Pediatric Research, 79*(1–2), 191–196. doi:10.1038/pr.2015.196

Stille, C., Turchi, R. M., Antonelli, R., Cabana, M. D., Cheng, T. L., Laraque, D., & Perrin, J. (2010). The family-centered medical home: Specific considerations for child health research and policy. *Academic Pediatrics, 10*(4), 211–217. https://www.academicpedsjnl.net/article/S1876-2859(10)00117-8/pdf

Subedi, D., DeBoer, M. D., & Scharf, R. J. (2017). Developmental trajectories in children with prolonged NICU stays. *Archives of Disease in Childhood, 102*(1), 29–34. doi:10.1136/archdischild-2016-310777

Talmi, A., Muther, E. F., Margolis, K., Buchholz, M., Asherin, R., & Bunik, M. (2016). The scope of behavioral health integration in a pediatric primary care setting. *Journal of Pediatric Psychology, 41*(10), 1120–1132. doi:10.1093/jpepsy/jsw065

Van Horne, B. S., Caughy, M. O., Canfield, M., Case, A. P., Greeley, C. S., Morgan, R., & Mitchell, L. E. (2018). First-time maltreatment in children ages 2–10 with and without specific birth defects: A population-based study. *Child Abuse and Neglect, 84*, 53–63. doi:10.1016/j.chiabu.2018.07.003

Vigod, S. N., Villegas, L., Dennis, C. L., & Ross, L. E. (2010). Prevalence and risk factors for postpartum depression among women with preterm and low-birth-weight infants: A systematic review. *BJOG: An International Journal of Obstetrics & Gynecology, 117*(5), 540–550. doi:10.1111/j.14710528.2009.02493.x

Wolraich, M. L., Hagan, J. F., Allan, C., Chan, E., Davison, D., Earls, M., Evans, S. W., Flinn, S. K., Froehlich, T., Frost, J., Holbrook, J. R., Lehmann, C. U., Lessin, H. R., Okechukwu, K., Pierce, K. L., Winner, J. D., Zurhellen, W.; Subcommittee on Children and Adolescents with Attention-Deficit/Hyperactivity Disorder. (2019). Clinical practice guideline for the diagnosis, evaluation, and treatment of attention-deficit/hyperactivity disorder in children and adolescents. *Pediatrics, 144*(4), e20192528. doi:10.1542/peds.2019-2528

For the benefit of digital users, indexed terms that span two pages (e.g., 52–53) may, on occasion, appear on only one of those pages.

Tables, figures, and boxes are indicated by *t*, *f*, and *b* following the page number.